High-Performance Concrete: Modification Methods, Sustainability, and Multifunctional Applications

High-Performance Concrete: Modification Methods, Sustainability, and Multifunctional Applications

Guest Editors

Yekai Yang
Weiqiang Wang
Yiwei Weng
Zhaoyao Wang
Qiao Wang
Ruizhe Shao

MDPI

Basel • Beijing • Wuhan • Barcelona • Belgrade • Novi Sad • Cluj • Manchester

Guest Editors

Yekai Yang
School of Building
Engineering and Mechanics
Yanshan University
Qinhuangdao
China

Weiqiang Wang
College of Water
Conservancy and
Hydropower Engineering
Hohai University
Nanjing
China

Yiwei Weng
Department of Building and
Real Estate
The Hong Kong Polytechnic
University
Hong Kong
China

Zhaoyao Wang
School of Science
Xi'an University of
Architecture and Technology
Xi'an
China

Qiao Wang
School of Civil and
Transportation Engineering
Hebei University of
Technology
Tianjin
China

Ruizhe Shao
School of Civil and
Environmental Engineering
University of Technology
Sydney (UTS)
Sydney
Australia

Editorial Office
MDPI AG
Grosspeteranlage 5
4052 Basel, Switzerland

This is a reprint of the Special Issue, published open access by the journal *Buildings* (ISSN 2075-5309), freely accessible at: https://www.mdpi.com/journal/buildings/special_issues/06LOR0AY0N.

For citation purposes, cite each article independently as indicated on the article page online and as indicated below:

Lastname, A.A.; Lastname, B.B. Article Title. *Journal Name* **Year**, *Volume Number*, Page Range.

ISBN 978-3-7258-4221-6 (Hbk)
ISBN 978-3-7258-4222-3 (PDF)
https://doi.org/10.3390/books978-3-7258-4222-3

Cover image courtesy of Yekai Yang

Contents

buildings

MDPI

Article

The Generation of the Target Aftershock Spectrum Based on the Conditional Mean Spectrum of Aftershocks

Ruiguang Zhu [1], Bohan Du [2], Yekai Yang [2] and Dagang Lu [3,*]

1 Key Lab of Green Construction and Intelligent Maintenance for Civil Engineering of Hebei Province, Yanshan University, Qinhuangdao 066000, China; zrg179@163.com
2 School of Civil Engineering and Mechanics, Yanshan University, Qinhuangdao 066000, China; dbh3616@163.com (B.D.); yekai.yang@ysu.edu.cn (Y.Y.)
3 School of Civil Engineering, Harbin Institute of Technology, Harbin 150001, China
* Correspondence: ludagang@hit.edu.cn

Abstract: Numerous studies have examined the responses of various structures to the mainshock–aftershock (MS–AS) ground motion, and the MS–AS ground motions are very important as the input. Therefore, in the absence of aftershock information, it is particularly critical to construct a reasonable MS–AS seismic sequence. This paper aims to provide a new reasonable method for generating the target aftershock response spectrum, which can be used to select or artificially simulate aftershock ground motion, given the seismic information of the main shock. Firstly, the magnitude, fault size, and location of the aftershock are determined. Then, other parameters required for the aftershock ground motion prediction equation (GMPE) are calculated. Subsequently, the correlation of the spectral shape to the MS–AS ground motion is used to modify the response spectrum predicted using the GMPE to obtain the conditional mean spectrum of aftershocks (CMS_A). Finally, the relative errors of the predicted spectrum via the ASK14 model and CMS_A are compared for four different assumptions. The results show that the simulated aftershock parameters and the actual ones accord well, and the relative errors of the CMS_A can be controlled within 20%. Meanwhile, the discrete property of the target aftershock response spectrum is closer to the real recorded response spectrum.

Keywords: MS–AS ground motion; target aftershock response spectrum; ground motion prediction model; conditional mean spectrum of aftershocks; spectral shape

1. Introduction

After an earthquake, many aftershocks often occur within a short period of time. Generally, the magnitude of aftershocks and their intensities are smaller than those of the main earthquake. However, the intensity of ground shaking caused by aftershocks at some sites may be greater than that of the main earthquake, such as the Christchurch aftershocks in New Zealand on 22 February 2011 [1]. Due to the randomness of various factors such as the focal location, focal depth, fault strike in the earthquake, and site conditions, the disaster caused by the aftershock is more catastrophic than the main earthquake. Therefore, some researchers have shifted more attention to the responses of various structures under the main shock and aftershocks [2–7], such as the special steel moment frame structures, corroded steel moment-resisting frames, etc. As a result, structural performance indexes such as vulnerability and recoverability under main shock and aftershock have been widely studied [8–10].

In studying structural reactions to MS–AS seismic sequences, researchers discovered that the input MS–AS ground motions significantly impact structural reactions. The most used types of MS–AS ground motions are repetitive and random ground motion sequences [11,12]. Torres et al. [13] improved the seismic performance of steel frames in MS–AS sequences, of which its aftershock ground motions were made by scaling the other mainshock ground motions. This method can reflect the relationship between the main shock and aftershocks in response spectrum amplitude to a certain extent. However, this method could be improved if the correlation and randomness of the main shock and aftershocks for the source mechanism, spectral shape, etc., are also considered. The same limitation was also observed in other studies [14]. Wei et al. [15] pointed out that the concrete-filled steel tubular composite columns with ultra-high performance concrete plates demonstrated good seismic performances with MS–AS sequences. If the above MS–AS sequences could reflect the correlation and randomness between the mainshock ground motions and their real aftershock ground motions, then the result might be more reasonable. For that reason, the real MS–AS ground motions were widely selected from different regional databases of strong motions [16] and then scaled to the target level based on local seismic hazards [17–19]. However, the real MS–AS ground motions may underestimate the aftershock impacts because the selected real seismic records cannot fully reflect the randomness of aftershock seismic sequences [20]. It may be difficult to fully reflect the randomness of the main shock and aftershocks in focal location, fault type, etc., for a small amount of real main shock and aftershock ground motions.

Therefore, it is necessary to construct an artificial main aftershock sequence to consider the correlation and randomness between the mainshock and aftershock ground motions [21,22]. Wang et al. [23] used the stochastic simulation of the main aftershock sequence to analyze the permanent displacement reliability of soil slopes based on the physical random function. The function could reflect the characteristics of the local site of the project by modeling the source, propagation path, and local site. The epidemic-type aftershock sequence (ETAS) model [24] and the branching aftershock sequence (BASS) model [25] are also widely used to simulate the regional aftershock sequences. Wang et al. [23] analyzed the stochastic simulation of the main aftershock sequences based on the physical random function and established the relationship between the main shock and aftershocks according to the theoretical copula model. The above method considers the correlation between some parameters of the main shock and aftershocks. Moreover, some researchers use an aftershock seismic hazard analysis to select ground tremors [26], which requires detailed seismic information. In recent years, some researchers [27] have begun to predict the parameters of aftershocks using machine learning methods, which may not fully explain the relevant mechanism.

This study strives to present a novel target aftershock spectrum that can, to the greatest extent feasible, capture the correlation and randomness between the MS–AS ground motions. The simulation approach fills in all the missing data for the GMPE of the aftershock ground motions based on the correlation and randomness between the main shock and its aftershocks, given the main earthquake. The aftershock magnitude and the hypocenter position should be established first to gather the necessary data. The location and size of aftershock faults are then estimated using the statistical relationship between magnitude and fault size and other relevant hypotheses. All other factors, including the rupture distance and hanging wall effect, are then calculated following their definitions. With the help of the aforementioned information, the GMPE was able to anticipate the response spectrum of the aftershock ground motions. On this foundation, it is possible to change the prediction spectrum of GMPE and achieve the target response spectrum of the aftershock using the prediction model of spectral shape parameters between the main shock and aftershocks. Therefore, this study could provide a new aftershock target response spectrum for studying high-performance concrete [28,29] and other structures subjected to the MS–AS seismic sequences.

2. The Target Aftershock Spectrum

The conditional mean spectrum of the aftershock (CMS_A) is selected to generate the target aftershock spectrum given the mainshock ground motion. The CMS_A could reflect the correlation of the spectral shapes between the mainshock ground motion and its aftershock ground motions. Given the response spectrum of the mainshock ground motion, the conditional mean of the response spectrum of the aftershock ground motion for the same period could be calculated as follows:

$$\mu_{\ln S_{a,A}(T_i)|\ln S_{a,M}(T_i)} = \mu_{\ln S_{a,A}}(M_A, R_A, T_i) + \mu_{\varepsilon_A(T_i)|\varepsilon_M(T_i)}\sigma_{\ln S_{a,A}}(T_i) \quad (1)$$

where M_A and R_A are the magnitude and source-to-site distance of an aftershock, respectively; $S_{a,A}$ and $S_{a,M}$ are the spectral accelerations of the aftershocks and their corresponding mainshock, respectively; $\mu_{\ln S_{a,A}}$ and $\sigma_{\ln S_{a,A}}$ are the mean and standard deviation of $\ln S_{a,A}$ predicted via the GMPE, respectively; ε_A and ε_M are the epsilon values of the aftershocks and their corresponding mainshock, respectively; $\mu_{\varepsilon_A(T_i)|\varepsilon_M(T_i)}$ is the conditional mean of $\varepsilon_A(T_i)$ conditioned on $\varepsilon_M(T_i)$ for the same period T_i,

$$\mu_{\varepsilon_A(T_i)|\varepsilon_M(T_i)} = \mu_{\varepsilon_A(T_i)} + \rho[\varepsilon_A(T_i), \varepsilon_M(T_i)] \cdot \frac{\sigma_{\varepsilon_A(T_i)}}{\sigma_{\varepsilon_M(T_i)}} \cdot [\varepsilon_M(T_i) - \mu_{\varepsilon_M(T_i)}] \quad (2)$$

where $\mu_{\varepsilon_A(T_i)}$, $\sigma_{\varepsilon_A(T_i)}$, $\mu_{\varepsilon_M(T_i)}$, and $\sigma_{\varepsilon_M(T_i)}$ are the means and standard deviations of ε_A and ε_M for the period T_i, respectively; $\rho[\varepsilon_A(T_i), \varepsilon_M(T_i)]$ is the correlation coefficient between ε_A and ε_M for the period T_i. For more details regarding the values of the above parameters, interested readers are encouraged to refer to the work of Zhu et al. [30]. The exponent of $\mu_{\ln S_{a,\,A}(T_i)|\ln S_{a,\,M}(T_i)}$ is the conditional mean spectrum of aftershocks.

According to the above section, the CMS_A is based on the GMPE of the aftershock and the correlation of the spectral shapes of the MS–AS ground motions. In this study, the ASK14 model [31] is selected to calculate the prediction spectrum of the aftershock ground motions because the ASK14 model could be used to predict the response spectrum of both mainshock and aftershock ground motions. Therefore, reasonably determining the aftershock seismic parameters for the ASK14 model becomes one of the key steps to calculating CMS_A. Meanwhile, the complexity in calculating the conditional mean spectrum of aftershocks depends on how rich the parameters are for the aftershock ground motions, given the mainshock ground motions. The conditional mean spectrum of aftershocks can be calculated directly with all the required parameters of the aftershock ground motions. For example, the station for recording the ground motion is broken after the main shock. In this case, the aftershock ground motions are not recorded, but its seismic parameters are collected. However, the statistical relationship between the main shock and its aftershocks and the corresponding assumption can be used to supplement the missing data for regions with partially missing data from the aftershocks or where the data from the aftershocks is completely absent.

3. Determination of Aftershock Seismic Parameters

In proposing the conditional mean spectrum of aftershocks, the calculation procedure for generating CMS_A is also provided in previous research [30]. Knowing how to reasonably determine the seismic parameters of the aftershock ground motions is an essential step, given the mainshock ground motions. This section will propose the method and assumptions for determining the seismic parameters of the aftershock ground motions based on the existing research results.

3.1. The Parameters Related to the Source

The mainshock is usually followed by a series of aftershocks, and only the maximum aftershock in terms of magnitude will be considered in this paper. The mean of the magnitude difference (Δm) between the mainshock and its largest aftershocks is about 1.2, and Δm ranges between about 0 and 3. Han et al. [32] point out that the beta distribution is the best candidate to describe the distribution of Δm. The beta distribution can be expressed as

$$p(\Delta m) = \begin{cases} \frac{1}{B(2.2,2.3)} \cdot \frac{\Delta m^{1.2}(3-\Delta m)^{2.3}}{3^{4.5}} & 0 \le \Delta m \le 3 \\ 0 & \text{otherwise} \end{cases} \quad (3)$$

where $p(\Delta m)$ is the probability density function (PDF) of the selected beta distribution, as shown in Figure 1, in which $B(2.2, 2.3)$ is the beta function for the corresponding elements 2.2 and 2.3. With the distribution of Δm determined, the magnitude of the largest aftershock can be obtained by subtracting Δm from the mainshock magnitude.

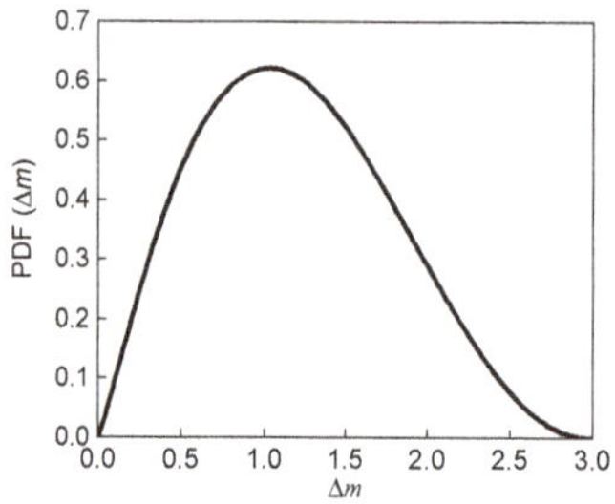

Figure 1. The probability density function of Δm.

The simplest assumption is that the aftershocks and its mainshock occur at the same place, but it will lead to bias [20]. Another assumption is that the epicenters of the aftershocks are uniformly distributed along the rupture length of the fault of their mainshock [33], as shown in Figure 2. Furthermore, it is also assumed that the epicenters of the aftershocks occur around the epicenter of their mainshock uniformly [34], as shown in Figure 3. The area of the circular region is related to the magnitude of their main shock and can be determined as follows:

$$\log_{10} A = M_M - 3.7 \tag{4}$$

where A is the area of the circular region (km^2), and M_M is the magnitude of their mainshock. With the determination of A, the radius of the circular region (R in Figure 3) can be calculated further.

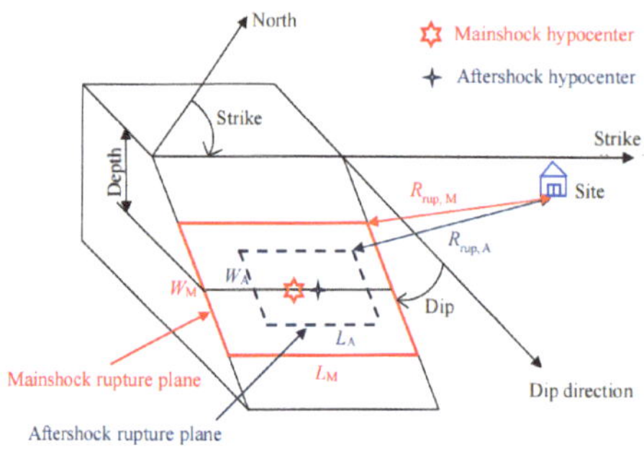

Figure 2. Hypocenter and rupture of the largest aftershock under linear assumption.

The depths of the hypocenters of the aftershocks are assumed to be the same as that of the mainshock, and the rupture planes of the aftershocks are parallel to the rupture plane of the mainshock. In other words, the strike angles and dip angles of the fault planes of the aftershocks are assumed to be the same as those of the mainshock. The size of the rupture plane of the aftershock can be determined as follows [35]:

$$\log(L) = a + b \cdot M \tag{5}$$

$$\log(W) = a + b \cdot M \tag{6}$$

where L and W are the rupture length and width, respectively. The coefficients a and b are listed in Table 1. L_M and W_M are the rupture length and width of the mainshock, and L_A and W_A are the rupture length and width of the aftershock, as shown in Figures 2 and 3.

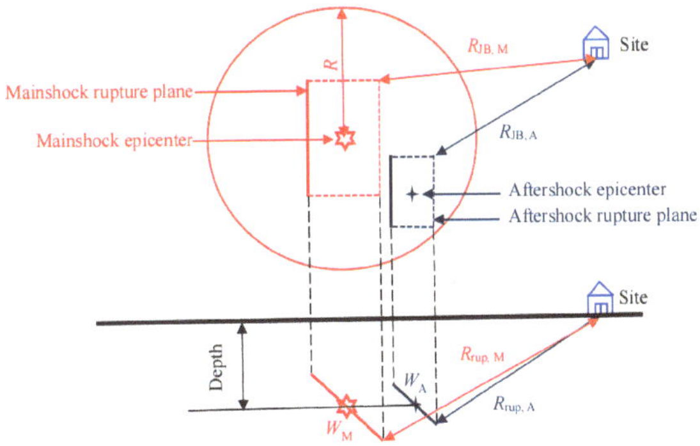

Figure 3. Hypocenter and rupture of the largest aftershock under the circular assumption.

Table 1. Regressions of the rupture length (L) and rupture width (W).

L (km)			*W* (km)		
Type of the Rupture	*a*	*b*	**Type of the Rupture**	*a*	*b*
Strike slip	−2.57	0.62	Strike slip	−0.76	0.27
Reverse	−2.42	0.58	Reverse	−1.61	0.41
Normal	−1.88	0.50	Normal	−1.14	0.35
All	−2.44	0.59	All	−1.01	0.32

3.2. The Parameters Related to the Distance

Many parameters are related to the distance in the ASK14 model, for example, the rupture distance, the Joyner–Boore distance, etc. By determining the rupture plane of the aftershock, including the location and size, these parameters related to the distance can be determined according to their definitions.

Figure 4 shows the definition of the centroid Joyner–Boore distance (CR_{JB}), which is the closed distance between the centroid of the Joyner–Boore rupture surface of the aftershock and the closest point on the edge of the Joyner–Boore rupture surface of the mainshock [36]. CR_{JB} is equal to zero under the assumption that the aftershocks occur on the same place as the mainshock or that the epicenters of the aftershocks are distributed uniformly along the rupture length of the fault of the mainshock. CR_{JB} must be determined according to its definition only in the case that the epicenters of the aftershocks are assumed to occur around the epicenter of the mainshock uniformly.

Figure 5 shows the schematic diagram of the rupture distance (R_{rup}) and Joyner–Boore distance (R_{JB}). As shown in Figures 2 and 3, $R_{rup,\,M}$ and $R_{JB,\,M}$ are the rupture distance and Joyner–Boore distance of the mainshock, and $R_{rup,\,A}$ and $R_{JB,\,A}$ are the rupture distance and Joyner–Boore distance of the aftershock. R_X is the distance measured perpendicular to the fault strike from the surface projection of the up-dip edge of the fault plane, as shown in Figure 6 [36].

3.3. Other Parameters

In this study, the site types of the aftershock ground motions are assumed to be the same as that of the mainshock ground motion. This means some parameters about the site model in the ASK14 model, such as the shear-wave velocity over the top 30 m (V_{S30}), depth to V_S = 1.0 km/s at the site (m) (Z_1), etc., are assumed to be the same as the mainshock ground. As mentioned previously, three fault types are involved in the ASK14 model: (1) reverse, (2) normal, and (3) others. After the mainshock, determining which fault type of aftershocks is likely to happen is complicated and beyond the scope of this study. According to the research by Han et al. [37], these fault types are assumed to happen randomly and have equal probability. As for the parameters related to the hanging wall site, whether the site is within the hanging wall region is determined according to Figure 7 [36]. HW, FW, and NU mean that the site is within the hanging wall region, the footwall region, or the neutral region, respectively. Even if the site is within the hanging wall region, whether the hanging wall effect exists also relates to the fault type [38]. The hanging wall effect is assumed to exist for all fault types to simplify the procedure. If the site is located in the hanging wall region, the hanging wall effect is considered to exist.

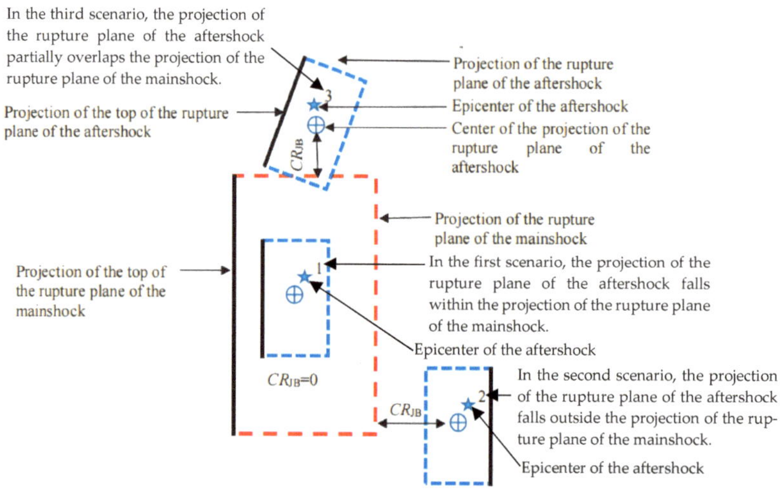

Figure 4. Definition of CR_{JB} [36].

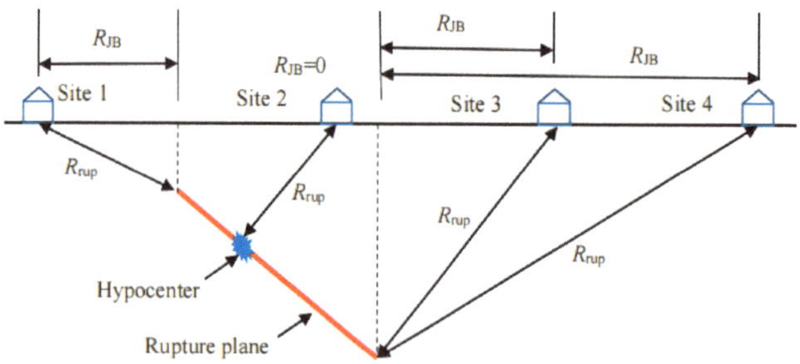

Figure 5. Definition of CR_{JB} [36].

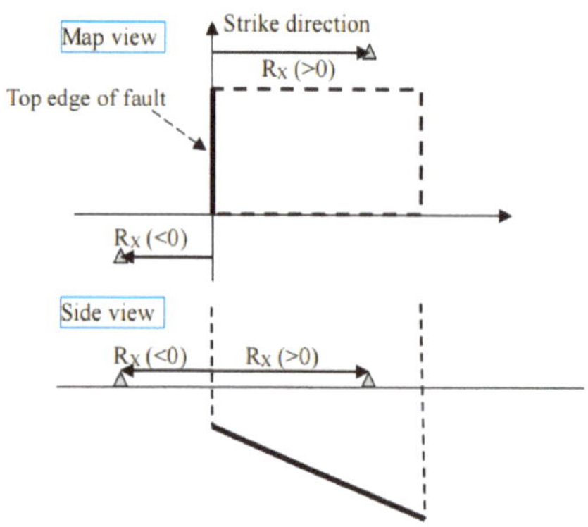

Figure 6. Schematic diagram of R_X [36].

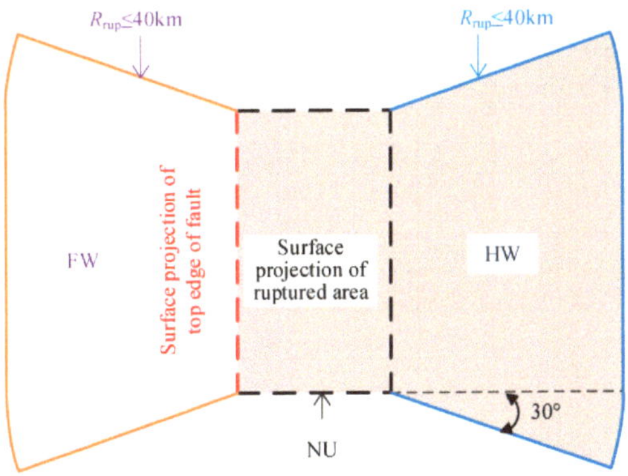

Figure 7. Schematic diagram of the hanging wall effect [36].

4. Conditional Mean Spectrum of the Aftershocks

The seismic parameters of the aftershock ground motions can be simulated according to the statistical relationship between the mainshock and its largest aftershock, given the mainshock ground motion.

4.1. The Aftershock Magnitude Is Known

4.1.1. The Simulated Seismic Parameters for the Aftershock Ground Motions

Given the magnitude of the aftershock, the other seismic parameters of the aftershock must be simulated using the above assumption. The above section gives three assumptions about where the aftershock occurred. Moreover, some researchers assume that the seismic parameters of the aftershock ground motions, except the magnitude, are identical to that of the corresponding mainshock ground motion. Therefore, this study uses four assumptions to determine the seismic parameters of the aftershock ground motions. The first assumption is that the aftershocks occur at the same location as their mainshock. The second and third assumptions are that the aftershocks are distributed uniformly along the rupture length of the fault of their mainshock [33] or uniformly distributed in a circular region [32]. The fourth assumption is that the seismic parameters of the aftershock ground motions are identical to those of the mainshock ground motions, except for the magnitude of the aftershocks [20]. For the second and third assumptions, the hypocenters of the aftershocks can be obtained via Latin hypercube sampling (LHS). The fault type of the aftershocks is simulated randomly. Then, the rupture lengths and widths of the rupture planes of the aftershocks are calculated according to Equations (5) and (6). The details of the rupture planes of the aftershocks are determined using the assumption that the strike angles and dip angles of the rupture planes of the aftershocks are identical to those of the mainshock. As a result, the other seismic parameters of the aftershocks, such as the rupture distance, the depth of the rupture, etc., can be determined further according to the definition of these parameters. Figure 8 shows the depths to the hypocenters of the aftershocks and their corresponding mainshocks. As shown in Figure 8, the data dots are distributed near the diagonal uniformly. Therefore, it is reasonable to assume that the depths of the hypocenters of the aftershocks and the one of their mainshocks are identical.

Figure 9 shows the down-dip rupture widths of the aftershocks with different assumptions, given the mainshocks. As shown in Figure 9, there are no essential distinctions between Figure 9a–c. The magnitudes of the aftershocks are equal to their actual values because only the magnitude and fault type are responsible for the down-dip rupture width. The only difference between them is the fault type of the aftershocks, which is simulated using the Monte Carlo method. Therefore, the subtle differences are caused by the different fault types of the aftershocks. The down-dip rupture widths of the aftershocks are assumed to be the same as that of the corresponding mainshock in Figure 9d. It can be found that the down-dip rupture width of the mainshocks is larger than those of their aftershocks, so the above assumption is not reasonable. A large magnitude usually leads to a large rupture because the magnitude of the mainshock is larger than those of its aftershocks.

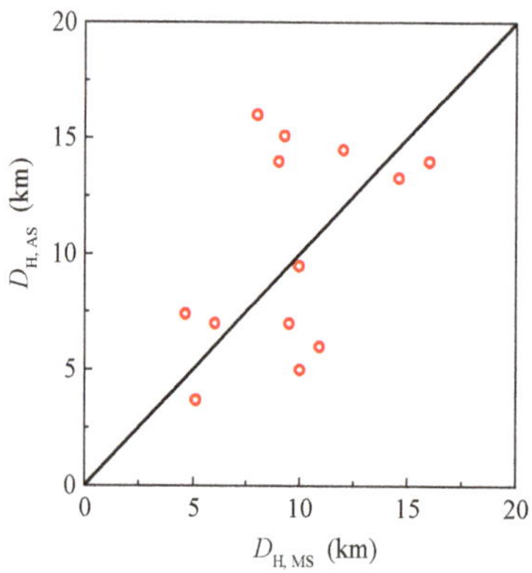

Figure 8. The hypocenter depths of the selected MS–AS seismic sequences.

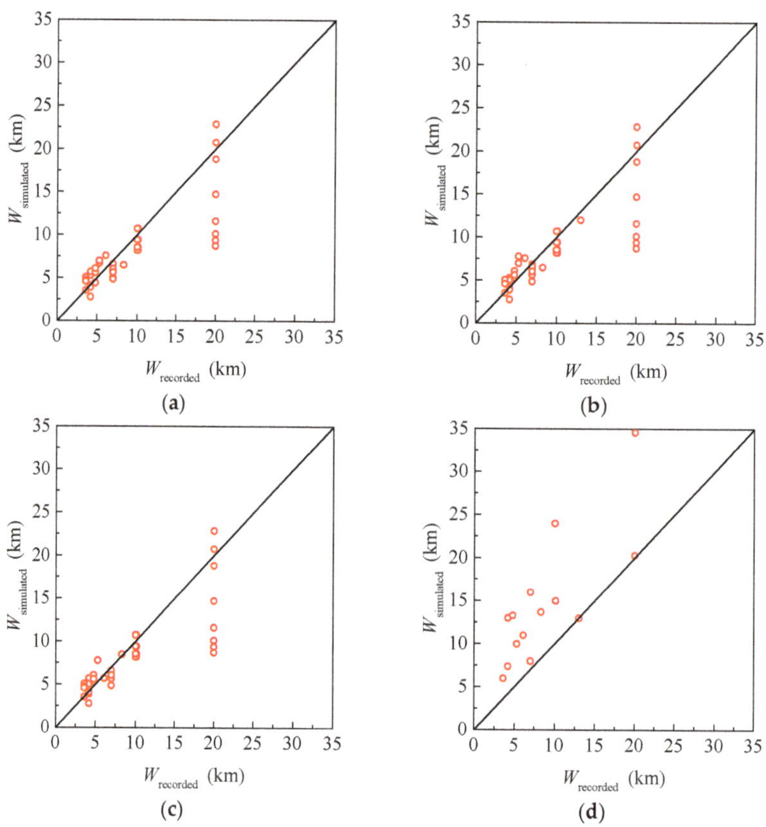

Figure 9. Down-dip rupture widths of the aftershocks with different assumptions listed as follows: (**a**) occurring at the same hypocenter; (**b**) linear assumption; (**c**) circular assumption; (**d**) identical to the mainshock.

Figure 10 shows the simulated rupture distances of the aftershocks with different assumptions. When the aftershock hypocenters are simulated using the linear model or the circular model, the results are similar, and the data points are evenly distributed around the diagonal. Figure 10a shows that simulated data points are clustered around the diagonal, but most simulated results are smaller than the real ones. As shown in Figure 10d, almost all the data points are distributed below the diagonal, which means that the simulation results are far from the real situations. The real rupture distances of the aftershocks are greater than that of the mainshock in general. Therefore, the assumption that the rupture distances of the aftershock are equal to that of the mainshock is unreasonable.

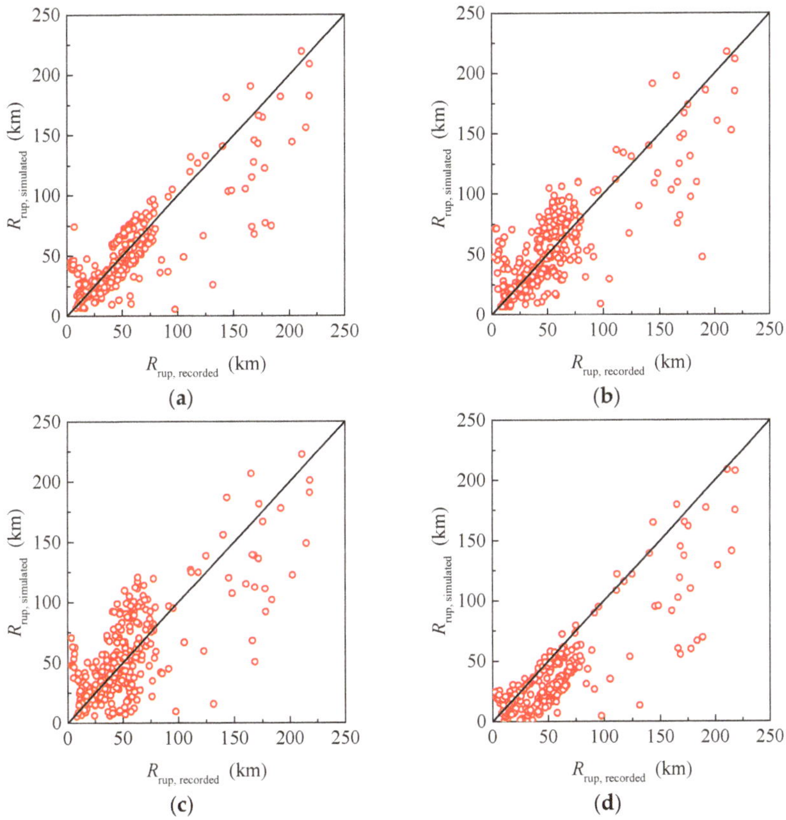

Figure 10. Rupture distances of the aftershock ground motions with different assumptions listed as follows: (**a**) occurring at the same hypocenter; (**b**) linear assumption; (**c**) circular assumption; (**d**) identical to the mainshock.

Figure 11 shows the Joyner–Boore distances of the aftershocks simulated under different assumptions. Overall, the results are consistent with those of the rupture distances of the aftershocks. Compared with the other assumptions, the first assumption has the best result. The results of the linear model and the circular model are similar. The result of the fourth assumption is deeply unreasonable.

Figure 12 shows the horizontal distances from the top edges of the rupture of the aftershock ground motions simulated with different assumptions. The results of the first assumption are very similar to those of the second assumption. The values simulated according to the first and second assumptions are larger than the actual values of the aftershock ground motions in general. The data points in Figure 12c are uniformly distributed on two sides of a diagonal line, but their dispersions are relatively high. In Figure 12d, the horizontal distances from the top edges of the rupture of the aftershock ground motions are assumed to be the same as those of the mainshock ground motions. As shown in Figure 12d, the horizontal distance from the top edge of the rupture of the mainshock ground motions is larger than those of the aftershock ground motions. Therefore, the fourth assumption will introduce bias compared with the other assumptions.

4.1.2. The Response Spectrum of the Aftershock Ground Motions

With the determination of the seismic parameters of the aftershock ground motions, the median response spectrum can be predicted using the ASK14 model [31]. Then, the conditional mean spectrum of aftershocks can be computed according to Equation (1). Figure 13a shows the response spectrum predicted using the ASK14 model and the conditional mean spectrum of aftershocks with the assumption that the aftershocks and mainshock occur at the same hypocenter. Meanwhile, the recorded response spectrum of the aftershock ground motions is also shown in Figure 13a. As shown in Figure 13a, the response spectrum predicted using the ASK14 model and the conditional mean spectrum of aftershocks are lower than the recorded spectra in the short and median periods in general, but it is just the opposite in long periods. Compared with the response spectrum predicted using the ASK14 model, the conditional mean spectrum of aftershocks matches the recorded spectrum better, no matter the median or the percentiles.

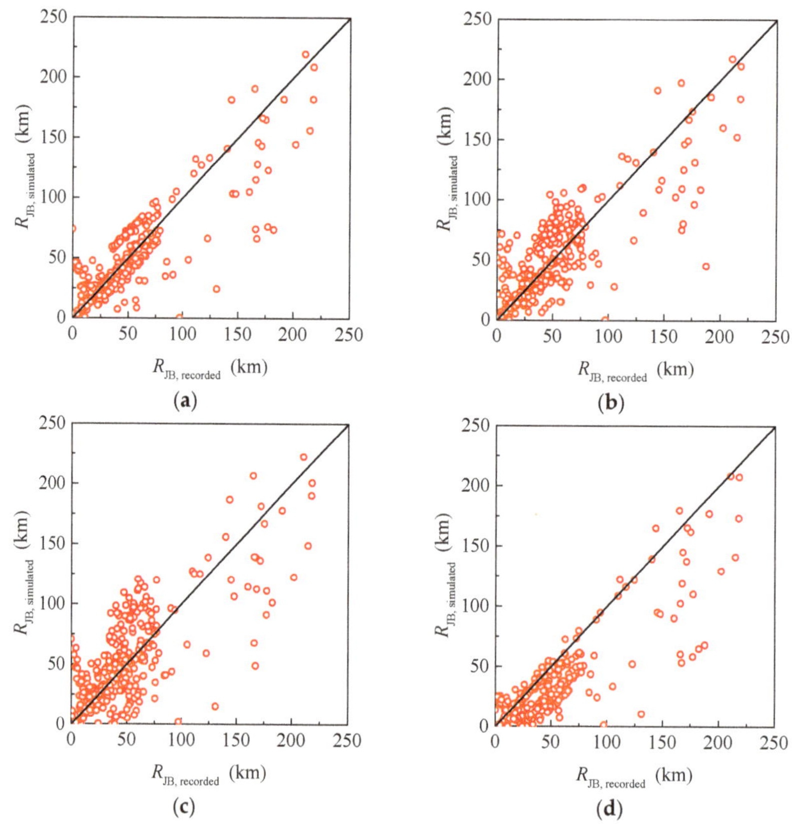

Figure 11. Joyner–Boore distances of the aftershock ground motions with different assumptions, listed as follows: **(a)** occurring at the same hypocenter; **(b)** linear assumption; **(c)** circular assumption; **(d)** identical to the mainshock.

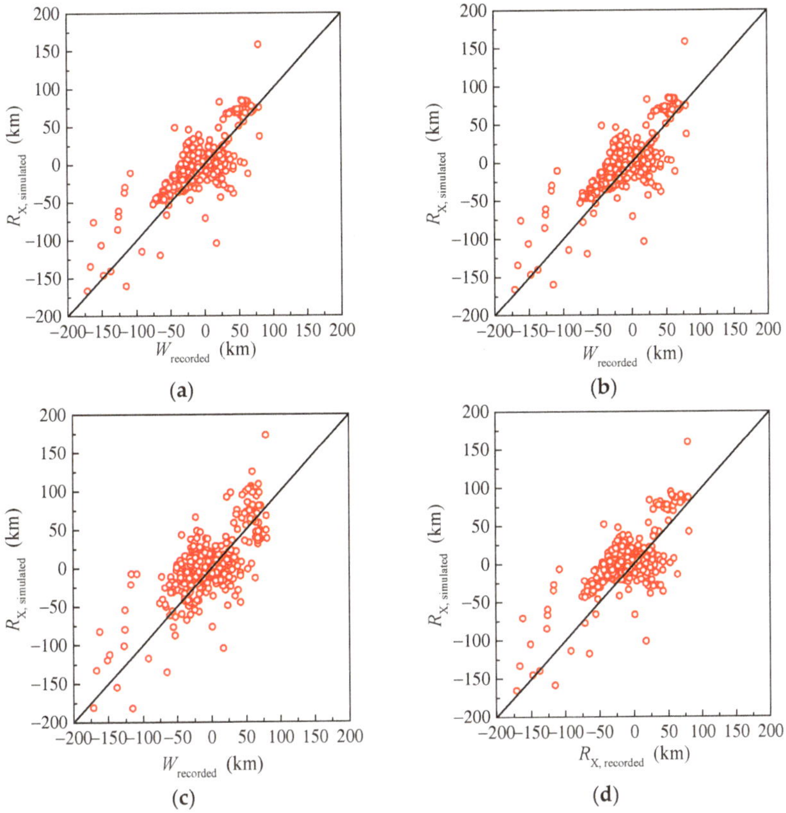

Figure 12. Horizontal distances from the top edges of the rupture of the aftershock ground motions with different assumptions listed as follows: (**a**) occurring at the same hypocenter; (**b**) linear assumption; (**c**) circular assumption; (**d**) identical to the mainshock.

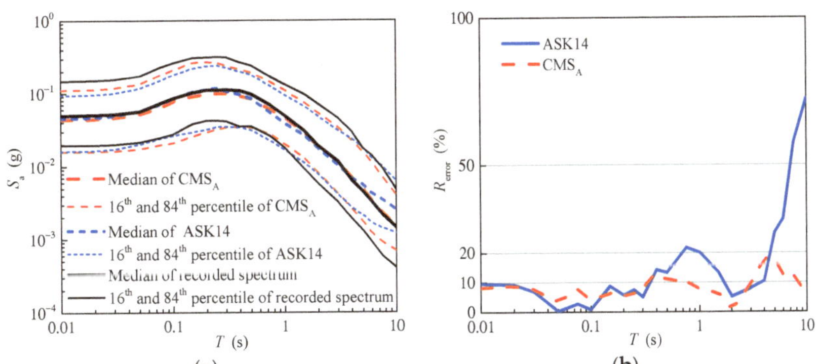

Figure 13. Conditional mean spectrum of aftershocks, with the assumption that the aftershocks and its mainshock occur at the same hypocenter and its relative errors, listed as follows: (**a**) conditional mean spectrum of aftershocks and (**b**) relative error.

The relative error (R_{error}) is calculated as follows:

$$R_{\text{error}} = \left| \frac{\mu_{\ln S_a}^{\text{Predict}} - \mu_{\ln S_a}^{\text{As-record}}}{\mu_{\ln S_a}^{\text{As-record}}} \right| \tag{7}$$

where $\mu_{\ln S_a}^{\text{Predict}}$ is the mean of the logarithm of the predicted response spectrum, which is the response spectrum predicted using the ASK14 model or the conditional mean spectrum of aftershocks, and $\mu_{\ln S_a}^{\text{As-record}}$ is the mean of the logarithm of the recorded response spectrum for the aftershock ground motions.

Figure 13b shows the relative errors of the median of the response spectrum predicted using the ASK14 model and the conditional mean spectrum of aftershocks. As shown in Figure 13b, the relative errors of the conditional mean spectrum of aftershocks are smaller than those of the response spectrum predicted using the ASK14 model in general. For the short and median periods, the relative errors of the conditional mean spectrum of aftershocks are nearly less than 10%, and range between 10% and 20% for the long periods. In contrast, the relative errors of the response spectrum predicted using the ASK14 model increase gradually, even reaching up to 70%.

Figure 14 shows the median and percentiles of the response spectrum predicted using the ASK14 model, the conditional mean spectrum of aftershocks with the linear model, showing that the epicenters of the aftershocks are uniformly distributed along the rupture length of the fault of their mainshock. The general trends with the linear model are similar to those with the assumption that the aftershock and its mainshock occur at the same hypocenter. For comparison purposes, Figure 15 shows the median and percentiles of the response spectrum predicted using the ASK14 model with the actual seismic parameters of the aftershock ground motions and the conditional mean spectrum of aftershocks. In contrast, the general trends in Figures 13 and 14 are in accordance with those in Figure 15, especially the relative errors of the response spectrum predicted using the ASK14 model. Therefore, the seismic parameters of the aftershock ground motions can be reasonably simulated with the assumption that the aftershocks and mainshock occur at the same hypocenter or that the epicenters of the aftershocks are uniformly distributed along the rupture length of the fault of their mainshock.

Figure 16 shows the median and percentiles of the response spectrum predicted using the ASK14 model and the conditional mean spectrum of aftershocks with the circular model and their relative errors. The response spectrum predicted using the ASK14 model with the circular model differs from those calculated according to the actual seismic parameters of the aftershock ground motions, especially for the median and long periods. Even so, the relative errors of the response spectrum predicted using the ASK14 are still at a low level. Meanwhile, the conditional mean spectrum of aftershocks can remain below 20% and match the recorded spectrum better than the response spectrum predicted using the ASK14 model. The only difference between the circular model and the above two assumptions is the location of the hypocenter or location of the rupture of the aftershock. Beyond that, the depth of the aftershock hypocenter, the strike and dip direction, etc., are identical to those of the first or second assumption. Therefore, the difference in the locations of the aftershock hypocenters leads to a difference in the other seismic parameters of the aftershock ground motions related to the aftershock rupture, which can lead to a difference in the response spectrum of the aftershock ground motions. For example, the simulated rupture distance and the Joyner–Boore distance with the circular model are larger than those with the first and second assumptions, as shown in Figures 10 and 11. The larger rupture distance and the Joyner–Boore distance further lead to the lower response spectrum predicted using the ASK14 model. In this case, it does not mean that the circular model is unreasonable, but only that it is not suitable for the aftershock ground motions selected in this paper. The selected aftershock ground motions are only from 13 mainshock–aftershock earthquake sequences; therefore, the circular model is determined using the number of mainshock–aftershock earthquakes.

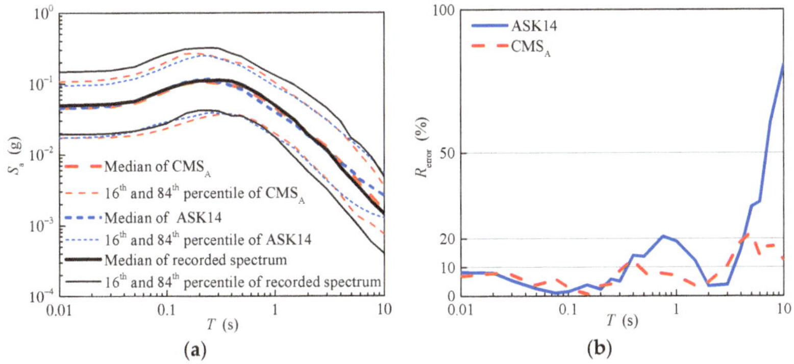

Figure 14. Conditional mean spectrum of aftershocks generated according to the linear model and its relative errors listed as follows: (**a**) conditional mean spectrum of aftershocks and (**b**) relative errors.

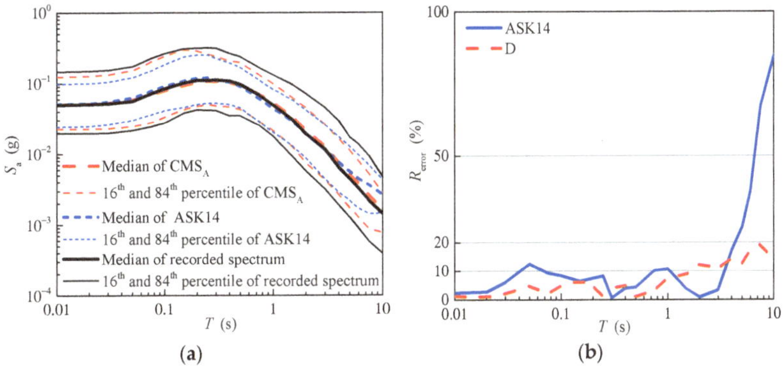

Figure 15. Conditional mean spectrum of aftershocks generated according to the actual seismic parameters of the aftershock ground motions and their relative errors listed as follows: (**a**) conditional mean spectrum of aftershocks and (**b**) relative errors.

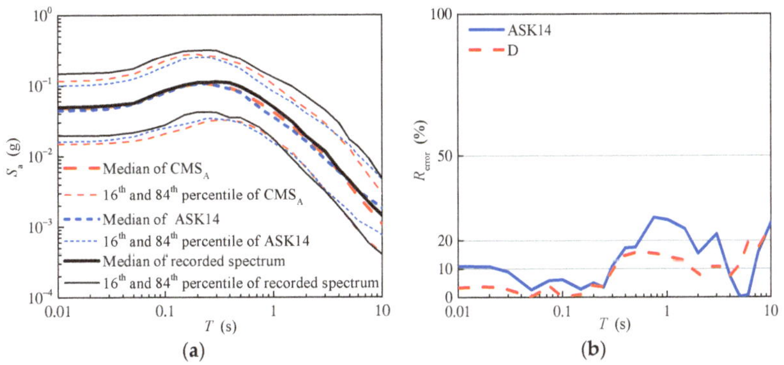

Figure 16. Conditional mean spectrum of aftershocks generated according to the circular model and its relative errors listed as follows: (**a**) conditional mean spectrum of aftershocks and (**b**) relative error.

Figure 17 shows the response spectrum of the aftershock ground motions predicted using the ASK14 model and the conditional mean spectrum of aftershocks under the fourth assumption that the magnitude of the aftershock is equal to its actual value and the other seismic parameters are set to those for its mainshock. As shown in Figure 17, the response spectrum predicted using the ASK14 model is higher than the recorded spectrum of the aftershock ground motions for the whole period. The response spectrum has relative errors of 10% to 50% when the period is less than 3 s. After that, the relative errors become larger and larger, even reaching up to about 280%. In this case, the conditional mean spectrum of aftershocks cannot match the recorder spectrum very well.

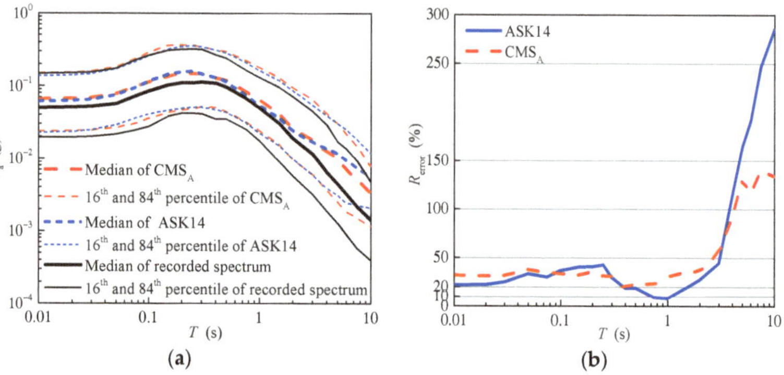

Figure 17. Conditional mean spectrum of aftershocks, with the assumption that the seismic parameters of the aftershocks and the mainshock ground motions are identical except the magnitude and their relative errors, listed as follows: (**a**) conditional mean spectrum of aftershocks and (**b**) relative error.

The major reason for the above results is that the seismic parameters of the aftershock ground motions are different from those of the mainshock ground motions, especially the rupture distance and Joyner–Boore distance. The rupture distance and Joyner–Boore distance of the mainshock ground motion are shorter than those of the aftershock ground motions, which leads to a larger response spectrum predicted using the ASK14 model. When calculating the response spectrum using the ASK14 model, the flag for aftershocks is set to one, and the parameter CR_{JB} is set to zero for the aftershock ground motions.

4.2. The Aftershock Magnitude Is Unknown

This paper gives a reasonable response spectrum of the aftershock ground motion with the actual magnitude of an aftershock and other simulated seismic parameters. If the magnitude of the aftershock is unknown, the major problem becomes reasonably determining the magnitude of the aftershock. In past research, the magnitudes of the aftershocks have been widely studied. The magnitudes of the aftershocks can be supposed to have certain values for some specific research purposes. Furthermore, the magnitudes of the aftershocks could be determined via the generalized Omori's law. Moreover, the magnitude difference between the mainshock and its largest aftershock can be determined according to some distributions. Then, the magnitude difference can be subtracted from the mainshock magnitude to obtain the magnitude of the largest aftershock.

In this paper, the magnitude difference is generated via the beta distribution, with a mean of the magnitude difference of 1.2. However, the mean of the magnitude difference is about 0.8 for the selected 662 MS–AS ground motions. In this case, it will introduce bias if the beta distribution is used to generate the magnitude difference for the selected MS–AS ground motions. Thus, this paper selects 150 MS–AS ground motions from the 662 MS–AS ground motions to ensure the magnitude difference of the reselected MS–AS ground motions is about 1.2. Table 2 shows the list of the reselected MS–AS earthquake sequences. The number of stations is set to 0.5 because the magnitudes of the Friuli and Coalinga earthquake sequences are the same, and only one station is reselected from them. Table 2 gives the number of the reselected stations for a certain MS–AS earthquake sequence. For example, 40 stations are reselected from 147 stations for the Chi-Chi earthquake, and the choice is completely random.

Table 2. List of the reselected MS–AS earthquake sequences.

EQID	Earthquake Name	Number of Stations	M_W	Class	CR_{JB} (km)
40	Friuli, Italy-01	0.5	6.5	C1	0
43	Friuli, Italy-02	0.5	5.91	C2-0040	8.79
50	Imperial Valley-06	12	6.53	C1	0
51	Imperial Valley-07	12	5.01	C2-0050	0
53	Livermore-01	1	5.8	C1	0
54	Livermore-02	1	5.42	C2-0053	10.75
56	Mammoth Lakes-01	1	6.06	C1	0
61	Mammoth Lakes-06	1	5.94	C2-0056	5.24
68	Irpinia, Italy-01	2	6.9	C1	0
69	Irpinia, Italy-02	2	6.2	C2-0068	2.41
76	Coalinga-01	0.5	6.36	C1	0
80	Coalinga-05	0.5	5.77	C2-0076	0
103	Chalfant Valley-02	1	6.19	C1	0
104	Chalfant Valley-03	1	5.65	C2-0103	4.01
113	Whittier Narrows-01	1	5.99	C1	0
114	Whittier Narrows-02	1	5.27	C2-0113	0
136	Kocaeli, Turkey	5	7.51	C1	0
138	Duzce, Turkey	5	7.14	C2-0136	15.68
137	Chi-Chi, Taiwan	40	7.62	C1	0
175	Chi-Chi, Taiwan-06	40	6.3	C2-0137	0
234	Umbria Marche, Italy	4	6	C1	0
237	Umbria Marche (aftershock 1), Italy	4	5.5	C2-0234	0
274	L'Aquila, Italy	4	6.3	C1	0
275	L'Aquila (aftershock 1), Italy	4	5.6	C2-0274	0
281	Darfield, New Zealand	3	7	C1	0
346	Christchurch, New Zealand	3	6.2	C2-0281	23.68

4.2.1. The Simulated Seismic Parameters for the Aftershock Ground Motions

Every mainshock ground motion is treated as an isolated earthquake, and the magnitude difference is simulated for every mainshock ground motion in the LHS. As a result, the different ground motions from the same mainshock will have a unique aftershock with a different magnitude, as shown in Figure 18. The magnitudes of the simulated aftershocks are slightly less than their actual values because the magnitude differences in the reselected MS–AS are slightly less than 1.2.

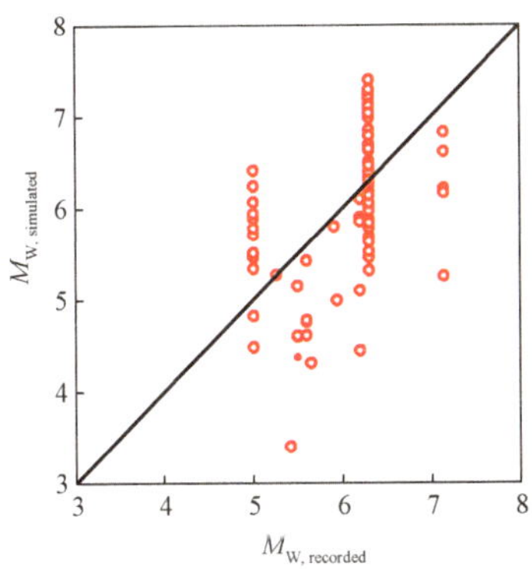

Figure 18. The magnitudes of the aftershock ground motions utilizing LHS.

With the determination of the aftershock magnitudes, the other seismic parameters, such as the width of the rupture, the rupture distance, etc., are simulated with different assumptions about where the aftershock hypocenter will occur. Figure 19 shows the simulated rupture distances and their actual values for the reselected MS–AS ground motions. As shown in Figure 19a–c, the data dots are distributed uniformly on both sides of the 45° diagonal line. The data dots in Figure 19c are more dispersed than those in Figure 19a,b, in which the distribution of the data dots is similar. It still cannot give a reasonable result when the rupture of the aftershocks is assumed to be the same as that of the mainshock, as shown in Figure 19d. The results of the other simulated parameters are similar to those when the aftershock magnitude is known. Therefore, this paper does not provide all the details about the other simulated seismic parameters.

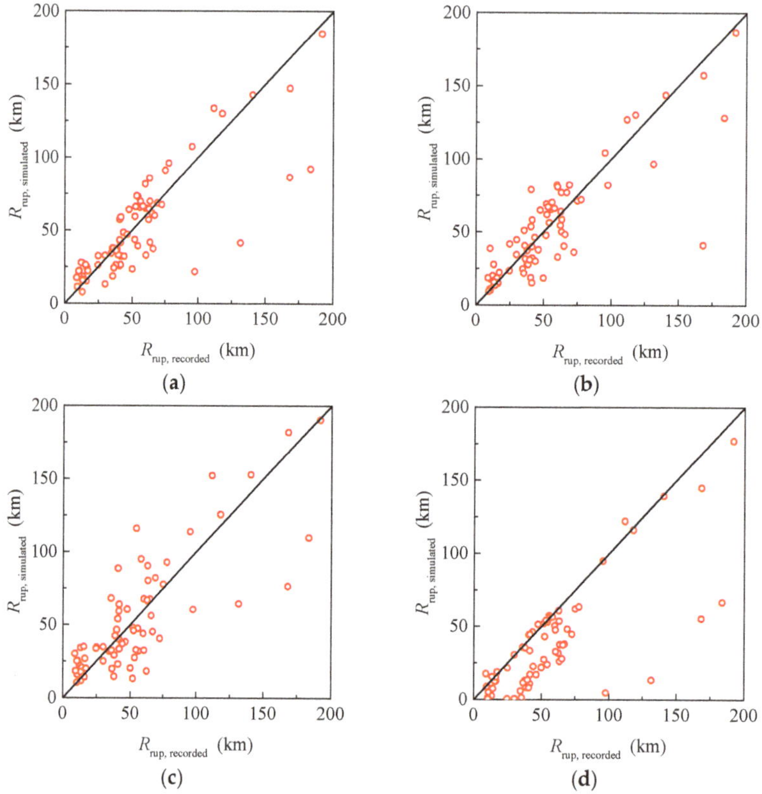

Figure 19. Rupture distances of the aftershock ground motions, with different assumptions when the seismic information of the aftershock is unknown, listed as follows: (**a**) occurring at the same hypocenter; (**b**) linear assumption; (**c**) circular assumption; (**d**) identical to the mainshock.

4.2.2. The Response Spectrum of the Aftershock Ground Motions

With the simulated magnitudes and different assumptions about the locations of the aftershock hypocenters, the response spectrum predicted using the ASK14 model and the conditional mean spectrum of aftershocks are calculated given the reselected mainshock ground motions, as shown in Figures 20–23. The simulated magnitudes of the aftershock ground motions with the different assumptions come from the same sample, which are shown in Figure 18. The results show that all the assumptions, except the last one, can provide a similar response spectrum predicted using the ASK14 model. Moreover, the conditional mean spectrum of aftershocks matches the recorded spectrum better, and its relative errors are less than 20%. The best results come from the linear model under the first three assumptions. When the seismic parameters of the aftershocks are set to those of the mainshock, except the magnitude, the response spectrum predicted using the ASK14 model is very different from the recorded spectrum and has a large relative error. In this case, the conditional mean epsilon of the aftershocks cannot modify the response spectrum predicted using the ASK14 model to make the conditional mean spectrum of the aftershocks match the recorded spectrum well.

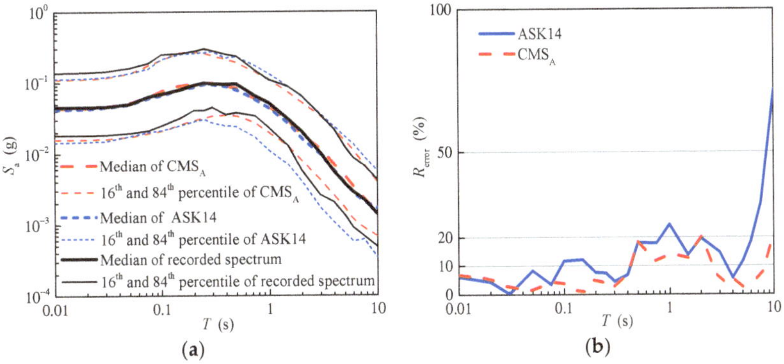

Figure 20. Conditional mean spectrum of aftershocks, with the assumption that the aftershocks and their mainshock occur at the same hypocenter and their relative errors when the seismic information of the aftershock is unknown, listed as follows: (**a**) conditional mean spectrum of aftershocks and (**b**) relative errors.

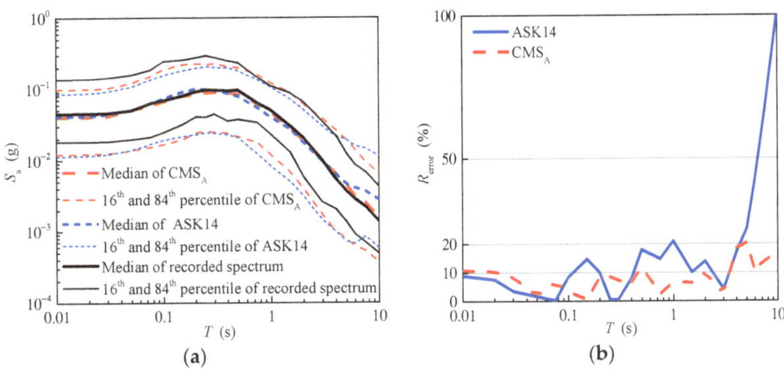

Figure 21. Conditional mean spectrum of aftershocks generated according to the linear model and its relative errors when the seismic information of the aftershocks is unknown listed as follows: (**a**) conditional mean spectrum of aftershocks and (**b**) relative errors.

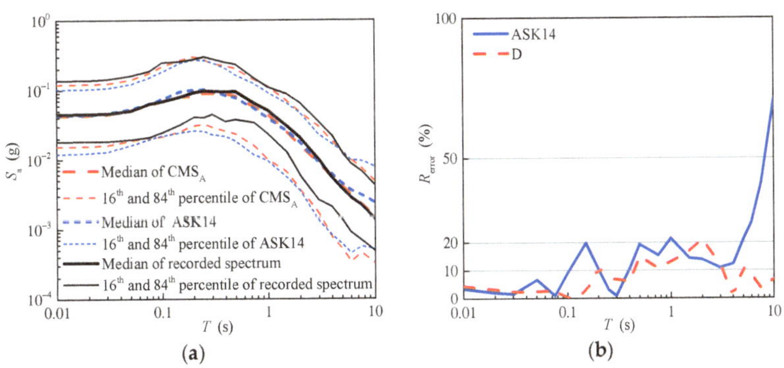

Figure 22. Conditional mean spectrum of aftershocks generated according to the circular model and its relative error when the seismic information of the aftershocks is unknown listed as follows: (**a**) conditional mean spectrum of aftershocks and (**b**) relative errors.

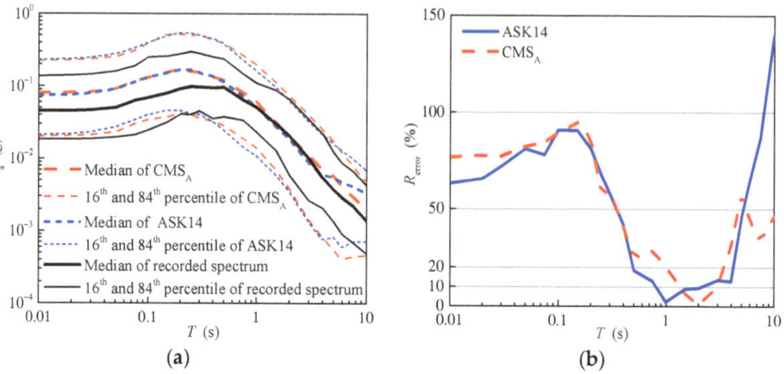

Figure 23. Conditional mean spectrum of aftershocks, with the assumption that the seismic parameters of the aftershocks and the mainshock ground motions are identical except the magnitudes and their relative errors when the seismic information of the aftershock is unknown, listed as follows: (**a**) conditional mean spectrum of aftershocks and (**b**) relative errors.

5. Conclusions

In this paper, a new method of generating the aftershock target spectrum according to the conditional mean spectrum of aftershocks is established, given information about the main shock. The target aftershock spectrum is compared with that predicted using the ground motion prediction model, and the relative errors are also analyzed under four assumptions. The following main conclusions can be drawn.

(1) In addition to the last assumption, the relative errors of the conditional mean spectra of aftershocks are relatively small, basically controlled within the range of 20%, and its discrete properties are closer to the real recorded response spectra. This is because the correlation between the spectral shapes of the mainshock and aftershock ground motion is further considered based on the ground motion prediction equation.

(2) For the first three assumptions, the method proposed in this paper can reasonably simulate the parameters of aftershock ground motions under the given main earthquake information. Under these assumptions, the sizes of the aftershock faults can be considered, and other parameters are solved according to the definition to ensure that the simulated parameters are close to the real parameters. The parameters simulated under the first assumption are relatively concentrated, although some of its parameters, such as R_{JB}, may be relatively larger than their real value.

In this research, a new method was developed to generate the target aftershock spectrum. The key parts are the simulation of the aftershock magnitude, the location and size of the aftershock rupture, and the correlation model of the spectral shape (epsilon) between the MS–AS ground motions. The target aftershock spectrum could be used to select aftershock ground motions from the real ground motion database or generate artificial aftershock grounds, given the mainshock ground motion.

Author Contributions: Conceptualization, D.L.; methodology, D.L.; software, R.Z. and B.D.; validation, D.L.; investigation, R.Z., B.D. and Y.Y.; writing—original draft preparation, R.Z. and B.D.; writing—review and editing, D.L. and Y.Y.; visualization, R.Z. and B.D.; supervision, D.L. All authors have read and agreed to the published version of the manuscript.

Funding: This study is founded by the Hebei Provincial Department of Human Resources and Social Security (Grant No. B2019003025).

Data Availability Statement: The selected ground motions were from the NGA-West2 ground motion database of the PEER ground motion database http://ngawest2.berkeley.edu/site (accessed on 5 October 2016).

Acknowledgments: The authors would like to gratefully acknowledge the support of the Hebei Provincial Department of Human Resources and Social Security (Personnel Department). For its work in ground motion database, the Pacific Earthquake Engineering Research Center (PEER) is also acknowledged.

Conflicts of Interest: The authors declare no conflict of interest.

List of Abbreviations and Symbols

Abbreviations:	(Alphabetically!!)
AS	Aftershock
ASK14	GMPE proposed by Abrahamson et al. in 2014 [31]
CMS_A	Conditional mean spectrum of aftershocks
ETAS	Epidemic-type aftershock sequence
GMPE	Ground motion prediction equation
MS	Main shock
PDF	Probability density function
Symbols:	(Alphabetically!!)
A	Area of the circular region (km^2)
a, b	Regression coefficients of the rupture length and rupture width
$B(2.2, 2.3)$	Beta function for the corresponding elements 2.2 and 2.3
CR_{JB}	Centroid Joyner–Boore distance
FW	Site within the footwall region
HW	Site within the hanging wall region
L	Rupture length
L_A	Rupture length of the aftershock
L_M	Rupture length of the main shock
M_A	Magnitude of the aftershock
M_M	Magnitude of the main shock
NU	Site within the neutral region
$p(\Delta m)$	PDF of the selected beta distribution
R_A	Source-to-site distance of an aftershock
R_{error}	Relative error
$R_{rup,A}$	Rupture distance of the aftershock
$R_{rup,M}$	Rupture distance of the main shock
R_X	Distance measured perpendicular to the fault strike from the surface projection of the up-dip edge of the fault plane
$S_{a,A}$	Spectral accelerations of the aftershock
$S_{a,M}$	Spectral accelerations of the mainshock
T_i	The ith period of the response spectrum
W	Rupture width
W_A	Rupture width of the aftershock
W_M	Rupture width of the main shock
Δm	Magnitude difference between the mainshock and its largest aftershock
ε_A	Epsilon values of the aftershock
ε_M	Epsilon values of the mainshock
$\mu_{\ln S_{a,A}}$	Mean of $\ln S_{a,A}$ predicted using the GMPE
$\mu_{\ln S_{a,A}(T_i)\|lnS_{a,M}(T_i)}$	Conditional mean of the $\ln S_{a,A}$ conditioned on the $\ln S_{a,M}$ at the period T_i
$\mu_{\ln S_a}^{As-record}$	Mean of the logarithm of the recorded response spectrum for the aftershock ground motions
$\mu_{\ln S_a}^{Predict}$	Mean of the logarithm of the predicted response spectrum
$\mu_{\varepsilon_A(T_i)}$	Means of ε_A at the period T_i
$\mu_{\varepsilon_A(T_i)\|\varepsilon_M(T_i)}$	Conditional mean of $\varepsilon_A(T_i)$ conditioned on $\varepsilon_M(T_i)$ at the period T_i
$\mu_{\varepsilon_M(T_i)}$	Means of ε_M at the period T_i
$\rho[\varepsilon_A(T_i), \varepsilon_M(T_i)]$	Correlation coefficient between ε_A and ε_M at the period T_i
$\sigma_{\ln S_{a,A}}$	Standard deviation of $\ln S_{a,A}$ predicted using the GMPE
$\sigma_{\varepsilon_A(T_i)}$	Standard deviations of ε_A at the period T_i
$\sigma_{\varepsilon_M(T_i)}$	Standard deviations of ε_M at the period T_i

References

1. Kam, W.Y.; Pampanin, S.; Elwood, K. Seismic performance of reinforced concrete buildings in the 22 February Christchurch (Lyttleton) earthquake. *Bull. N. Z. Soc. Earthq. Eng.* **2011**, *44*, 239–278. [CrossRef]
2. Torfehnejad, M.; Sensoy, S. Aftershock collapse capacity assessment of special steel moment frame structures. *Structures* **2023**, *56*, 105046. [CrossRef]
3. Saed, G.; Balomenos, G.P. Fragility framework for corroded steel moment-resisting frame buildings subjected to mainshock-aftershock sequences. *Soil Dyn. Earthq. Eng.* **2023**, *171*, 107975. [CrossRef]

4. Rajabi, E.; Golestani, Y. Study of steel buildings with LCF system under critical mainshock-aftershock sequence: Evaluation of fragility curves and estimation of the response modification factor by artificial intelligence. *Structures* **2023**, *56*, 105044. [CrossRef]
5. Huang, X.; Liu, J.; Wang, N.; Xu, S. Pseudo-dynamic experimental study on seismically isolated prefabricated RC structure with roller-bearing subjected to mainshock-aftershock sequences. *J. Build. Eng.* **2023**, *65*, 105775. [CrossRef]
6. Tesfamariam, S.; Goda, K. Risk assessment of CLT-RC hybrid building: Consideration of earthquake types and aftershocks for Vancouver, British Columbia. *Soil Dyn. Earthq. Eng.* **2022**, *156*, 107240. [CrossRef]
7. Pang, R.; Zai, D.; Xu, B.; Liu, J.; Zhao, C.; Fan, Q.; Chen, Y. Stochastic dynamic and reliability analysis of AP1000 nuclear power plants via DPIM subjected to mainshock-aftershock sequences. *Reliab. Eng. Syst. Saf.* **2023**, *235*, 109217. [CrossRef]
8. Fang, C.; Ping, B.; Zheng, Y.; Ping, Y.; Ling, H. Seismic fragility and loss estimation of self-centering steel braced frames under mainshock-aftershock sequences. *J. Build. Eng.* **2023**, *73*, 106433. [CrossRef]
9. Du, M.; Zhang, S.; Wang, C.; She, L.; Li, J.; Lu, T. Seismic fragility assessment of aqueduct bent structures subjected to mainshock-aftershock sequences. *Eng. Struct.* **2023**, *292*, 116505. [CrossRef]
10. Pang, R.; Xu, B.; Zhou, Y.; Zhang, X.; Wang, X. Fragility analysis of high CFRDs subjected to mainshock-aftershock sequences based on plastic failure. *Eng. Struct.* **2020**, *206*, 110152. [CrossRef]
11. Hatzigeorgiou, G.D.; Beskos, D.E. Inelastic displacement ratios for SDOF structures subjected to repeated earthquakes. *Eng. Struct.* **2009**, *31*, 2744–2755. [CrossRef]
12. Li, Y.; Song, R.; Van De Lindt, J.W. Collapse fragility of steel structures subjected to earthquake mainshock-aftershock sequences. *J. Struct. Eng.* **2014**, *140*, 04014095. [CrossRef]
13. Torres, J.R.; Bojórquez, E.; Bojórquez, J.; Leyva, H.; Ruiz, S.E.; Reyes-Salazar, A.; Palemón-Arcos, L.; Rivera, J.L.; Carvajal, J.; Reyes, H.E. Improving the seismic performance of steel frames under mainshock–aftershock using post-tensioned connections. *Buildings* **2023**, *13*, 1676. [CrossRef]
14. Furinghetti, M.; Lanese, I.; Pavese, A. Experimental hybrid simulation of severe aftershocks chains on buildings equipped with curved surface slider devices. *Buildings* **2022**, *12*, 1255. [CrossRef]
15. Wei, J.; Ying, H.; Yang, Y.; Zhang, W.; Yuan, H.; Zhou, J. Seismic performance of concrete-filled steel tubular composite columns with ultra high performance concrete plates. *Eng. Struct.* **2023**, *278*, 115500. [CrossRef]
16. Zheng, X.; Shen, Y.; Zong, X.; Su, H.; Zhao, X. Vulnerability analysis of main aftershock sequence of aqueduct based on incremental dynamic analysis method. *Buildings* **2023**, *13*, 1490. [CrossRef]
17. Ruiz-García, J.; Ramos-Cruz, J.M. Collapse strength ratios for structures under mainshock-aftershock subduction seismic sequences. *Structures* **2023**, *56*, 104864. [CrossRef]
18. Nugroho, L.Z.; Chiu, C.-K. Damage-controlling seismic design of low- and mid-rise RC buildings considering mainshock-aftershock sequences. *Structures* **2023**, *57*, 105099. [CrossRef]
19. Yakhchalian, M.; Yakhchalian, M. An advanced intensity measure for aftershock collapse fragility assessment of structures. *Structures* **2022**, *44*, 933–946. [CrossRef]
20. Goda, K.; Taylor, C.A. Effects of aftershocks on peak ductility demand due to strong ground motion records from shallow crustal earthquakes. *Earthq. Eng. Struct. Dyn.* **2012**, *41*, 2311–2330. [CrossRef]
21. Kim, B.; Shin, M. A model for estimating horizontal aftershock ground motions for active crustal regions. *Soil Dyn. Earthq. Eng.* **2017**, *92*, 165–175. [CrossRef]
22. Hu, S.; Gardoni, P.; Xu, L. Stochastic procedure for the simulation of synthetic main shock-aftershock ground motion sequences. *Earthq. Eng. Struct. Dyn.* **2018**, *47*, 2275–2296. [CrossRef]
23. Wang, G.; Pang, R.; Yu, X.; Xu, B. Permanent displacement reliability analysis of soil slopes subjected to mainshock-aftershock sequences. *Comput. Geotech.* **2023**, *153*, 105069. [CrossRef]
24. Pu, W.; Li, Y. Evaluating structural failure probability during aftershocks based on spatiotemporal simulation of the regional earthquake sequence. *Eng. Struct.* **2023**, *275*, 115267. [CrossRef]
25. Khalil, C.; Lopez-Caballero, F. Lifetime response of a liquefiable soil foundation-embankment system subjected to sequences of mainshocks and aftershocks. *Soil Dyn. Earthq. Eng.* **2023**, *173*, 108107. [CrossRef]
26. Ghotbi, A.R.; Taciroglu, E. Conditioning criteria based on multiple intensity measures for selecting hazard-consistent aftershock ground motion records. *Soil Dyn. Earthq. Eng.* **2020**, *139*, 106345. [CrossRef]
27. Ding, Y.; Chen, J.; Shen, J. Prediction of spectral accelerations of aftershock ground motion with deep learning method. *Soil Dyn. Earthq. Eng.* **2021**, *150*, 106951. [CrossRef]
28. Chaiyasarn, K.; Buatik, A.; Mohamad, H.; Zhou, M.; Kongsilp, S.; Poovarodom, N. Integrated pixel-level CNN-FCN crack detection via photogrammetric 3D texture mapping of concrete structures. *Autom. Constr.* **2022**, *140*, 104388. [CrossRef]
29. Abadel, A.A. Physical, mechanical, and microstructure characteristics of ultra-high-performance concrete containing lightweight aggregates. *Materials* **2023**, *16*, 4883. [CrossRef]
30. Zhu, R.G.; Lu, D.G.; Yu, X.H.; Wang, G.Y. Conditional mean spectrum of aftershocks. *Bull. Seismol. Soc. Am.* **2017**, *107*, 1940–1953. [CrossRef]
31. Abrahamson, N.A.; Silva, W.J.; Kamai, R. Summary of the ASK14 ground motion relation for active crustal regions. *Earthq. Spectra* **2014**, *30*, 1025–1055. [CrossRef]
32. Han, R.; Li, Y.; van de Lindt, J. Assessment of seismic performance of buildings with incorporation of aftershocks. *J. Perform. Constr. Facil.* **2015**, *29*, 04014088. [CrossRef]

33. Yeo, G.L.; Cornell, C.A.A. probabilistic framework for quantification of aftershock ground-motion hazard in California: Methodology and parametric study. *Earthq. Eng. Struct. Dyn.* **2009**, *38*, 45–60. [CrossRef]
34. Kumitani, S.; Takada, T. Probabilistic assessment of buildings damage considering aftershocks of earthquakes. *J. Struct. Constr. Eng.* **2009**, *74*, 459–465. [CrossRef]
35. Wells, D.L.; Coppersmith, K.J. New empirical relationships among magnitude, rupture length, rupture width, rupture area, and surface displacement. *Bull. Seismol. Soc. Am.* **1994**, *84*, 974–1002.
36. Ancheta, T.D.; Darragh, R.B.; Stewart, J.P.; Seyhan, E.; Silva, W.J.; Chiou, B.S.-J.; Wooddell, K.E.; Graves, R.W.; Kottke, A.R.; Boore, D.M. NGA-West2 database. *Earthq. Spectra* **2014**, *30*, 989–1005. [CrossRef]
37. Han, R.; Li, Y.; van de Lindt, J. Seismic risk of base isolated non-ductile reinforced concrete buildings considering uncertainties and mainshock–aftershock sequences. *Struct. Saf.* **2014**, *50*, 39–56. [CrossRef]
38. Abrahamson, N.; Silva, W.J. Empirical response spectral attenuation relations for shallow crustal earthquakes. *Seismol. Res. Lett.* **1997**, *68*, 94–127. [CrossRef]

buildings

MDPI

Article

Enhancing Volumetric Stability of Metakaolin-Based Geopolymer Composites with Organic Modifiers WER and SCA

Mo Zhang [1], Yongquan Zang [1] and Lingyan Shan [2,*]

[1] School of Civil and Transportation Engineering, Hebei University of Technology, 5340 Xiping Road, Tianjin 300401, China; mozhang@hebut.edu.cn (M.Z.); 202121601059@stu.hebut.edu.cn (Y.Z.)

[2] Fundamental Research Innovation Center, Research Institute of Highway Ministry of Transport, 8 Xitucheng Road, Beijing 100088, China

* Correspondence: ly.shan@rioh.cn

Abstract: Shrinkage during hardening and curing is one of the largest challenges for the widespread application of metakaolin-based geopolymers (MKGs). To solve this problem, a silane coupling agent (SCA) and waterborne epoxy resin (WER) were used to synthesize MKG composites. The individual and synergistic effects of the SCA and WER on chemical, autogenous, and drying shrinkage were assessed, the modification mechanisms were investigated by microstructural characterization, and shrinkage resistance was evaluated by the chloride ion permeability of MKG composite coatings. The results showed that the SCA and WER significantly decreased the chemical shrinkage, autogenous shrinkage, and drying shrinkage of the MKG, with the highest reductions of 46.4%, 131.2%, and 25.2% obtained by the combination of 20 wt% WER and 1 wt% SCA. The incorporation of the organic modifiers densified the microstructure. Compared with the MKG, the total volume of mesopores and macropores in MKG-WER, MKG-SCA, and MKG-WER-SCA decreased by 11.5%, 8.7%, and 3.8%, respectively. In particular, the silanol hydrolyzed from the SCA can react with the opened epoxy ring of the WER and the aluminosilicate oligomers simultaneously to form a compact network and resist shrinkage during the hardening and continuous reaction of the geopolymer. Furthermore, the apparently lowered chloride ion diffusion coefficient of concrete (i.e., reduction of 51.4% to 59.5%) by the WER- and SCA-modified MKG coatings verified their improved shrinkage resistance. The findings in this study provide promising methods to essentially solve the shrinkage problem of MKGs at the microscale and shed light on the modification mechanism by WERs and SCAs, and they also suggest the applicability of MKG composites in protective coatings for marine concrete.

Keywords: metakaolin-based geopolymer; chemical shrinkage; autogenous shrinkage; drying shrinkage; organic modification

1. Introduction

Geopolymers are a type of cementitious material synthesized through the alkali activation of aluminosilicate materials, such as metakaolin [1], granulated blast furnace slag [2], steel slag [3], etc. Due to the reuse capability of industrial by-products and low carbon emissions of the production process, geopolymers have received wide research interest [4]. In recent years, the applicability of geopolymers as protective coating materials has been increasingly investigated due to their high toughness [5], high thermal stability [6], good corrosion resistance [7], and water impermeability [8]. A metakaolin-based geopolymer (MKG) coating presented excellent resistance to seawater corrosion and high adhesion strength to concrete and steel substrates [9], while the intrinsic shrinkage nature can induce serious cracking problems and limit the application of MKGs [10–12]. High shrinkage gave rise to microcracks in the MKG coating and accelerated the intrusion and penetration of aggressive ions into the concrete, rendering the geopolymer coating functionally ineffective [13].

Many efforts have endeavored to reduce shrinkage cracking risks [14]. Incorporating shortcut fibers is one of the most widely applied methods, which controls the development and expansion of cracks during different types of shrinkage [15,16]. Al et al. revealed that steel fibers and glass fibers reduced the drying shrinkage of fly ash-based geopolymer composites by 16–24% after curing for 28 days [17]. Vilaplana et al. showed that 0.2 wt% of 3 mm carbon fibers (CFs) was sufficient to reduce the maximum strain of drying shrinkage to less than 1.5 mm/m [15]. However, the workability and mechanical strength of the geopolymer were significantly impacted by the dispersity and type of fiber [18,19]. At the same time, the fibers cannot participate in geopolymerization, and thus, they can barely reduce shrinkage at the microscale and essentially dissolve shrinkage problems [20,21]. Other studies have focused on modifications with liquid organic solvents, such as silane coupling agents (SCAs) and waterborne epoxy resins (WERs), to reduce the shrinkage of geopolymers. Liquid organic solvents could be evenly dispersed in the geopolymer gels, thus enhancing the compactness of the geopolymer and inhibiting the propagation of microcracks in the geopolymer [22]. Wang et al. found that the incorporation of an SCA reduced the drying shrinkage of MKGs by 18% after curing for 28 days [23]. Zhang et al. found that the incorporation of an SCA improved the compressive strength of an MKG by 14.99% and the flexural strength by 11.24%. The structure of the MKG became more compact, and the closed pore size was reduced from 13.16 nm to 8.11 nm [24]. The improved mechanical and shrinkage properties were likely to have resulted from the involvement of the SCA in the polymerization of the MKG, generating enriched N-A-S-H gels and thus refining the pore structure of the SCA-MKG composites [25]. Epoxy resin is another organic solvent that can be well dispersed in geopolymers [26]. In contrast to the bond strength of geopolymer gels, epoxy resin had a strong interaction with the inorganic matrix of the geopolymer, as epoxy resin molecules opened their rings during the cross-linking process and formed a dense network of hydrogen bonds with each other, thus improving the strength of the geopolymer [27,28]. Apriany et al. found that epoxy resin reduced the drying shrinkage of fly ash–slag-based geopolymer composites by 5.2–12.2% [29]. Du et al. found that the compressive strength of a metakaolin-granulated blast furnace slag geopolymer increased by 30% with the incorporation of 20 wt% epoxy resin [30]. The improvement of the mechanical properties and durability of geopolymers suggested the wide application of liquid organic solvent modification. However, the performance and underlying mechanisms of shrinkage reduction in geopolymers by incorporating multiple organic solvents have rarely been reported.

Due to the distinctive reaction processes and microstructures of geopolymers compared with ordinary Portland cement (OPC), the shrinkage mechanism of geopolymers is quite different from that of OPC [31]. For geopolymers, autogenous shrinkage is the volume reduction caused by the combined action of self-desiccation and chemical shrinkage without water transferring to the external environment [32]. Among them, self-desiccation is caused by the dissolution process of geopolymers, continuously consuming pore water in the capillary pores, thus leading to the development of pores inside the geopolymer and generating capillary pressure [33]. Chemical shrinkage is caused by the variation in the density of geopolymer products before and after geopolymerization [34]. Li et al. found that MKGs underwent three stages of chemical shrinkage, i.e., chemical shrinkage, chemical expansion, and chemical shrinkage again [35]. However, chemical shrinkage is less likely to occur during the hydration of cement because of the great toughness and particle skeleton of cement [36]. In an open environment, drying shrinkage is caused by the evaporation of water from the pore structure of the geopolymer [37], which can be much greater than that of OPC [38,39]. Therefore, autogenous shrinkage, chemical shrinkage, and drying shrinkage correspond to the volume changes in the geopolymer during dissolution, pre-hardening, and post-hardening processes, respectively. Under the combined effect of autogenous shrinkage, chemical shrinkage, and drying shrinkage, the macroscopic volume of the geopolymer changes, leading to tensile stresses, inhomogeneous deformations, and damaging cracks, which can seriously affect the mechanical properties of the geopolymer and thus its durability [40]. By adding additives to suppress the change in the geopolymer volume during the different reaction times of the geopolymer, the shrinkage of the geopolymer can be significantly reduced, and the strength of the geopolymer can be increased. Yang et al. found that the reaction of geopolymers based on fly ash and metakaolin drove the pore fluids to the autogenous shrinkage sites and reduced the capillary stresses, and autogenous shrinkage showed a negative trend (i.e., expansion) before it became positive (shrinkage) [41]. Ruan et al. [42] found that the hydrophobic chemical groups introduced by polydimethylsiloxane (PDMS) and sodium methylsilicate (SMS) could be strongly bound to the geopolymer gel, giving the MKG a good water-repellent effect and thus reducing autogenous shrinkage by 91.1% and 41.8%, respectively. In terms of chemical shrinkage, PDMS improved the dispersion of the solid precursors, and SMS increased the alkalinity of the MKG, allowing the MKG to form a denser and more amorphous Si-rich gel, which reduced the chemical expansion of the MKG. Tian et al. [43] found that the addition of 5 wt% silicon acrylic (Si-A) reduced the drying shrinkage of fly ash- and slag-based geopolymers by 63.5%. This was due to the film formed by the Si-A polymer on the hydration products, which sealed the water in the geopolymer and prevented its evaporation. However, the existing studies only focus on the effects of organic solvent modification on the shrinkage of geopolymers. There are few studies on the effects of organic solvents on the whole reaction process of geopolymers, i.e., autogenous shrinkage, chemical shrinkage, and drying shrinkage [44].

As shown in Figure 1, a waterborne epoxy resin (WER), a silane coupling agent (SCA), and a mixture of the above two were used to synthesize an organically modified MKG to reduce shrinkage in this study. The influence of the individual addition and synergistic mixture of the WER and SCA on the chemical shrinkage, autogenous shrinkage, and drying shrinkage of the MKG was investigated. The modification mechanism of the WER, SCA, and WER-SCA on the shrinkage properties of the MKG was analyzed using microstructural characterization by scanning electron microscopy (SEM), energy-dispersive spectroscopy (EDS), Fourier-transform infrared spectroscopy (FTIR), X-ray diffraction (XRD), mercury intrusion porosimetry (MIP), and nuclear magnetic resonance (NMR). An appropriate reaction process among the WER, SCA, and MKG was proposed. Finally, the resistance of the WER-SCA-modified MKG coating to chloride ion penetration was evaluated by rapid chloride migration (RCM) tests to illustrate its applicability in marine protective coatings.

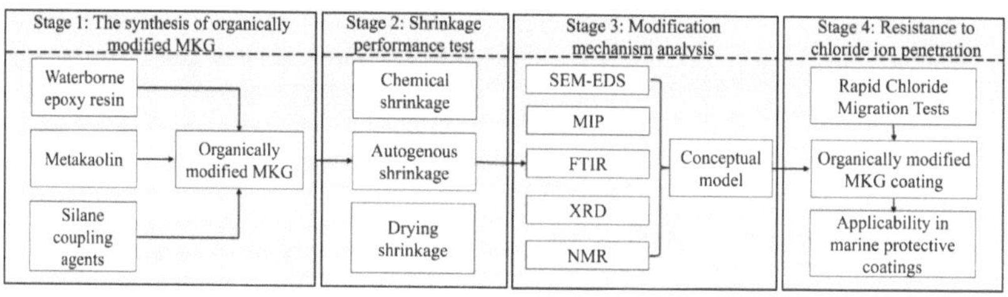

Figure 1. Research methodology of metakaolin-based geopolymer composites enhanced with organic modifiers WER and SCA.

2. Materials and Methods

2.1. Materials

Metakaolin (MK) with a mesh size of 1250 was provided by Jiaozuo Yukun Co., Ltd., in Jiaozuo, China. The average particle size of MK is 10 μm, and the specific surface area is 128,710 cm^2/g. The main chemical composition of MK is listed in Table 1, and the mineralogical properties are presented in the form of XRD patterns, as shown in Figure 2d. The alkaline activator solution used in the experiment was prepared with sodium metasilicate solution ($Na_2O{\cdot}2SiO_2$, $Na_2O/SiO_2 = 2.0$, and a solid content of 42%) and 50 wt% sodium hydroxide (NaOH) solution. Deionized water was used throughout the experiments. E51 epoxy resin and the Q17 waterborne hardener (diethylenetriamine

(DETA) as the main ingredient) were selected as the main components to prepare the waterborne epoxy resin (WER). The n-Octyl triethoxy silane coupling agent (SCA) was selected as another type of organic modifier. E51 epoxy resin and the Q17 waterborne hardener were purchased from Yingyi Environmental Protection Technology Co., Ltd. in Weifang, China, and the silane coupling agent was purchased from Nanjing Feiteng Technology Co., Ltd., in Nanjing, China. The chemical structures of E51 epoxy resin, the SCA, and DETA are shown in Figure 2.

Table 1. Chemical composition of metakaolin.

Metakaolin	SiO_2	Al_2O_3	TiO_2	Fe_2O_3	Na_2O	CaO	K_2O	MgO
Chemical Composition (wt%)	49.67	42.54	2.14	1.32	0.68	0.19	0.18	0.14

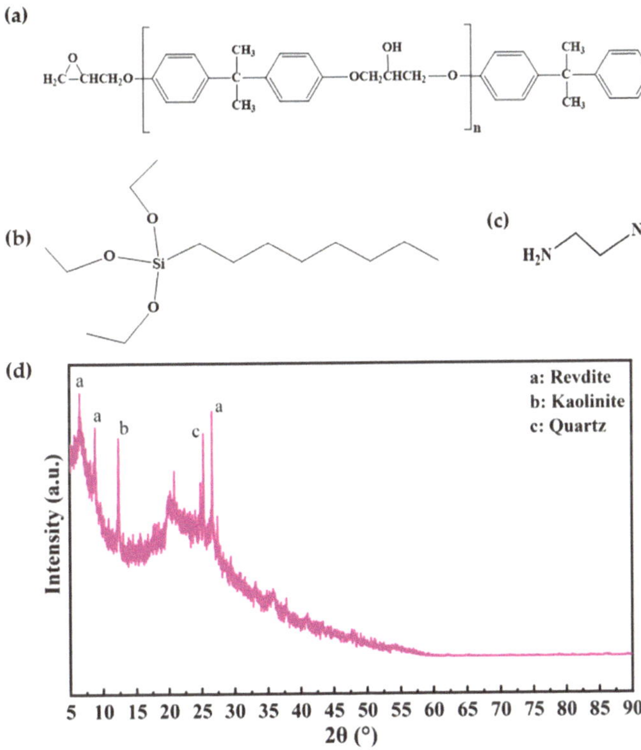

Figure 2. The chemical structures of (**a**) E51 epoxy resin, (**b**) the n-Octyl triethoxy SCA, and (**c**) DETA and (**d**) the XRD pattern of metakaolin.

2.2. Sample Preparation

The mix proportions of all MKG sample sets in this experiment are listed in Table 2 and were determined on the basis of previous studies [45,46]. A 50 wt% NaOH solution was prepared 24 h in advance and cooled to room temperature. The 50 wt% NaOH solution and $Na_2O{\cdot}SiO_2$ solution were mixed in a volume ratio of 5:1 to obtain the alkali activator solution. MK and the alkali activator solution were mixed for 3 min to obtain an MKG paste using a cement mortar mixer. At the same time, the waterborne curing agent Q17 and E51 epoxy resin were mixed in a mass ratio of 5:3 to obtain the waterborne epoxy resin (WER). For the WER-modified MKG (MKG-WER), the WER was mixed with the MKG paste in a mass ratio of 20%. The SCA was mixed with the MKG paste at a mass ratio of 1%

by direct dropping for the SCA-modified MKG (MKG-SCA). For the SCA-WER-modified MKG (MKG-WER-SCA), the SCA was slowly mixed with fresh MKG-WER paste at a mass ratio of 1% and stirred for 3 min. The prepared MKG and MKG-WER coatings are shown in Figure 3.

Table 2. Material compositions of organic-liquid-modified geopolymer.

Sample	Metakaolin (g)	$Na_2O{\cdot}2SiO_2$ (mL)	50 wt% NaOH (mL)	E51 Epoxy Resin (g)	Q17 Hardener (g)	SCA (g)
MKG	100	90	18	-	-	-
MKG-WER	100	90	18	32.9	19.8	-
MKG-SCA	100	90	18	-	-	2.6
MKG-WER-SCA	100	90	18	32.9	19.8	3.2

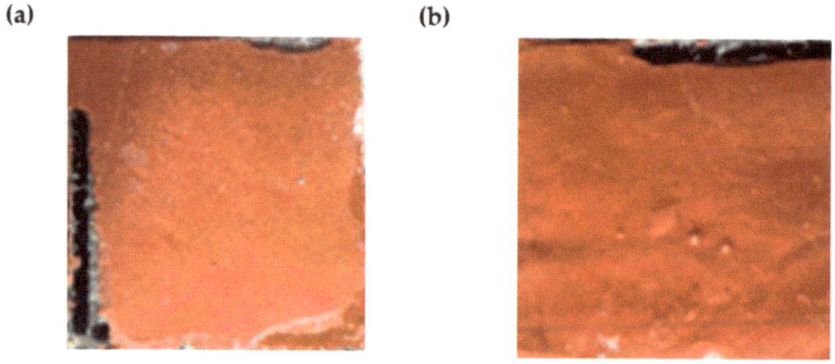

Figure 3. (**a**) MKG coating and (**b**) MKG–WER coating on cement concrete.

2.3. Testing Program

2.3.1. Drying Shrinkage Test

According to the Chinese standard GB/T 50082-2009 [47], 25 mm × 25 mm × 280 mm prism specimens were prepared and demolded after sealed curing for 24 h. The lengths of the specimens along the longitudinal axis were determined with a BC-300d bench comparator, with an accuracy of 0.001 mm. The specimens were cured in sealed bags at room temperature for 7 days. The first readings were recorded immediately after demolding, and then the daily length changes of the specimens were recorded to calculate the drying shrinkage.

2.3.2. Chemical Shrinkage Test

According to the ASTM standard C1608-2017 [48], dilatometry was used to measure the chemical shrinkage of the MKG, MKG-WER, MKG-SCA, and MKG-WER-SCA. The prepared pastes were injected into vials to a height of 7 mm. The paste level was then sealed with droplets of vegetable oil, and the vial was plugged using a rubber stopper with a graduated capillary tube inserted through it. The level of the vegetable oil in the graduated tube was within the graduation line. The vials were left to stand in a water bath to maintain the temperature at 23 °C. The initial readings of the bottom of the meniscus in the capillary tube were recorded after 1 h of curing, and then the level changes (hi) in the glass tube were recorded every hour for the first 8 h and every day thereafter. Chemical shrinkage was calculated according to Equation (1) [48]:

$$S_i = \frac{(h_i - h_0)}{m_c} \quad (1)$$

where S_i is the chemical shrinkage value in mL/g; h_0 is the initial height of the liquid level in the scale tube in mL; h_i is the change in the liquid level in the capillary tube in mL; and m_c is the mass of the pastes in the vials in g.

2.3.3. Autogenous Shrinkage Test

The autogenous shrinkage of four types of geopolymer composite pastes was measured continuously over a period of 7 days according to the ASTM standard C1698-2009 (2014) [49]. The prepared geopolymer composite paste was filled into a corrugated tube, of which the length change was monitored automatically with a digital gauge every hour from the final setting time (i.e., 6.5 h, 4 h, 6 h, and 3.5 h for MKG, MKG-SCA, MKG-WER, and MKG-WER-SCA, respectively) until the 24th h, and then every day for the following 6 days. Autogenous shrinkage was calculated according to Equations (2) and (3) [49]:

$$L_0 = L_{ref} + R_t - 2L_{plug} \tag{2}$$

$$\varepsilon = \frac{R_t - R_i}{L_0} \times 10^6 \tag{3}$$

where L_0 is the initial length of the sample measured at the final setting time in mm; L_{ref} is the length of the reference rod in mm; R_t is the reading of the dial gauge at each measurement moment in mm; L_{plug} is the length of one stopper plugged in one end of the corrugated tube in mm; ε is the autogenous shrinkage in µm/mm; and R_i is the dial gauge reading at the final setting time in mm.

2.3.4. Microstructural Characterization

The microstructural evolution of the four types of geopolymer composites was characterized using an S4800 scanning electron microscope at an accelerating voltage of 5 kV, and EDS was conducted to determine the chemical compositions of the resins and geopolymer gels. The pore size distribution and pore volume of the composites were measured by mercury intrusion porosimetry with a Micromeritics Autopore IV, and cubic specimens of about 27 mm^3 were used. The bonding structure of the specimens was characterized by a TENSOR 27 FTIR device in the wavelength range from 600 cm^{-1} to 4000 cm^{-1}. The mineral composition of the specimens was determined using a Smartlab 9KW XRD diffractometer with CuKα radiation at a voltage of 40 kV and a current of 100 mA. The scan rate was 6°/min from 5° to 40° (2θ) at 0.02/step. The chemical reaction between the organic modifier and the geopolymer was characterized by solid-state 27Al and ^{29}Si nuclear magnetic resonance (NMR) using a Bruker 400M NMR spectrometer with a probe diameter of 4 mm and a MAS spin rate of 10 KHz. The parameters of ^{27}Al NMR and ^{29}Si NMR were as follows:

For ^{27}Al MAS NMR, the resonance frequency was 104.26 MHz, single-pulse sampling was adopted, the pulse width was 0.97 µs, the relaxation delay time was 1 s, the number of scans was 800 times, and the chemical shift was referenced to aqueous $NaAlO_2$.

For ^{29}Si MAS NMR, the resonance frequency was 79.49 MHz, single-pulse sampling was adopted, the pulse width was 4.97 µs, the relaxation delay time was 5 s, the number of scans was 512 times, and the chemical shift was referenced to tetramethyl orthosilicate at 0 ppm.

2.3.5. Rapid Chloride Migration Test

According to the Chinese standard GB/T 50082-2009 [47], the chloride ion penetration resistance of geopolymer coatings was measured by the rapid chloride migration (RCM) test. Cylindrical concrete specimens with a size of φ100 mm × 50 mm after curing for 14 days were used for this experiment. A 2~3 mm thick geopolymer paste coating was applied to the top and bottom surfaces of the specimens. The sides of the specimens were coated with a petroleum wax sealant and then cured at room temperature for 7 days. During the test, the applied voltage was set to 30 V to record the initial current. Based on the initial current, the applied voltage was adjusted according to the relationship between the initial current and voltage in Table 3, and a new initial current and voltage were recorded. At the end of the assigned test duration, the initial and final temperatures of the anode solution were recorded by electrocouples, and the duration of the experiment was recorded. The diffusion coefficient of the chloride ion was calculated according to Equation (4) [47]:

$$D_{RCM} = \frac{0.0239 \times (273 + T)L}{(U - 2)t} \left(X_d - 0.0238\sqrt{\frac{(273 + T)LX_d}{U - 2}} \right) \quad (4)$$

where D_{RCM} is the chloride ion migration coefficient in $\times 10^{-12}$ m^2/s; U is the absolute value of the applied voltage according to Table 3 in V; T is the average value of the initial and final temperature of the anode solution in °C; L is the thickness of the geopolymer specimens in mm; X_d is the average value of the chloride ion penetration depth in mm; and t is the test duration in h.

Table 3. The relationship between the initial current, voltage, and test time [47].

Initial Current (I_{30V}/mA)	Applied Voltage (U/V)	Possible New Initial Current (I_0/mA)	Duration of Test (t/h)
$I_0 < 5$	60	$I_0 < 10$	96
$5 \leq I_0 < 10$	60	$10 \leq I_0 < 20$	48
$10 \leq I_0 < 15$	60	$20 \leq I_0 < 30$	24
$15 \leq I_0 < 20$	50	$25 \leq I_0 < 35$	24
$20 \leq I_0 < 30$	40	$25 \leq I_0 < 40$	24
$30 \leq I_0 < 40$	35	$35 \leq I_0 < 50$	24
$40 \leq I_0 < 60$	30	$40 \leq I_0 < 60$	24

3. Results and Discussion

3.1. Chemical, Autogenous, and Drying Shrinkage

The drying shrinkage, chemical shrinkage, and autogenous shrinkage of the WER-, SCA-, and SCA-WER-modified MKG composites were tested and are illustrated in Figure 4. As shown in Figure 4a, the drying shrinkage of the MKG and MKG composites increased sharply in the first 10 days, then slowed down, and gradually tended to be stable on the 21st day. The drying shrinkage of MKG-SCA, MKG-WER, and MKG-WER-SCA was much lower than that of the MKG. In particular, the shrinkage of MKG-WER-SCA was even lower than that of MKG-SCA and MKG-WER. Compared to the MKG, the drying shrinkage of MKG-SCA, MKG-WER, and MKG-WER-SCA on the 28th day decreased by 24.5%, 23.5%, and 25.2%, respectively. Since only a small amount of water existed in the form of bonding water in geopolymers, a large amount of unbound water or free water evaporated during the curing process, resulting in large drying shrinkage in the early stage. Consistently, the chemical shrinkage of all four samples developed rapidly in the early stage and then became slower after 1 to 2 days, as shown in Figure 4b. The four sets of samples showed generally increasing trends and increasing rates of chemical shrinkage in the first 8 h, while MKG-SCA showed slightly lower chemical shrinkage at the end of 8 h than the other three composites. In the following testing period, the chemical shrinkage of the MKG increased much faster than that of the organically modified geopolymer composites, with a higher increase than that of the three organically modified geopolymer composites. Compared to the MKG, the chemical shrinkage of MKG-SCA, MKG-WER, and MKG-WER-SCA on the 7th day decreased by 58.8%, 47.9%, and 46.4%, respectively. Different from drying shrinkage and chemical shrinkage, the autogenous shrinkage of the MKG showed a linear upward trend in the period from the final setting to the 18th h and then gradually stabilized, as illustrated in Figure 4c,d. MKG-SCA, MKG-WER, and MKG-WER-SCA showed negligible autogenous shrinkage in the first 9 h after the final setting and then developed with different trends. The autogenous shrinkage of MKG-WER increased from the 9th h to 18th h and then tended to be stable. The autogenous shrinkage of MKG-SCA and MKG-WER-SCA had similar trends, increasing from the 9th to the 16th hr, then decreasing to 82.19 and 43.55 μm/m at the 24th h and further to −110.32 and

−296.39 μm/m at the 48th h (see Figure 4c), and finally stabilizing. This indicated that MKG-SCA and MKG-WER-SCA had slight volumetric expansion after the first 24 h. After 7 days of curing, all organically modified geopolymers showed a decrease in autogenous shrinkage, with MKG-SCA and MKG-WER-SCA exhibiting expansion. Compared to the MKG, the autogenous shrinkage of MKG-SCA, MKG-WER, and MKG-WER-SCA decreased by 111.4%, 64.7%, and 131.2%, respectively.

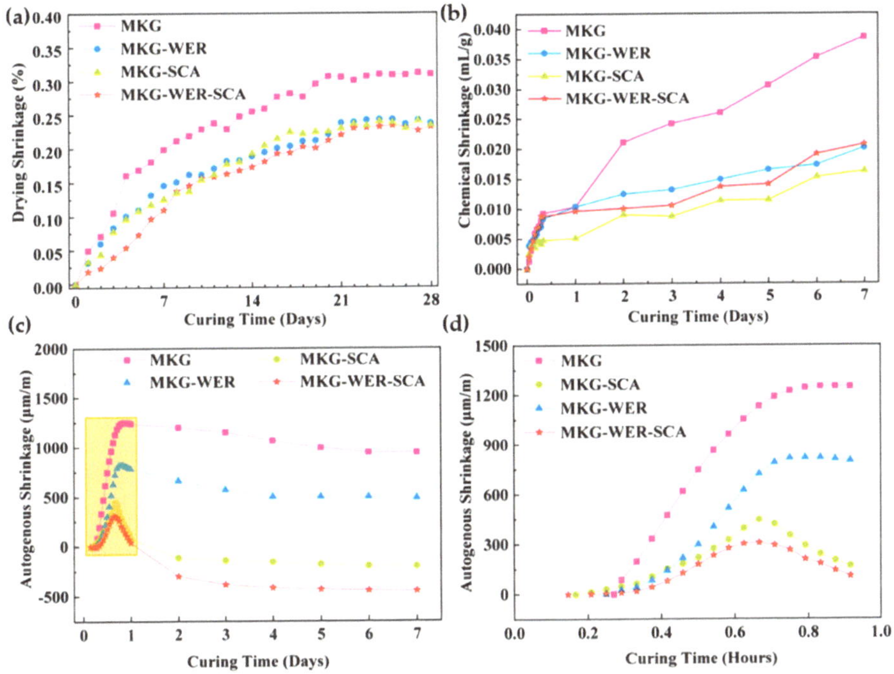

Figure 4. The (**a**) drying shrinkage, (**b**) chemical shrinkage, and (**c**) autogenous shrinkage during the curing of 7 days and (**d**) autogenous shrinkage during the curing of the first 24 h of MKG, MKG-SCA, MKG-WER, and MKG-WER-SCA composites.

Metakaolin underwent a dissolution–polymerization–polycondensation process with alkali activation [50]. First, metakaolin was rapidly dissolved in the alkaline aqueous solution, generating a large number of silicate and aluminate oligomers [42]. During this process, the density of the material decreased, and the chemical shrinkage of the MKG had a monotonically increasing period. Since autogenous shrinkage includes both chemical shrinkage and self-desiccation, the autogenous shrinkage of the MKG showed the same trend. Afterward, the aluminate oligomers further polymerized with the silicate oligomers in the pore water and formed a silica-rich amorphous geopolymer network [51]. MK underwent drastic self-desiccation and gradually hardened, and the autogenous shrinkage of the MKG further developed. However, part of the WER and SCA in the organically modified geopolymer composites covered the surface of the metakaolin to form a coating film and hinder the reaction process [52,53]. As a result, MKG-SCA, MKG-WER, and MKG-WER-SCA had lower chemical shrinkage and slower autogenous shrinking rates than the MKG in the early stage.

On the other hand, the WER and SCA reacted with the geopolymer gel to form a more ductile micro-network and fix more water molecules [54,55]. Some of the WER in the form of spheres and films can also partially fill or simply seal the capillary pores, contributing to a denser porous structure [56]. The SCA has the structure of R_n-S-$X_{(4-n)}$ (n = 1, 2), where X stands for alkoxy, and R stands for an organo-functional group, enabling it to react with the geopolymer gel and the WER simultaneously [57,58]. The SCA acted as a bridge between the organic agent and the inorganic substances, resulting in a more compact three-dimensional network structure of the MKG composites. At the same time, water molecules were more stably retained in the networks of MKG composites. This would significantly reduce the drying shrinkage, which is induced by the evaporation of unbound or free water from the geopolymer matrix [59]. As a result, MKG-SCA, MKG-WER, and MKG-WER-SCA had lower drying shrinkage than the MKG. At the same time, the incorporation of the WER and SCA produced more a-Anatase, b-Phlogopite-1M, and c-Calcite in the geopolymer, leading to a slight expansion and a decrease in the autogenous shrinkage of the geopolymer, as shown in Figure 4c. These will be further discussed in Section 3.2.

It was revealed that the incorporation of 1 wt% SCA and 20 wt% WER reduced the drying shrinkage of the MKG significantly, particularly the combination of the SCA and WER. As the chemical shrinkage and the autogenous shrinkage of the MKG composites were decreased, the drying shrinkage is suggested to have been reduced by the modification of the microstructure of the geopolymerization products by the organic liquids.

3.2. Microstructure and Modification Mechanism

3.2.1. Micromorphology and Porosity

The effects of the WER and SCA on the microstructure of the MKG were investigated by characterizing the micromorphology and porosity of the SCA- and WER-modified MKG. As shown in Figure 5a, relatively wide and long microcracks were found in the MKG. Compared with the MKG, the microstructures of MKG-SCA, MKG-WER, and MKG-WER-SCA were denser, and the microcracks were fewer and narrower, indicating that the addition of organic modifiers increased the microstructural compactness of the MKG and reduced the generation of microcracks. The denser microstructure means less pore water and a more closed pore structure, which will reduce the consumption of pore water in the process of geopolymer dissolution and reduce the capillary stress generated by the evaporation of pore water into the external environment, thus improving the resistance to autogenous shrinkage and drying shrinkage. In addition, the resin in MKG-WER and MKG-WER-SCA was embedded in the matrix with a close connection to the surrounding geopolymer gel. As shown in the enlarged portion inserted in Figure 5c,d, the surface of the resin spheres in MKG-WER was smooth, while that in MKG-WER-SCA had many "pits", which might be caused by the chemical reaction between the SCA and WER.

As shown in Figure 6, the interface between the WER and the geopolymer matrix was characterized by SEM-EDS. The content of carbon (C) greatly changed along the scanning line, which gradually changed from a matrix to a resin and from a resin to a matrix (see Figure 6b). This indicates great compatibility between the resin and the geopolymer gel. Sodium (Na) and aluminum (Al) showed an overall stable trend along the scan line, while oxygen (O) was higher in the resin region than in the matrix region, and silicon (Si) was lower in the matrix region. This indicates that Al and Na are evenly distributed across the resin and the matrix, with more O in the resin region and more Si in the matrix region. In addition, a point of interest on the resin and geopolymer matrix was selected and characterized by EDS, the spectrum of which is illustrated in Figure 6c,d, respectively. The main elements of Point 1 (on the resin) and Point 2 (on the geopolymer) both contain the elements C, Si, Al, Na, and O. For the WER (Point 1), C and O were the main elements in the resin, and the high content of Si could come from the SCA and the adhered geopolymer and Al from the adhered geopolymer. On the other hand, the C and Si in the spectrum of Point 2 (on the geopolymer) could partially originate from the SCA and WER linked in the geopolymer matrix. In this case, the SCA acted as a bridge between the WER and MKG, reacting with both the resin and the aluminosilicate products and strengthening the connection between these two materials [57].

To verify the densification effect of the organic–inorganic interaction on the microstructure of the MKG composites, the porosity of the MKG, MKG-WER, MKG-SCA, and MKG-

WER-SCA was characterized by MIP. The pore size distribution of the composites after curing for 28 days and a diagram of the pore volume in different size ranges are shown in Figure 7. The pores of the four samples were mainly in the micropore (<100 nm) range. The proportions of mesopores (100 nm–1000 nm) and macropores (>1000 nm) were relatively small. The volume of the micropores of MKG-WER, MKG-SCA and MKG-WER-SCA was higher than that of the MKG, while the mesopore and macropore volume showed the opposite trend. Compared to the MKG, the total volume of mesopores and macropores in MKG-WER, MKG-SCA, and MKG-WER-SCA decreased by 11.5%, 8.7%, and 3.8%, respectively. The total pore volume of the SCA- and WER-modified geopolymer composites was higher than that of the MKG, with MKG-WER-SCA having the highest pore volume due to the significantly increased volume of micropores and the higher pore size of the dominant micropore, as shown in Figure 7a,b. The chain-like organic resin molecules of MKG-WER-SCA and MKG-WER filled the voids and converted macropores into micropores, resulting in a more compact microstructure, although the total pore volume increased. In addition, "small pits" formed on the surface of MKG-WER-SCA (see Figure 5d), which can be another reason for the large increase in micropores in MKG-WER-SCA. The main diameters of the micropores in MKG-WER-SCA and MKG-WER were larger than those of the MKG and MKG-SCA (see Figure 7a). The film formed by the WER blocked a portion of the hollow pore channels, creating closed pores and affecting the migration of water. However, under the high pressure of the mercury intrusion test, the film would break, and the presence of these pores still remained detectable, increasing the porosity and pore diameter of MKG-WER-SCA and MKG-WER [60].

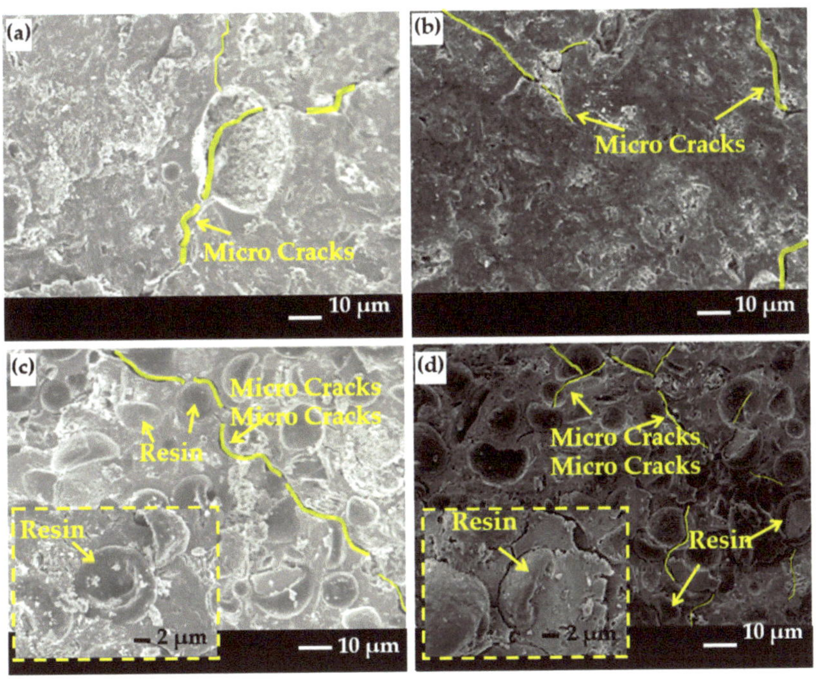

Figure 5. The SEM images of (**a**) MKG, (**b**) MKG-SCA, (**c**) MKG-WER, and (**d**) MKG-WER-SCA cured for 28 days.

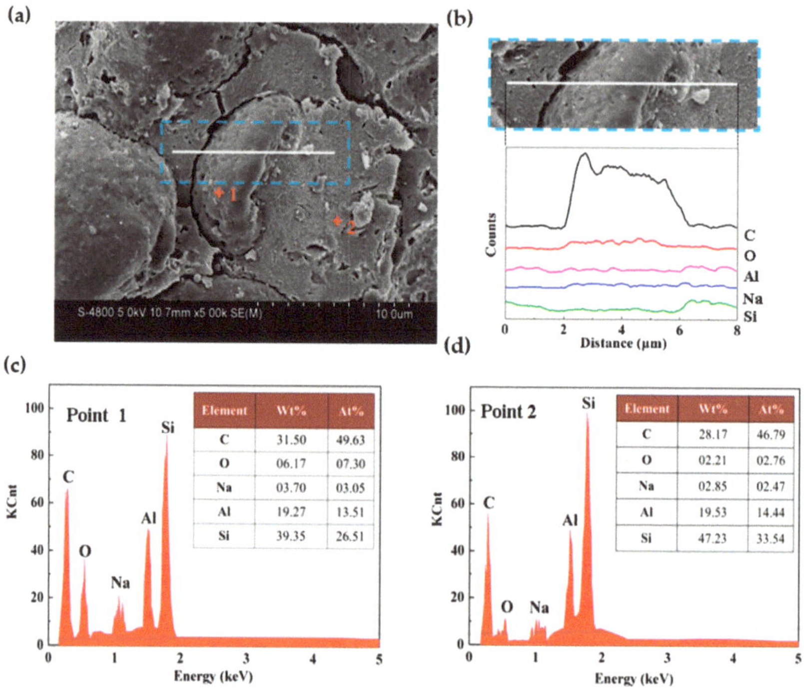

Figure 6. (**a**) The SEM image of MKG−WER−SCA and the EDS spectra of (**b**) the line scanned across the WER and geopolymer matrix, (**c**) Point 1, and (**d**) Point 2 in (**a**).

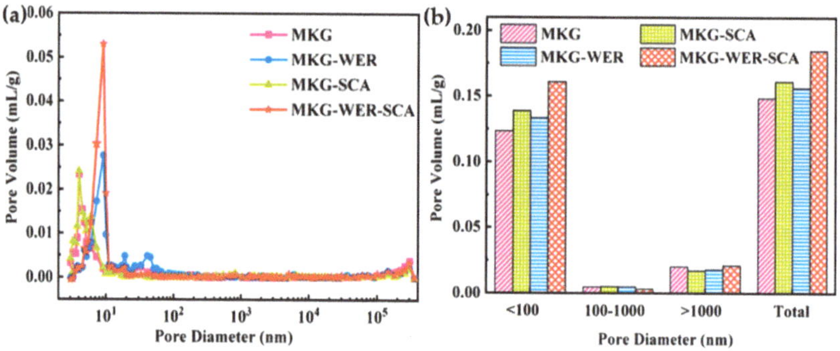

Figure 7. The (**a**) pore size distribution volume and (**b**) the volume of the pores in different size ranges of composites.

3.2.2. Characteristic Bonds and Mineralogy

As shown in Figure 8a, the characteristic bonds of the MKG, MKG-SCA, MKG-WER, and MKG-WER-SCA composite pastes were characterized by FTIR. The bands at 3450~3570 cm^{-1} and 1650 cm^{-1} in the patterns of all four samples were attributed to O-H stretching vibrations and bending vibrations, respectively [28]. The peak centered at 1040 cm^{-1} was attributed to the stretching vibration of Si-O-X (X represents Al or Si) [61], and the band at 703 cm^{-1} was attributed to the symmetric stretching vibration of Si-O-X [28,62], indicating the polymerization of Si-O oligomers and the formation of geopolymer gels. Moreover, the intensities of these two peaks in MKG-SCA, MKG-WER, and MKG-WER-SCA were higher than their counterparts in the MKG, indicating that the addition of organic modifiers promotes the formation of geopolymer gels. In particular, the spectra of MKG-WER and MKG-WER-SCA were similar, and a peak at 1240 cm^{-1} with low intensity was found, which was caused by the stretching vibration of aromatic hydrocarbons in the main chain of the epoxy resin [63]. A small peak was also found at 1515 cm^{-1}, which was caused by N–H bending vibrations [26].

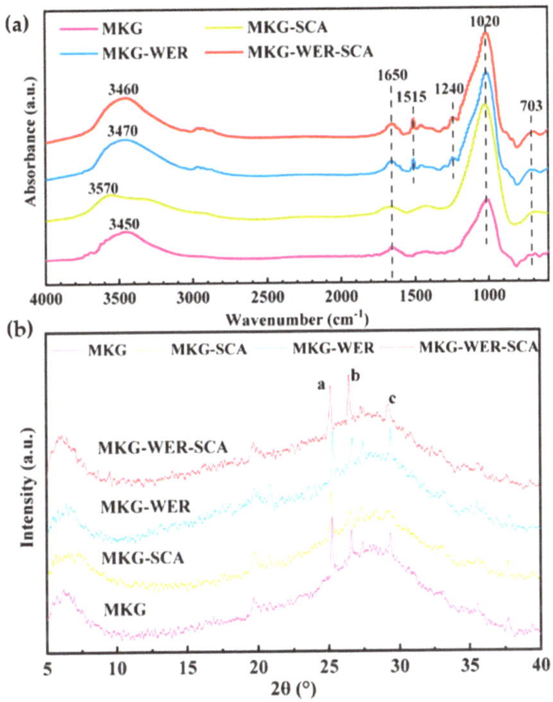

Figure 8. The (**a**) FTIR spectra and (**b**) XRD patterns of the MKG, MKG-SCA, MKG-WER, and MKG-WER-SCA after 28 days of curing (a: Anatase; b: Phlogopite-1M; c: Calcite).

As shown in Figure 8b, the mineral composition of the MKG, MKG-SCA, MKG-WER, and MKG-WER-SCA cured for 28 days was characterized by XRD. A hump in the range of 20~35° 2θ was found in the patterns of all MKG and MKG composites, indicating the formation of geopolymer gels. The strength and width of this hump of MKG-SCA were approximated to those of the MKG, indicating that the addition of the SCA in the small amount used (1wt%) had little influence on the mineralogy of the MKG. In addition, the mineral crystalline phases, including anatase (a-Anatase), phlogopite (b-Phlogopite-1M), and calcite (c-Calcite), were found in the four composites.

3.2.3. Molecular Structure

As shown in Figure 9a, the ^{27}Al MAS NMR spectra of the MKG, MKG-SCA, MKG-WER, and MKG-WER-SCA all had only one peak at 57.5 ppm, which was the typical signal of IV-coordinated Al, indicating that the Al polymerization of $[Al(OH)_4]^-$ in the MKG and the MKG composites was complete [64]. This was mainly due to the faster and higher reaction rate of polymerization between aluminate and silicate than polymerization between silicates. During the reaction, $[Al(OH)_4]^-$ groups with a negative charge were more stable than Si due to the larger atomic size and higher local charge of the Al atom. Meanwhile, polymerization involving aluminate oligomers might occur more easily due to the four hydroxyl groups of $[Al(OH)_4]^-$ [51,65]. The intensity of the signal at 57.5 ppm of

MKG-WER and MKG-WER-SCA was obviously higher than that of the MKG. This might be due to the fact that the strong basicity of DETA introduced by the WER improved the alkalinity of the MKG matrix and promoted the dissolution of MK, releasing more $[Al(OH)^4]^-$, $[SiO(OH)^3]^-$, and $[SiO_2(OH)^2]^{2-}$ [51] and improving the degree of polymerization. On the other hand, the SCA increased the number of Si-O bridging bonds, which would suppress the polycondensation of Al to a certain extent, and decreased the intensity of this peak in MKG-SCA and MKG-WER-SCA compared to the MKG and MKG-WER, respectively [66]. As shown in Figure 9b, the ^{29}Si MAS NMR spectra of the MKG, MKG-SCA, MKG-WER, and MKG-WER-SCA all had a wide hump in the range of $-120\sim-60$ ppm, indicating that a stable Si coordination sphere had formed [35]. However, the humps of MKG-SCA and MKG-WER-SCA were shifted to more negative wavenumbers compared to the MKG and MKG-WER, respectively. It might be due to the fact that the Si-O- of the SCA bonded with -Si-O-Si- and -Si-O-Al- in the MKG matrix, changing the stable Si coordination.

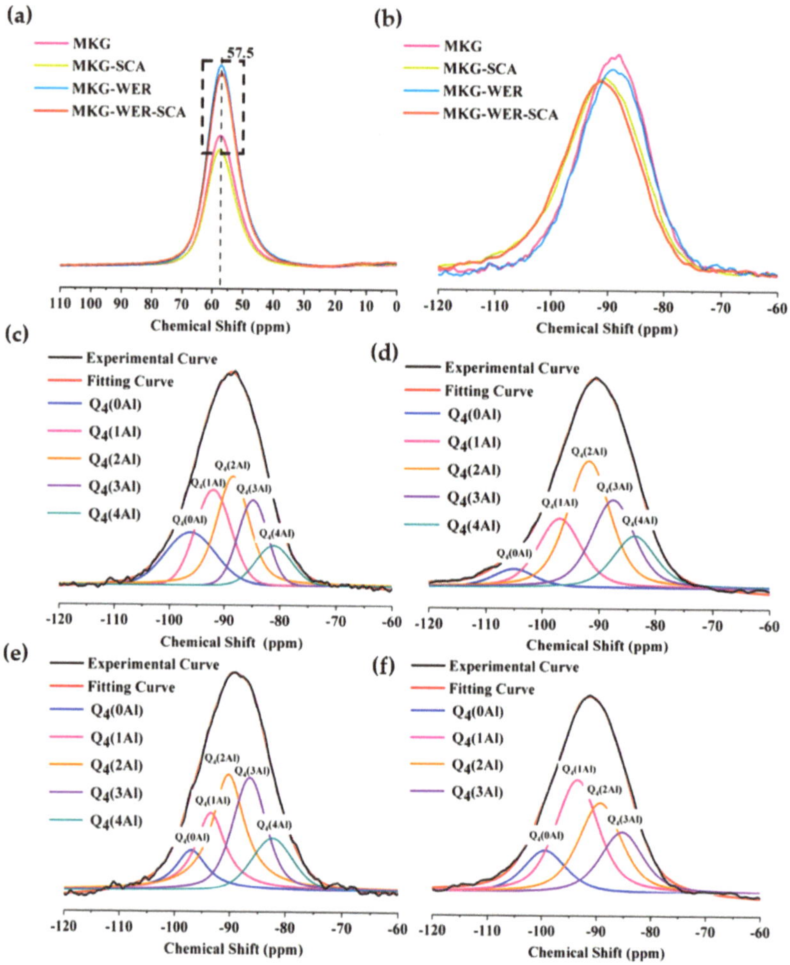

Figure 9. The (**a**) ^{27}Al and (**b**) ^{29}Si MAS NMR spectra of the MKG, MKG-SCA, MKG-WER, and MKG-WER-SCA. The deconvolution fitting of ^{29}Si MAS NMR spectrum of (**c**) the MKG, (**d**) MKG-SCA, (**e**) MKG-WER, and (**f**) MKG-WER-SCA (note: the black lines represent experimental curves; the red lines represent the fitting curves; the remaining lines represent the fitting peaks).

To investigate the coordination environment of Si more comprehensively, deconvolution analysis was performed on the 29Si MAS NMR spectra of the composites. As shown in Figure 9c–f, the peak in the 29Si MAS NMR spectrum in the range of −70~−120 ppm was deconvoluted to Q4(mAl), where Q4 is the Si tetrahedron connected to four bridging O atoms, and m is the number of aluminum atoms connected to [SiO4] units via bridging oxygen [65,67]. The fitted peaks were assigned to Q4(0Al), Q4(1Al), Q4(2Al), Q4(3Al), and Q4(4Al), indicating that a highly polymerized three-dimensional structure was formed in the MKG and all organically modified MKG composites. In addition, the proportion of each type of Q4(mAl) was calculated by dividing the area of the deconvoluted Gaussian peak by the total area of the experimental curve, as listed in Table 4 [67]. The peaks of different Q4(mAl) coordinates in MKG-SCA, MKG-WER, and MKG-WER-SCA all shifted in a more negative direction than in the MKG, indicating that the number of polymers including monomers and small oligomers of the MKG decreased after the incorporation of organic modifiers, and the degree of polymerization of organically modified MKGs increased [35]. The proportion of Q4(2Al), Q4(3Al), and Q4(4Al) in MKG-SCA and MKG-WER increased compared to the MKG, indicating that the addition of the WER and SCA promoted the formation of higher-polymerized -Si-O-Al- and -Si-O-Si-. At the same time, the fraction of Q4(1Al) in MKG-WER-SCA was higher than in MKG-WER and MKG-SCA, while Q4(2Al) and Q4(3Al) showed the opposite trend. This indicates that more -Si-O-Al- bonds tend to form in the geopolymer when the WER and SCA are used synergistically [68]. This is consistent with the XRD results, where the Phlogopite-1M peak of MKG-WER-SCA was clearly higher than those of MKG-WER and MKG-SCA (see Figure 8b).

Table 4. Signal positions and ratios of deconvoluted peaks.

Peaks	MKG		MKG-WER		MKG-SCA		MKG-WER-SCA	
	Signal Position (ppm)	Ratio (%)	Signal Position (ppm)	Ratio (%)	Signal Position (ppm)	Ratio (%)	Signal Position (ppm)	Ratio (%)
Q_4(0Al)	−96.2	18.68	−96.9	10.64	−105.1	5.12	−99.4	13.97
Q_4(1Al)	−92.0	24.04	−93.4	19.46	−97.0	19.46	−93.6	36.78
Q_4(2Al)	−88.5	29.77	−90.3	31.19	−91.9	35.89	−89.3	29.38
Q_4(3Al)	−84.9	17.57	−86.5	25.59	−87.6	24.82	−85.3	19.97
Q_4(4Al)	−81.2	9.94	−82.4	13.12	−83.7	14.70	--	--

3.2.4. Polymerization Mechanism

Based on the above results and observations, we propose a reasonable reaction process among the SCA, WER, and MKG, as illustrated in Figure 10. In the first step, the aluminosilicate mineral components in MK dissolved in the alkali solution and released $Si(OH)_4$ and $Al(OH)_4^-$. Secondly, the released $Si(OH)_4$ and $Al(OH)_4^-$ in the alkali solution polymerized and formed aluminosilicate oligomers, while the WER opened the epoxy ring of the epoxy resin to form hydroxyl groups, and the SCA hydrolyzed to form silanol groups (≡Si-OH). In the third step, the hydroxyl groups formed by the WER were hydrogen-bonded by reacting with the hydroxyl groups in the aluminosilicate oligomers and water molecules. Furthermore, the silanol groups formed by the SCA and the Si-OH and Al-OH groups in the aluminosilicate oligomers polymerized to form -Si-O-Si- and -Si-O-Al- bonds. At the same time, the alkoxy groups (–OCH_3 or –OC_2H_5) in the SCA were bound to the opened rings of the WER, resulting in a dense organic–inorganic WER-SCA-MKG network formed by the bridging SCA between the WER and MKG gel [55,69].

The dissolution of metakaolin in the first stage was the most important factor influencing the chemical shrinkage of the MKG. The chemical shrinkage of MKG-WER-SCA and MKG-WER was larger than that of MKG-SCA, which can be attributed to the strong base (i.e., DETA) introduced by the WER, which promotes the dissolution of metakaolin [51]. Later, the WER opened its ring, and the SCA was hydrolyzed to form silanol groups. At this point, the products of the WER and SCA might attach to the aluminosilicate oligomers generated by the alkali activation of metakaolin, forming a film that prevents further polymerization [43]. This is consistent with the almost disappearance of autogenous shrinkage in MKG-WER-SCA, MKG-WER, and MKG-SCA in the early stage. Eventually, a dense organic–inorganic was formed to fix more water molecules, and MKG-WER-SCA exhibited the lowest drying shrinkage [59]. From the microstructural point of view, the intensity of MKG-WER-SCA, MKG-WER, and MKG-SCA peaks in FTIR (see Figure 8a) at 1040 cm^{-1} and 703 cm^{-1} was higher than that of the MKG. The total pore volume of MKG-WER-SCA, MKG-WER, and MKG-SCA was larger than that of the pure geopolymer (see Figure 7b). This indicates that a denser resin–gel structure was formed, which is confirmed by the SEM images of MKG-WER-SCA (see Figure 6d). These findings elucidate the formation of the organic–inorganic WER-SCA-MKG network.

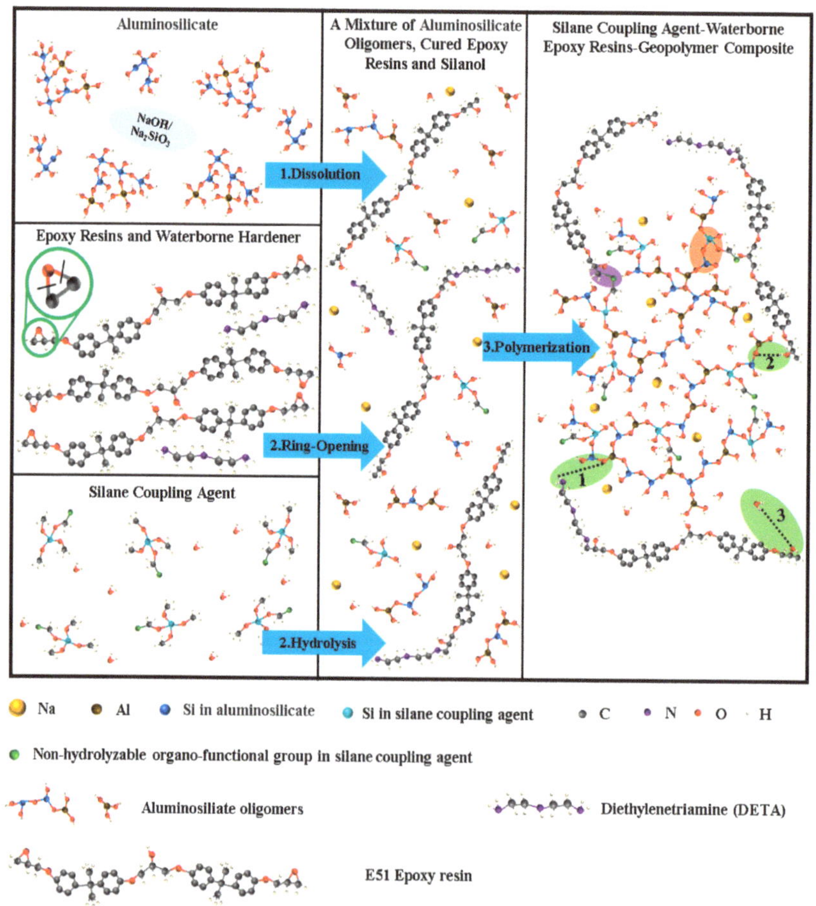

Figure 10. A conceptual model of the reaction of MKG-WER-SCA (note: dashed lines "1, 2, 3" represent the hydrogen bonds formed between the amino and hydroxyl groups in the WER and the hydroxyl and water molecules in the MKG; the purple area is the bonding of the WER to the SCA; the orange area is the SCA bonded to the MKG network).

3.3. Resistance to Chloride Ion Penetration

The shrinkage and induced cracks at different scales have a significant influence on the permeability of cementitious materials. The higher shrinkage of the MKG can lead to surface cracks in the specimen, which are susceptible to chloride ion penetration, thus promoting the diffusion of chloride ions [70]. In this case, the chloride ion penetration of the MKG and MKG composites was assessed. The 2~3 mm thick coatings of the MKG, MKG-WER, MKG-SCA, and MKG-WER-SCA were applied to the concrete samples and tested with the RCM test to evaluate the resistance of the MKG and MKG composites to chloride ion penetration. After the RCM test, a $AgNO_3$ solution was sprayed on the section of the concrete samples, and the color of the Cl^--penetrated area turned white. The boundary of the white area was marked with a red dotted line, as shown in Figure 11. The penetration depth of Cl^- in the three composite-coated concrete samples was lower than that in the uncoated concrete and MKG-coated concrete specimens. As shown in Figure 12, the diffusion coefficient of Cl^- (D_{RCM}) of each sample was calculated according to the diffusion depth. The D_{RCM} of the MKG-coated concrete was 2.6×10^{-12} m^2/s, 29.7% lower than that of the uncoated concrete, which was 3.7×10^{-12} m^2/s. The D_{RCM} of the three MKG composite-coated concrete samples varied in the range of 1.5×10^{-12} to 1.8×10^{-12} m^2/s, which was 51.4% to 59.5% lower than that of the control group and 30.8% to 42.3% lower than that of the MKG-coated sample. This showed that the protective coatings of the MKG and MKG composites effectively inhibited the diffusion of Cl^-, with MKG-SCA having the best apparent protective effect. On the other hand, the D_{RCM} values of the control group and MKG-coated concrete were between 2×10^{-12} and 8×10^{-12} m^2/s, which showed that the concrete had good resistance to the penetration of Cl^- according to the standard (see Table 5) proposed by Tang [71]. The chloride ion diffusion coefficients of MKG-WER-, MKG-SCA-, and MKG-WER-SCA-coated concrete were all less than 2×10^{-12} m^2/s, indicating that the WER and SCA-modified MKG had better resistance to Cl^- penetration, verifying their lower shrinkage and denser microstructure.

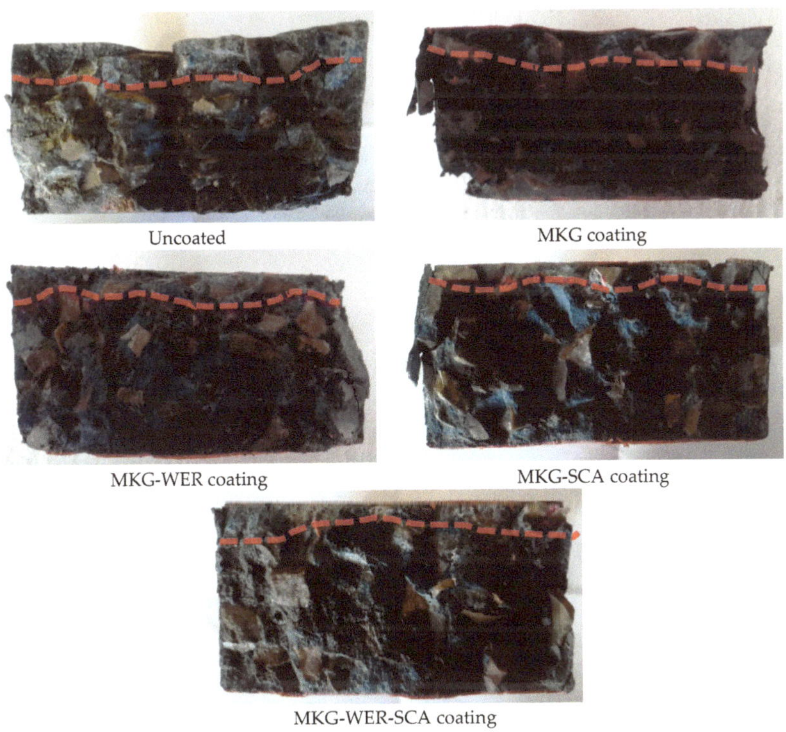

Figure 11. The cross-sections of all samples tested with the RCM method (note: the white area above the red dashed line is the Cl^- penetration depth).

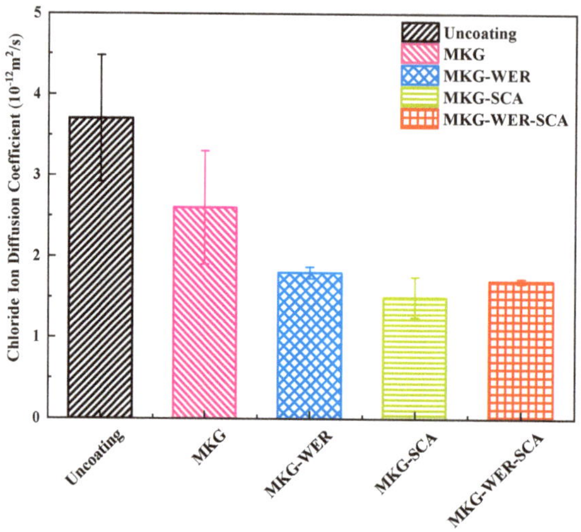

Figure 12. Chloride ion diffusion coefficients of concrete with and without MKG composite coatings.

Table 5. Reference standard for chloride ion diffusion coefficient [71].

Apparent Diffusion Coefficient of Chloride ions ($D_a/10^{-12}$ m^2/s)	Concrete Properties
<2	Very good resistance to chloride ion penetration
<8	Good resistance to chloride ion penetration
<16	General resistance to chloride ion penetration
>16	Not suitable for harsh environments

4. Conclusions

The shrinkage properties of the MKG were modified with a WER, an SCA, and a synergistic modifier consisting of the WER and SCA. The chemical shrinkage, autogenous shrinkage, and drying shrinkage of the organic-agent-modified MKG were tested, and the modification mechanisms were investigated. Finally, the improved volumetric stability of MKG composites was verified by assessing the resistance of chloride ion penetration of the MKG composite coatings. Accordingly, the following conclusions can be drawn:

1. The addition of the SCA, WER, and mixture of these two agents significantly reduced the drying shrinkage, chemical shrinkage, and autogenous shrinkage of the MKG. The chemical shrinkage and shrinkage rate of the SCA-modified MKG were the lowest, while the synergistic modification by the WER and SCA led to the highest reduction in the autogenous shrinkage and drying shrinkage of the MKG. In particular, the MKG modified by the SCA and SCA-WER showed slight micro-expansion, which might be due to modified porosity caused by the SCA and newly formed products that increased the volume of the composites.
2. MKG-WER-SCA had the most promising performance in reducing drying shrinkage, chemical shrinkage, and autogenous shrinkage, which is mainly attributed to the densified microstructure and the "restriction" effect of the organic modifiers. The microstructure of MKG-WER-SCA was densified by the compact organic–inorganic network formed by the bridging SCA between MKG and the WER. The denser microstructure reduced the consumption of pore water during the dissolution of the geopolymer and the evaporation of pore water into the external environment, thereby reducing the drying shrinkage, chemical shrinkage, and autogenous shrinkage. Furthermore, the coating film of WER-SCA restricted the chemical shrinkage and autogenous shrinkage of the MKG.

3. The improved chloride permeability of concrete with the organically modified MKG coating further confirmed the improved shrinkage resistance of MKG-WER, MKG-SCA, and MKG-WER-SCA. The chloride ion diffusion coefficient of organically modified geopolymer-coated concrete was 2×10^{-12} m^2/s and 51.4~59.5% lower than that without a coating compared with the control group. This indicates that MKG composite coatings can effectively inhibit the diffusion of chloride ions and be applied in concrete protective coatings for marine engineering.

Author Contributions: M.Z.: conceptualization, writing—review and editing. Y.Z.: Data curation, investigation, writing—original draft. L.S.: methodology, resources, writing—review and editing. All authors have read and agreed to the published version of the manuscript.

Funding: Central Public-Interest Scientific Institution Basal Research Fund: Research on Deflection Differences of Wide Stiffness Domain Structures under Repeated Loads (2017-9032).

Data Availability Statement: The raw data supporting the conclusions of this article will be made available by the authors on request.

Conflicts of Interest: The authors declare that they have no known competing financial interests or personal relationships that could have appeared to influence the work reported in this paper.

References

1. Kim, B.; Lee, S. Review on characteristics of metakaolin-based geopolymer and fast setting. *J. Korean Ceram. Soc.* **2020**, *57*, 368–377. [CrossRef]
2. Patil, S.; Karikatti, V.; Chitawadagi, M. Granulated Blast-Furnace Slag (GGBS) based Geopolymer Concrete–Review. *Int. J. Adv. Sci. Eng* **2018**, *5*, 879–885. [CrossRef]
3. Abdel-Ghani, N.T.; Elsayed, H.A.; AbdelMoied, S. Geopolymer synthesis by the alkali-activation of blastfurnace steel slag and its fire-resistance. *Hbrc J.* **2018**, *14*, 159–164. [CrossRef]
4. Yang, H.; Liu, L.; Yang, W.; Liu, H.; Ahmad, W.; Ahmad, A.; Aslam, F.; Joyklad, P. A comprehensive overview of geopolymer composites: A bibliometric analysis and literature review. *Case Stud. Constr. Mater.* **2022**, *16*, e00830. [CrossRef]
5. Guo, X.; Yang, J. Intrinsic properties and micro-crack characteristics of ultra-high toughness fly ash/steel slag based geopolymer. *Constr. Build. Mater.* **2020**, *230*, 116965. [CrossRef]
6. Nair, B.; Zhao, Q.; Cooper, R. Geopolymer matrices with improved hydrothermal corrosion resistance for high-temperature applications. *J. Mater. Sci.* **2007**, *42*, 3083–3091. [CrossRef]
7. Tong, L.; Zhao, J.; Cheng, Z. Chloride ion binding effect and corrosion resistance of geopolymer materials prepared with seawater and coral sand. *Constr. Build. Mater.* **2021**, *309*, 125126. [CrossRef]
8. Najafi, E.K.; Chenari, R.J.; Arabani, M. The potential use of clay-fly ash geopolymer in the design of active-passive liners: A review. *Clays Clay Miner.* **2020**, *68*, 296–308. [CrossRef]
9. Jiang, C.; Wang, A.; Bao, X.; Ni, T.; Ling, J. A review on geopolymer in potential coating application: Materials, preparation and basic properties. *J. Build. Eng.* **2020**, *32*, 101734. [CrossRef]
10. Jindal, B.B.; Alomayri, T.; Hasan, A.; Kaze, C.R. Geopolymer concrete with metakaolin for sustainability: A comprehensive review on raw material's properties, synthesis, performance, and potential application. *Environ. Sci. Pollut. Res.* **2023**, *30*, 25299–25324. [CrossRef]
11. Duan, P.; Yan, C.; Luo, W. A novel waterproof, fast setting and high early strength repair material derived from metakaolin geopolymer. *Constr. Build. Mater.* **2016**, *124*, 69–73. [CrossRef]
12. Zarina, Y.; Al Bakri Abdullah, M.M.; Kamarudin, H.; Nizar, I.K.; Razak, R.A. Reviews on the geopolymer materials for coating application. *Adv. Mater. Res.* **2013**, *626*, 958–962. [CrossRef]
13. Zhang, Z.; Yao, X.; Wang, H. Potential application of geopolymers as protection coatings for marine concrete III. Field experiment. *Appl. Clay Sci.* **2012**, *67*, 57–60. [CrossRef]
14. Li, N.; Zhang, Z.; Shi, C.; Zhang, J. Some progresses in the challenges for geopolymer. *IOP Conf. Ser. Mater. Sci. Eng.* **2018**, *431*, 022003. [CrossRef]
15. Vilaplana, J.L.; Baeza, F.J.; Galao, O.; Alcocel, E.; Zornoza, E.; Garcés, P. Mechanical properties of alkali activated blast furnace slag pastes reinforced with carbon fibers. *Constr. Build. Mater.* **2016**, *116*, 63–71. [CrossRef]
16. Ma, H.; Zhu, H.; Chen, H.; Ni, Y.; Xu, X.; Huo, Q. Shrinkage-reducing measures and mechanisms analysis for alkali-activated coal gangue-slag mortar at room temperature. *Constr. Build. Mater.* **2020**, *252*, 119001. [CrossRef]
17. Al-Mashhadani, M.M.; Canpolat, O.; Aygörmez, Y.; Uysal, M.; Erdem, S. Mechanical and microstructural characterization of fiber reinforced fly ash based geopolymer composites. *Constr. Build. Mater.* **2018**, *167*, 505–513. [CrossRef]
18. Junior, J.; Saha, A.K.; Sarker, P.K.; Pramanik, A. Workability and Flexural Properties of Fibre-Reinforced Geopolymer Using Different Mono and Hybrid Fibres. *Materials* **2021**, *14*, 4447. [CrossRef]

19. Farhan, N.A.; Sheikh, M.N.; Hadi, M.N. Engineering Properties of Ambient Cured Alkali-Activated Fly Ash–Slag Concrete Reinforced with Different Types of Steel Fiber. *Am. Soc. Civ. Eng.* **2018**, *30*, 04018142. [CrossRef]
20. Rashad, A.M. Effect of steel fibers on geopolymer properties–the best synopsis for civil engineer. *Constr. Build. Mater.* **2020**, *246*, 118534. [CrossRef]
21. Samal, S.; Blanco, I. An Application Review of Fiber-Reinforced Geopolymer Composite. *Fibers* **2021**, *9*, 23. [CrossRef]
22. Colangelo, F.; Roviello, G.; Ricciotti, L.; Ferone, C.; Cioffi, R. Preparation and characterization of new geopolymer-epoxy resin hybrid mortars. *Materials* **2013**, *6*, 2989–3006. [CrossRef]
23. Wang, X.; Zhang, C.; Wu, Q.; Zhu, H.; Liu, Y. Thermal properties of metakaolin-based geopolymer modified by the silane coupling agent. *Mater. Chem. Phys.* **2021**, *267*, 124655. [CrossRef]
24. Zhang, C.; Wang, X.; Hu, Z.; Wu, Q.; Zhu, H.; Lu, J. Long-term performance of silane coupling agent/metakaolin based geopolymer. *J. Build. Eng.* **2021**, *36*, 102091. [CrossRef]
25. Liang, G.; Zhu, H.; Zhang, Z.; Wu, Q. Effect of rice husk ash addition on the compressive strength and thermal stability of metakaolin based geopolymer. *Constr. Build. Mater.* **2019**, *222*, 872–881. [CrossRef]
26. Ferone, C.; Roviello, G.; Colangelo, F.; Cioffi, R.; Tarallo, O. Novel hybrid organic-geopolymer materials. *Appl. Clay Sci.* **2013**, *73*, 42–50. [CrossRef]
27. Roviello, G.; Ricciotti, L.; Tarallo, O.; Ferone, C.; Colangelo, F.; Roviello, V.; Cioffi, R. Innovative fly ash geopolymer-epoxy composites: Preparation, microstructure and mechanical properties. *Materials* **2016**, *9*, 461. [CrossRef]
28. Roviello, G.; Ricciotti, L.; Ferone, C.; Colangelo, F.; Cioffi, R.; Tarallo, O. Synthesis and characterization of novel epoxy geopolymer hybrid composites. *Materials* **2013**, *6*, 3943–3962. [CrossRef]
29. Saludung, A.; Ogawa, Y.; Kawai, K. Microstructure and mechanical properties of epoxy resin-reinforced geopolymer exposed to high temperatures. *Mater. Lett.* **2023**, *331*, 133473. [CrossRef]
30. Du, J.; Bu, Y.; Shen, Z.; Hou, X.; Huang, C. Effects of epoxy resin on the mechanical performance and thickening properties of geopolymer cured at low temperature. *Mater. Des.* **2016**, *109*, 133–145. [CrossRef]
31. Ma, Y.; Ye, G. The shrinkage of alkali activated fly ash. *Cem. Concr. Res.* **2015**, *68*, 75–82. [CrossRef]
32. Neto, A.A.M.; Cincotto, M.A.; Repette, W. Drying and autogenous shrinkage of pastes and mortars with activated slag cement. *Cem. Concr. Res.* **2008**, *38*, 565–574. [CrossRef]
33. Lee, N.; Jang, J.G.; Lee, H.-K. Shrinkage characteristics of alkali-activated fly ash/slag paste and mortar at early ages. *Cem. Concr. Compos.* **2014**, *53*, 239–248. [CrossRef]
34. Mastali, M.; Kinnunen, P.; Dalvand, A.; Firouz, R.M.; Illikainen, M. Drying shrinkage in alkali-activated binders—A critical review. *Constr. Build. Mater.* **2018**, *190*, 533–550. [CrossRef]
35. Li, Z.; Zhang, S.; Zuo, Y.; Chen, W.; Ye, G. Chemical deformation of metakaolin based geopolymer. *Cem. Concr. Res.* **2019**, *120*, 108–118. [CrossRef]
36. Khatib, J.M.; Ramadan, R.; Ghanem, H.; Elkordi, A.; Sonebi, M. Effect of limestone fines as a partial replacement of cement on the chemical, autogenous, drying shrinkage and expansion of mortars. *Mater. Today Proc.* **2022**, *58*, 1199–1204. [CrossRef]
37. Thomas, R.; Lezama, D.; Peethamparan, S. On drying shrinkage in alkali-activated concrete: Improving dimensional stability by aging or heat-curing. *Cem. Concr. Res.* **2017**, *91*, 13–23. [CrossRef]
38. Luo, L.; Yao, W.; Liang, G.; Luo, Y. Workability, autogenous shrinkage and microstructure of alkali-activated slag/fly ash slurries: Effect of precursor composition and sodium silicate modulus. *J. Build. Eng.* **2023**, *73*, 106712. [CrossRef]
39. Kumarappa, D.B.; Peethamparan, S.; Ngami, M. Autogenous shrinkage of alkali activated slag mortars: Basic mechanisms and mitigation methods. *Cem. Concr. Res.* **2018**, *109*, 1–9. [CrossRef]
40. Li, Z.; Liang, X.; Chen, Y.; Ye, G. Effect of metakaolin on the autogenous shrinkage of alkali-activated slag-fly ash paste. *Constr. Build. Mater.* **2021**, *278*, 122397. [CrossRef]
41. Yang, T.; Zhu, H.; Zhang, Z. Influence of fly ash on the pore structure and shrinkage characteristics of metakaolin-based geopolymer pastes and mortars. *Constr. Build. Mater.* **2017**, *153*, 284–293. [CrossRef]
42. Ruan, S.; Chen, S.; Liu, Y.; Zhang, Y.; Yan, D.; Zhang, M. Early-age deformation of hydrophobized metakaolin-based geopolymers. *Cem. Concr. Res.* **2023**, *169*, 107168. [CrossRef]
43. Tian, Z.; Liu, X.; Zhang, Z.; Zhang, K.; Tang, X. Potential using of water-soluble polymer latex modified greener road geopolymeric grouts: Its preparation, characterization and mechanism. *Constr. Build. Mater.* **2021**, *273*, 121757. [CrossRef]
44. Reeb, C.; Pierlot, C.; Davy, C.; Lambertin, D. Incorporation of organic liquids into geopolymer materials-A review of processing, properties and applications. *Ceram. Int.* **2021**, *47*, 7369–7385. [CrossRef]
45. Zhang, M.; Xu, H.; Zeze, A.L.P.; Zhang, J. Metakaolin-based geopolymer composites modified by epoxy resin and silane: Mechanical properties and organic-inorganic interaction mechanism. *Appl. Clay Sci.* **2023**, *232*, 106767. [CrossRef]
46. Zhang, M.; Xu, H.; Zeze, A.L.P.; Liu, X.; Tao, M. Coating performance, durability and anti-corrosion mechanism of organic modified geopolymer composite for marine concrete protection. *Cem. Concr. Compos.* **2022**, *129*, 104495. [CrossRef]
47. *GB/T 50082-2009*; Standard for Test Methods of Long-Term Performance and Durability of Ordinary Concrete. China Building Industry Press: Beijing, China, 2009.
48. *US-ASTM 1608-17*; Standard Test Method for Chemical Shrinkage of Hydraulic Cement Paste. ASTM International: West Conshohocken, PA, USA, 2017.

49. *US-ASTM 1698-09*; Standard Test Method for Autogenous Strain of Cement Paste and Mortar. ASTM International: West Conshohocken, PA, USA, 2009.
50. Jaya, N.A.; Yun-Ming, L.; Cheng-Yong, H.; Abdullah, M.M.A.B.; Hussin, K. Correlation between pore structure, compressive strength and thermal conductivity of porous metakaolin geopolymer. *Constr. Build. Mater.* **2020**, *247*, 118641. [CrossRef]
51. Weng, L.; Sagoe-Crentsil, K. Dissolution processes, hydrolysis and condensation reactions during geopolymer synthesis: Part I—Low Si/Al ratio systems. *J. Mater. Sci.* **2007**, *42*, 2997–3006. [CrossRef]
52. Zhang, Z.; Yan, P. Hydration kinetics of the epoxy resin-modified cement at different temperatures. *Constr. Build. Mater.* **2017**, *150*, 287–294. [CrossRef]
53. Feng, H.; Le, H.; Wang, S.; Zhang, M.H. Effects of silanes and silane derivatives on cement hydration and mechanical properties of mortars. *Constr. Build. Mater.* **2016**, *129*, 48–60. [CrossRef]
54. Yao, J.Z.; Wang, Y.C.; Xu, D.L.; Sheng, L. Mechanical performance and hydration mechanism of geopolymer composite reinforced by resin. *Mater. Sci. Eng. A* **2010**, *527*, 6574–6580.
55. Zhang, C.; Hu, Z.; Zhu, H.; Wang, X.; Gao, J. Effects of silane on reaction process and microstructure of metakaolin-based geopolymer composites. *J. Build. Eng.* **2020**, *32*, 101695. [CrossRef]
56. Guo, S.-Y.; Zhang, X.; Chen, J.-Z.; Mou, B.; Shang, H.-S.; Wang, P.; Zhang, L.; Ren, J. Mechanical and interface bonding properties of epoxy resin reinforced Portland cement repairing mortar. *Constr. Build. Mater.* **2020**, *264*, 120715. [CrossRef]
57. Tesoro, G.; Wu, Y. Silane coupling agents: The role of the organofunctional group. *J. Adhes. Sci. Technol.* **1991**, *5*, 771–784. [CrossRef]
58. Xie, Y.; Hill, C.A.; Xiao, Z.; Militz, H.; Mai, C. Silane coupling agents used for natural fiber/polymer composites: A review. *Compos. Part A Appl. Sci. Manuf.* **2010**, *41*, 806–819. [CrossRef]
59. Qomi, M.J.A.; Brochard, L.; Honorio, T.; Maruyama, I.; Vandamme, M. Advances in atomistic modeling and understanding of drying shrinkage in cementitious materials. *Cem. Concr. Res.* **2021**, *148*, 106536. [CrossRef]
60. Zhang, Z.; Zhang, H.; Liu, T.; Lv, W. Study on the micro-mechanism and structure of unsaturated polyester resin modified concrete for bridge deck pavement. *Constr. Build. Mater.* **2021**, *289*, 123174. [CrossRef]
61. Mo, Z.; Zhao, M.; Zhang, G.; Sietins, J.M.; Sergio, G.F.; Pepi, M.S.; Yan, X.; Tao, M. Reaction kinetics of red mud-fly ash based geopolymers: Effects of curing temperature on chemical bonding, porosity, and mechanical strength. *Cem. Concr. Compos.* **2018**, *93*, 175–185.
62. Zaharaki, D.; Komnitsas, K.; Perdikatsis, V. Use of analytical techniques for identification of inorganic polymer gel composition. *J. Mater. Sci.* **2010**, *45*, 2715–2724. [CrossRef]
63. Zhang, J.; Zhang, W.; Lu, J.; Zhu, C.; Lin, W.; Feng, J. Aqueous epoxy-based superhydrophobic coatings: Fabrication and stability in water. *Prog. Org. Coat.* **2018**, *121*, 201–208. [CrossRef]
64. Wang, L.Q.; Mattigod, S.V.; Parker, K.E.; Hobbs, D.T.; Mccready, D.E. Nuclear magnetic resonance studies of aluminosilicate gels prepared in high-alkaline and salt-concentrated solutions. *J. Non-Cryst. Solids* **2005**, *351*, 3435–3442. [CrossRef]
65. Sagoe-Crentsil, K.; Weng, L. Dissolution processes, hydrolysis and condensation reactions during geopolymer synthesis: Part II. High Si/Al ratio systems. *J. Mater. Sci.* **2007**, *42*, 3007–3014. [CrossRef]
66. Brochier Salon, M.C.; Belgacem, M.N. Hydrolysis-Condensation Kinetics of Different Silane Coupling Agents. *Phosphorus* **2011**, *186*, 240–254. [CrossRef]
67. Zhu, X.; Yan, D.; Fang, H.; Chen, S.; Ye, H. Early-stage geopolymerization revealed by ^{27}Al and ^{29}Si nuclear magnetic resonance spectroscopy based on vacuum dehydration. *Constr. Build. Mater.* **2021**, *266*, 121114. [CrossRef]
68. Wan, Q.; Rao, F.; Song, S.; Cholico-González, D.F.; Ortiz, N.L. Combination formation in the reinforcement of metakaolin geopolymers with quartz sand. *Cem. Concr. Compos.* **2017**, *80*, 115–122. [CrossRef]
69. Djouani, F.; Chehimi, M.M.; Benzarti, K. Interactions of fully formulated epoxy with model cement hydrates. *J. Adhes. Sci. Technol.* **2013**, *27*, 469–489. [CrossRef]
70. Dellinghausen, L.; Gastaldini, A.; Vanzin, F.; Veiga, K. Total shrinkage, oxygen permeability, and chloride ion penetration in concrete made with white Portland cement and blast-furnace slag. *Constr. Build. Mater.* **2012**, *37*, 652–659. [CrossRef]
71. *JG/T 337-2011*; Agents of Surface Coating for Protection of Concrete Structures. China Communications Press: Beijing, China, 2011.

buildings

MDPI

Article

New Natural Frequency Studies of Orthotropic Plates by Adopting a Two-Dimensional Modified Fourier Series Method

Zhaoying Wu [1], An Li [2,*], Yu Wu [3], Zhiming Yin [2] and Salamat Ullah [4,*]

1 School of Civil Engineering, Changchun Institute of Engineering, Changchun 130012, China
2 PipeChina Construction Project Management Company, Langfang 065000, China
3 Beijing Urban Construction Exploration & Surveying Design Research Institute Co., Ltd., Beijing 100032, China
4 Key Lab of CAD & CG, Laboratory of Soft Machines and Smart Devices of Zhejiang Province & Department of Engineering Mechanics, Zhejiang University, Hangzhou 310027, China
* Correspondence: lian@pipechina.com.cn (A.L.); salamatkhattak@gmail.com (S.U.)

Abstract: The free vibration behavior of orthotropic thin plates, which are clamped at three edges and free at one edge, is a matter of great concern in the engineering field. Various numerical/approximate approaches have been proposed for the present problem; however, lack precise analytic benchmark solutions are lacking in the literature. In the present study, we propose a modified two-dimensional Fourier series method to effectively handle free vibration problems of plates under various edge conditions. In the given solution, the adopted trial function automatically satisfies several boundary conditions. After imposing Stoke's transformation in the trial function and letting it satisfy the remaining boundary conditions, we can change the present plate problem into calculating several systems of linear algebra equations which are easily handled. The present method can be regarded as an easily implemented, rational, and rigorous approach, as it can exactly satisfy both the governing equation and the associated edge conditions. Another advantage of the present method over other analytical approaches is that it has general applicability to various boundary conditions through the utilization of different types of Fourier series, and it can be extended for the further dynamic/static analysis of plates under different shear deformation theories. Finally, all the novel analytical solutions are confirmed to be sufficiently accurate since they match well with the FEM results. The new analytic solution obtained may serve as a benchmark for validating other numerical and approximate methods.

Keywords: free vibration behaviors; orthotropic rectangular thin plates; two-dimensional modified Fourier series method

1. Introduction

Rectangular orthotropic thin plates are increasingly being utilized in various engineering fields due to their outstanding mechanical performance such as the high stiffness-to-weight ratio and strength-to-weight [1–3]. Among the mechanical investigations of such structures, vibration problems have attracted continuous attention since they commonly cause early failure [4–6]. Within the framework of classical plate theory, the governing partial differential equation (PDE), as well as the boundary conditions, have been well established for a long time. Consequently, researchers have mainly focused on the solution methods of various plates. The solution procedure for plate problems falls into two categories: numerical/approximate approaches and analytical approaches. However, based on the authors' knowledge, precise mechanical analysis for plates subjected to different edge restraints, no matter numerical/approximate or analytic solutions, are far from complete.

Previous studies have indicated that numerous efforts have been devoted to developing various solution methods for plate problems. For instance, due to the development of computer technology, numerical/approximate methods, such as the finite element method [7–9], the bubble complex finite strip method [10], the discrete singular convolution method [11,12], the finite the difference method [13], the boundary element method [14], the classical Rayleigh–Ritz procedure [15], the differential cubature method [16], the discrete singular convolution–differential quadrature coupled methods [17], differential quadrature method [18], are becoming more and more popular in analyzing various plate problems. Several novel numerical approaches have also demonstrated enormous potential in analyzing plate mechanical problems [19–21]. It is true that the above mentioned methods can offer accurate results for free vibration behaviors of plates. However, numerical/approximate approaches also have some shortcomings, such as the huge input and output volume; the accuracy of the results heavily depends on the accuracy of the grid. Some other related studies have been conducted to investigate the properties of variable stiffness chain mail fabrics [22,23]. Additionally, experimental techniques have been employed to analyze a composite beam externally bonded with a carbon-fiber-reinforced plastic plate [24].

Due to the suitability of analytical approaches in optimizing structural design and providing precise theoretical data for examining numerical/approximate algorithms, it is still completely necessary to develop simple and effective analytical solution procedures. As for dynamic analysis of plate structures, obtaining analytic free vibration solutions is important for both theoretical understanding and engineering applications. The primary purpose of conducting free vibration analysis on plates is to acquire precise natural frequencies and the corresponding deformation shapes. These parameters usually serve as critical indicators for structural design. Due to the mathematical nature of plate problems, solving the BVPs (boundary value problems) of high-order PDEs (partial differential equations) is necessary. According to the history of solving plate problems, semi-inverse methods are the earliest and most conventional analytical solution procedures. Among these effective semi-inverse methods, the Navier's method [25–28] and Lévy's method [29,30] account for a large proportion. Similarly, Ray [31] established new governing PDEs for the static and dynamic problems of laminated plates on the basis of a new zeroth-order shear deformation theory (ZSDT). The author exactly predicted bending and free vibration solutions for both thin and thick laminate plates with all edges simply supported via taking the Navier's method. By means of adopting the Lévy's method, it is worth mentioning that the Lévy's method exhibits better convergent performance over the Navier's method. As for tapered plates subjected to SRSR (two opposite edges being simply supported and the other two edges being rotationally restrained) edge conditions, Kobayashi [32] also used the Lévy solutions procedure to provide new analytic solutions to determine the non-dimensional critical buckling load parameters and frequency coefficients of plates, in which the effect of boundary spring restraint and thickness variation on stability and dynamic performance of plates are well illustrated through numerical examples. Through the above studies, it can easily be seen that current semi-inverse free vibration solutions are primarily restricted to Navier-type plates whose edges are all simply supported, and Lévy-type plates whose two opposite edges are simply supported. Some other analytical methods have been developed for plate-related structures such as bridges [33–35]. However, in mainstream engineering practice, non-Levy-type plates are the most commonly encountered. The absence of precise analytic benchmark solutions for other types of edge restraints substantially narrows the range of application of orthotropic plates. For this reason, several representative analytical approaches for non-Lévy-type plates have been proposed. For instance, Zhang developed a finite integral transform method [36–42] to solve the mechanical problems of plates subjected to classical or non-classical edge conditions; the method was proven to be rigorous and effective in analyzing plate mechanical performance. Rahbar employed a semi-analytical method [43] to study the forced vibration responses of plates with clamped and simply supported edges. Li invented a new analytical approach [44–46], which is the combination of the symplectic elastic method and the superposition method, to handle non-Lévy-type thin/thick plate problems. Chen achieved efficient benchmark random vibration solutions for thin plates by using the discrete analytical method [47], in which the edge conditions involved a clamped edge, simply supported edge, and free edge. Xing evaluated the natural frequencies of plates with all combinations of simply supported and clamped edge restraints by employing an improved separation of variables method [48]. The dynamic formulation of a sandwich microshell considered modified couple stress and thickness–stretching [49]. With the consideration of the first-order shear deformation theory, Moghadam [50] provided analytic bending solutions for piezolaminated thick plates under simply supported/clamped edge conditions subjected to thermo-electro-mechanical loadings by applying the effective superposition solution procedure. All the given solutions demonstrated high accuracy and excellent convergence through comparison studies. Gorman [51] extended this method to investigate the dynamic and stability behaviors of plates subjected to rotational elastic edge support; accurate eigenvalues for both the critical buckling load and frequencies of squares are detailed for validating numerical/approximate approaches. Kiani [52] offered close-form solutions for the critical temperature of fully clamped FGM plates lying on elastic foundations by using three different types of approximate analytic methods. On the basis of the first shear deformation theory, Liew [53] formulated the governing vibration PDEs for Mindlin plates and chose boundary characteristic orthogonal polynomials as the trial function for three generalized displacements to solve dynamic problems of plates under several edge conditions, in which some deflection contour plots for plates under some special edge restraints were the first known. Focusing on rectangular orthotropic Mindlin plates under line elastic supports or point elastic supports and lying on non-homogeneous elastic foundations in a thermal environment, Zhou [54] developed an improved Fourier series approach to deal with free and forced vibration problems of plates. This method is believed to be an efficient tool for studying the mechanical performance of plates with non-classical boundary restraints due to the highly accurate solutions presented. By means of proposing a novel variational asymptotic approach, Peng [55] studied flexural vibration problems for sandwich plates with re-entrant honeycomb cores under some typical combinations of classical edge conditions. In this study, the effects of negative Poisson's ratios, core thickness ratio, and plate thickness on frequency parameters of plates are thoroughly discussed. Combining the Kantorovich method and the Galerkin method, Rostami [56] acquired precise analytical in-plane vibration solutions for rotating cantilever orthotropic plates, in which the obtained in-plane deformation shapes are heavily influenced when changing the plate's aspect ratio. It should be emphasized that despite the above methods providing precise analytical data for dynamic problems of non-Lévy-type plates, many of these approaches are only suitable for some specific non-Lévy-type plates. Consequently, to the best of the author's knowledge, there still very few available free vibration solutions for orthotropic plates with non-Lévy-type plates.

It is known that among the various analytic approaches for plate problems, Navier's method, based on Fourier series theory, is undoubtedly one of the most widely known of all. In the solution procedure of this classical method, the double Sine series is always treated as the trial function for plate deflection. However, such a trial function only automatically satisfies the Navier-type boundary condition. This solution procedure could be extended to deal with problems of plates subjected to more complex edge conditions by combining Stoke's transformation technique. For example, through the application of Stoke's transformation in the double Sine series form solution, Tang [57,58] developed a modified two-dimensional Fourier series method for conducting new thermal buckling investigations for plates under classical/non-classical edge conditions.

This method offers a significant advantage in overcoming boundary-continuous problems when employing Fourier series solutions for plate problems, making it promising for addressing plates subjected to diverse non-Levy-type boundary restraints. Its primary benefit lies in providing a unified solution procedure similar to classical Navier's solution, simplifying the process compared to the finite integral transform method by avoiding complex transformation steps. Additionally, by extending this procedure appropriately, researchers can easily explore new exact analytical solutions for various plate behaviors, including bending, free vibration, and buckling, based on different shear deformation theories. Notably, compared with other analytical methods, this approach offers several advantages: it simplifies precise plate free vibration analysis by avoiding complicated mathematical manipulations; it reduces the mathematical complexity by converting higher-order partial differential equations into linear algebra equations within the Fourier series framework; and it provides more precise solutions for moderately thick/thick plates under complex boundary conditions by utilizing different types of Fourier series. The trial function employed in this method precisely satisfies both the governing vibration formula and non-Levy-type boundaries after determining the unknown constants, which carry clear physical significance.

The primary objective of this study is to further extend the modified Fourier series method for new accurate free vibration analysis of orthotropic plates with one edge free and the other three edges clamped. These types of plate problems have the features of having both clamped edges and free edges in a plate, which increases the solving difficulties. In the present solution procedure, we first chose the two-dimensional Sine-half-sinusoidal series which automatically satisfies partial boundary conditions as the trial function for the deflection of plates. We then acquired new formulas for the first fourth-order partial derivatives by imposing Stoke's transformation on the deflection. We finally obtained four sets of easily solvable linear algebra equations after letting the deflection satisfy the governing PDE and the remaining edge conditions. In the present study, all the non-dimensional natural frequencies and the corresponding deformation shapes, which are accurately confirmed by FEM results and solutions available in the literature, are tabulated or plotted to serve as reference data for future studies.

2. Basic Equations

As demonstrated in Figure 1, the schematic figure of an orthotropic plate with one edge free and other three edges clamped is depicted. Employing the well-accepted classical Kirchhoff assumptions, the governing PDE for the free vibration of an orthotropic thin plate can be given as:

$$D_x \frac{\partial^4 W(x,y,t)}{\partial x^4} + 2H \frac{\partial^4 W(x,y,t)}{\partial x^2 \partial y^2} + D_y \frac{\partial^4 W(x,y,t)}{\partial y^4} + \rho h \frac{\partial^2 W(x,y,t)}{\partial t^2} = 0 \quad (1)$$

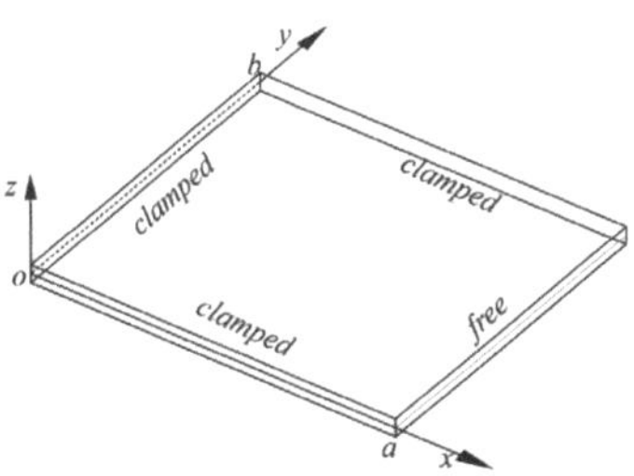

Figure 1. Orthotropic rectangular plates with one edge free and the other three edges clamped.

Here, ρ, h, and $W(x,y,t)$ are the density, thickness, and time-dependent deflection of plates, respectively. The flexural rigidities in Equation (1) are represented by the following formula:

$$D_x = \frac{E_x h^3}{12(1-\mu_x \mu_y)}, D_y = \frac{E_y h^3}{12(1-\mu_x \mu_y)}, D_{xy} = \frac{G_{xy} h^3}{12}, H = D_1 + 2D_{xy}, D_1 = \mu_y D_x = \mu_x D_y \quad (2)$$

where μ_x, μ_y, E_x, E_y and G_{xy} are the elastic constants of plates. The internal forces such as the bending moments M_x and M_y, and the equivalent shear forces V_x and V_y, can be expressed in terms of the above-mentioned constants as follows:

$$
\begin{aligned}
M_x &= -D_x\left(\frac{\partial^2 W}{\partial x^2} + \mu_y \frac{\partial^2 W}{\partial y^2}\right) \\
M_y &= -D_y\left(\frac{\partial^2 W}{\partial y^2} + \mu_x \frac{\partial^2 W}{\partial x^2}\right) \\
V_x &= -\left[D_x \frac{\partial^3 W}{\partial x^3} + (H + 2D_{xy}) \frac{\partial^3 W}{\partial y^2 \partial x}\right] \\
V_y &= -\left[D_y \frac{\partial^3 W}{\partial y^3} + (H + 2D_{xy}) \frac{\partial^3 W}{\partial x^2 \partial y}\right]
\end{aligned} \tag{3}
$$

Based on the vibration theory, taking $W(x,y,t) = W(x,y)\sin(\omega t)$, one can derive the following formula:

$$
D_x \frac{\partial^4 W(x,y)}{\partial x^4} + 2H \frac{\partial^4 W(x,y)}{\partial x^2 \partial y^2} + D_y \frac{\partial^4 W(x,y)}{\partial y^4} - \rho h \omega^2 W(x,y) = 0 \tag{4}
$$

When the orthotropic thin plate is clamped at $x = 0,\ y = 0,\ y = b$ and free at $x = a$, expressions for such type of boundary conditions are as follows:

$$
W|_{x=0} = 0,\ W|_{y=0} = W|_{y=b} = 0,\ V_x|_{x=a} = 0 \tag{5}
$$

$$
\begin{aligned}
&\left.\frac{\partial W}{\partial x}\right|_{x=0} = 0, -D_x\left.\left(\frac{\partial^2 W}{\partial x^2} + \mu_y \frac{\partial^2 W}{\partial y^2}\right)\right|_{x=a} = 0 \\
&\left.\frac{\partial W}{\partial y}\right|_{y=0} = 0,\ \frac{\partial W}{\partial y}_{y=b} = 0
\end{aligned} \tag{6}
$$

Aiming to solve the present plate problem, a two-dimensional Sine-half-sinusoidal series was chosen as the trial function of the plate deflection $W(x,y)$:

$$
W(x,y) = \sum_{m=1,3}^{\infty} \sum_{n=1}^{\infty} W_{mn} \sin \frac{\alpha_m x}{2} \sin(\beta_n y) \tag{7}
$$

In which $\alpha_m = \frac{m\pi}{a}$, $\beta_n = \frac{n\pi}{b}$; $W_{mn} = \frac{4}{ab}\int_0^a \int_0^b W(x,y) \sin \frac{\alpha_m x}{2} \sin(\beta_n y) \mathrm{d}x\mathrm{d}y$ is an unknown constant.

Imposing Stoke's transformation [57–60] over the trial function in Equation (7), one can obtain new Fourier expansions for the higher-order partial derivatives of plate deflections, which are shown below:

$$
\begin{aligned}
\frac{\partial W}{\partial x} &= \sum_{m=1,3}^{\infty} \sum_{n=1}^{\infty} \left(-\frac{2}{a} I_{1n} + \frac{\alpha_m}{2} W_{mn}\right) \cos \frac{\alpha_m x}{2} \sin(\beta_n y) \\
\frac{\partial^2 W}{\partial x^2} &= \sum_{m=1,3}^{\infty} \sum_{n=1}^{\infty} \left\{\frac{2}{a}\left[\frac{\alpha_m}{2} I_{1n} + (-1)^{\frac{m-1}{2}} I_{2n}\right] - \left(\frac{\alpha_m}{2}\right)^2 W_{mn}\right\} \sin \frac{\alpha_m x}{2} \sin(\beta_n y) \\
\frac{\partial^3 W}{\partial x^3} &= \sum_{m=1,3}^{\infty} \sum_{n=1}^{\infty} \left\{\frac{2}{a}\left[\left(\frac{\alpha_m}{2}\right)^2 I_{1n} + \frac{\alpha_m}{2}(-1)^{\frac{m-1}{2}} I_{2n} - I_{3n}\right] - \left(\frac{\alpha_m}{2}\right)^3 W_{mn}\right\} \cos \frac{\alpha_m x}{2} \sin(\beta_n y) \\
\frac{\partial^4 W}{\partial x^4} &= \sum_{m=1,3}^{\infty} \sum_{n=1}^{\infty} \left\{\frac{2}{a}\left[\begin{array}{l} -\left(\frac{\alpha_m}{2}\right)^3 I_{1n} - \left(\frac{\alpha_m}{2}\right)^2 (-1)^{\frac{m-1}{2}} I_{2n} \\ +\frac{\alpha_m}{2} I_{3n} + (-1)^{\frac{m-1}{2}} I_{4n} \end{array}\right] + \left(\frac{\alpha_m}{2}\right)^4 W_{mn}\right\} \sin \frac{\alpha_m x}{2} \sin(\beta_n y)
\end{aligned} \tag{8}
$$

$$
\begin{aligned}
\frac{\partial W}{\partial y} &= \sum_{m=1,3}\sum_{n=0}\left\{\frac{\varepsilon_n}{b}\left[(-1)^n J_{2m}-J_{1m}\right]+\beta_n W_{mn}\right\}\sin\frac{\alpha_m x}{2}\cos(\beta_n y)\\
\frac{\partial^2 W}{\partial y^2} &= \sum_{m=1,3}\sum_{n=1}\left\{-\frac{2}{b}\beta_n\left[(-1)^n J_{2m}-J_{1m}\right]-\beta_n^2 W_{mn}\right\}\sin\frac{\alpha_m x}{2}\sin(\beta_n y)\\
\frac{\partial^3 W}{\partial y^3} &= \sum_{m=1,3}\sum_{n=0}\left\{\frac{\varepsilon_n}{b}\left\{\begin{array}{l}(-1)^n J_{4m}-J_{3m}\\ -\beta_n^2\left[(-1)^n J_{2m}-J_{1m}\right]\end{array}\right\}-\beta_n^3 W_{mn}\right\}\sin\frac{\alpha_m x}{2}\cos(\beta_n y)\\
\frac{\partial^4 W}{\partial y^4} &= \sum_{m=1,3}\sum_{n=1}\left\{-\frac{2}{b}\beta_n\left\{\begin{array}{l}(-1)^n J_{4m}-J_{3m}\\ -\beta_n^2\left[(-1)^n J_{2m}-J_{1m}\right]\end{array}\right\}+\beta_n^4 W_{mn}\right\}\sin\frac{\alpha_m x}{2}\sin(\beta_n y)
\end{aligned}
\tag{9}
$$

$$
\begin{aligned}
\frac{\partial^2 W}{\partial x\partial y} &= \sum_{m=1,3}^{\infty}\sum_{n=0,1}^{\infty}\left\{\frac{\varepsilon_n}{b}\left[(-1)^n K_{2m}-K_{1m}\right]-\frac{2}{a}\beta_n I_{1n}+\frac{\alpha_m\beta_n}{2}W_{mn}\right\}\cos\frac{\alpha_m x}{2}\cos(\beta_n y)\\
\frac{\partial^3 W}{\partial x\partial y^2} &= \sum_{m=1,3}^{\infty}\sum_{n=1}^{\infty}\left\{-\frac{2}{a}L_{1n}+\frac{\alpha_m\beta_n}{2}\frac{2}{b}\left[(-1)^n J_{2m}-J_{1m}\right]-\frac{\alpha_m\beta_n^2}{2}W_{mn}\right\}\cos\frac{\alpha_m x}{2}\sin(\beta_n y)\\
\frac{\partial^3 W}{\partial x^2\partial y} &= \sum_{m=1,3}^{\infty}\sum_{n=0,1}^{\infty}\left\{\begin{array}{l}\frac{2}{a}\left[\frac{\alpha_m\beta_n}{2}I_{1n}+\beta_n(-1)^{\frac{m-1}{2}}I_{2n}\right]\\ +\frac{\varepsilon_n}{b}\left[(-1)^n K_{4m}-K_{3m}\right]-\left(\frac{\alpha_m}{2}\right)^2\beta_n W_{mn}\end{array}\right\}\sin\frac{\alpha_m x}{2}\cos(\beta_n y)\\
\frac{\partial^4 W}{\partial x^2\partial y^2} &= \sum_{m=1,3}^{\infty}\sum_{n=1}^{\infty}\left\{\begin{array}{l}-\frac{2}{a}\beta_n^2\left[\frac{\alpha_m}{2}I_{1n}+(-1)^{\frac{m-1}{2}}I_{2n}\right]\\ -\frac{2}{b}\beta_n\left[(-1)^n K_{4m}-K_{3m}\right]+\left(\frac{\alpha_m}{2}\right)^2\beta_n^2 W_{mn}\end{array}\right\}\sin\frac{\alpha_m x}{2}\sin(\beta_n y)
\end{aligned}
\tag{10}
$$

Denote

$$
\begin{aligned}
I_{1n} &= \frac{2}{b}\int_0^b W|_{x=0}\sin(\beta_n y)\mathrm{d}y, & I_{2n} &= \frac{2}{b}\int_0^b \left.\frac{\partial W}{\partial x}\right|_{x=a}\sin(\beta_n y)\mathrm{d}y\\
I_{3n} &= \frac{2}{b}\int_0^b \left.\frac{\partial^2 W}{\partial x^2}\right|_{x=0}\sin(\beta_n y)\mathrm{d}y, & I_{4n} &= \frac{2}{b}\int_0^b \left.\frac{\partial^3 W}{\partial x^3}\right|_{x=a}\sin(\beta_n y)\mathrm{d}y\\
J_{1m} &= \frac{2}{a}\int_0^a W|_{y=0}\sin\frac{\alpha_m x}{2}\mathrm{d}x, & J_{2m} &= \frac{2}{a}\int_0^a W|_{y=b}\sin\frac{\alpha_m x}{2}\mathrm{d}x\\
J_{3m} &= \frac{2}{a}\int_0^a \left.\frac{\partial^2 W}{\partial y^2}\right|_{y=0}\sin\frac{\alpha_m x}{2}\mathrm{d}x, & J_{4m} &= \frac{2}{a}\int_0^a \left.\frac{\partial^2 W}{\partial y^2}\right|_{y=b}\sin\frac{\alpha_m x}{2}\mathrm{d}x\\
K_{1m} &= \frac{2}{a}\int_0^a \left.\frac{\partial W}{\partial x}\right|_{y=0}\cos\frac{\alpha_m x}{2}\mathrm{d}x, & K_{2m} &= \frac{2}{a}\int_0^a \left.\frac{\partial W}{\partial x}\right|_{y=b}\cos\frac{\alpha_m x}{2}\mathrm{d}x\\
K_{3m} &= \frac{2}{a}\int_0^a \left.\frac{\partial^2 W}{\partial x^2}\right|_{y=0}\sin\frac{\alpha_m x}{2}\mathrm{d}x, & K_{4m} &= \frac{2}{a}\int_0^a \left.\frac{\partial^2 W}{\partial x^2}\right|_{y=h}\sin\frac{\alpha_m x}{2}\mathrm{d}x\\
L_{1n} &= \frac{2}{b}\int_0^b \left.\frac{\partial^2 W}{\partial y^2}\right|_{x=0}\sin(\beta_n y)\mathrm{d}y
\end{aligned}
\tag{11}
$$

According to the boundary conditions in Equation (5), we can clearly derive the following relationships:

$$
I_{1n}=L_{1n}=0,\ J_{1m}=J_{2m}=K_{1m}=K_{2m}=K_{3m}=K_{4m}=0,\ D_x I_{4n}=\left(H+2D_{xy}\right)\beta_n^2 I_{2n} \tag{12}
$$

Substituting the plate deflection, new expressions of $\partial^4 W/\partial x^4, \partial^4 W/\partial y^4$ and $\partial^4 W/\left(\partial x^2\partial y^2\right)$ of Equations (8)–(10), and constants relationships of Equation (12) into the governing PDE, we can derive Equation (13):

$$\sum_{m=1,3}^{\infty}\sum_{n=1}^{\infty}\left\{\begin{array}{l}\left(\frac{D_x\alpha_m^4}{16}+\frac{H\alpha_m^2\beta_n^2}{2}+D_y\beta_n^4-\rho h\omega^2\right)W_{mn}\\-D_y\frac{2}{b}\beta_n\left[(-1)^nJ_{4m}-J_{3m}\right]\\-D_x\frac{2}{a}\left[(-1)^{\frac{m-1}{2}}\left(\frac{\alpha_m^2}{4}+\mu_y\beta_n^2\right)I_{2n}-\frac{\alpha_m}{2}I_{3n}\right]\end{array}\right\}\sin\frac{\alpha_m x}{2}\sin(\beta_n y)=0 \quad (13)$$

Simplifying Equation (13), we can obtain the relationship between the W_{mn} and constants I_{2n}, I_{3n}, J_{3m}, and J_{4m}, as follows:

$$W_{mn}=A_{mn}\left\{\begin{array}{l}D_x\frac{2}{a}\left[(-1)^{\frac{m-1}{2}}\left(\frac{\alpha_m^2}{4}+\mu_y\beta_n^2\right)I_{2n}-\frac{\alpha_m}{2}I_{3n}\right]\\+D_y\frac{2}{b}\beta_n\left[(-1)^nJ_{4m}-J_{3m}\right]\end{array}\right\} \quad (14)$$

in which $A_{mn}=1\Big/\left(\frac{D_x\alpha_m^4}{16}+\frac{H\alpha_m^2\beta_n^2}{2}+D_y\beta_n^4-\rho h\omega^2\right)$.

Utilizing the obtained W_{mn}, we finally derived the formula for $W(x,y)$ in terms of I_{2n}, I_{3n}, J_{3m}, and J_{4m}, which is given as follows:

$$W(x,y)=\sum_{m=1,3}^{\infty}\sum_{n=1,3,}^{\infty}A_{mn}\left\{\begin{array}{l}D_y\frac{2}{b}\beta_n\left[(-1)^nJ_{4m}-J_{3m}\right]\\+D_x\frac{2}{a}\left[(-1)^{\frac{m-1}{2}}\left(\frac{\alpha_m^2}{4}+\mu_y\beta_n^2\right)I_{2n}-\frac{\alpha_m}{2}I_{3n}\right]\end{array}\right\}\sin\frac{\alpha_m x}{2}\sin(\beta_n y) \quad (15)$$

Through the above derivations, the obtained plate deflection has satisfied zero deflection at clamped edges, and zero equivalent shear forces at the free edge. The unknown constants, I_{2n}, I_{3n}, J_{3m}, and J_{4m}, will be determined by the matching edge conditions described in Equation (6). In combination with the orthogonal properties of the Fourier series, we can derive the following four infinite systems of linear algebra equations after using the expressions of plate's slopes and bending moment in Equations (8)–(10) to satisfy the boundary conditions in Equation (6):

$$\sum_{m=1,3}^{\infty}\frac{\alpha_m}{2}A_{mn}\left\{\begin{array}{l}D_y\beta_n\frac{2}{b}\left[(-1)^nJ_{4m}-J_{3m}\right]\\+D_x\frac{2}{a}\left[(-1)^{\frac{m-1}{2}}\left(\frac{\alpha_m^2}{4}+\mu_y\beta_n^2\right)I_{2n}-\frac{\alpha_m}{2}I_{3n}\right]\end{array}\right\} \quad n=1,2,3\cdots \quad (16)$$

$$\begin{array}{l}\sum\limits_{m=1,3}^{\infty}\left(\frac{\alpha_m^2}{4}+\mu_y\beta_n^2\right)(-1)^{\frac{m-1}{2}}A_{mn}\beta_nD_y\frac{2}{b}\left[(-1)^nJ_{4m}-J_{3m}\right]\\+\sum\limits_{m=1,3}^{\infty}\frac{2}{a}(-1)^{m-1}\left[D_xA_{mn}\left(\frac{\alpha_m^2}{4}+\mu_y\beta_n^2\right)^2-1\right]I_{2n}\\-\sum\limits_{m=1,3}^{\infty}\left(\frac{\alpha_m^2}{4}+\mu_y\beta_n^2\right)A_{mn}(-1)^{\frac{m-1}{2}}\frac{\delta_m}{2}D_x\frac{2}{a}I_{3n}=0 \qquad n=1,2,3\cdots\end{array} \quad (17)$$

$$\sum_{n=1}^{\infty}\beta_nA_{mn}\left\{\begin{array}{l}D_y\beta_n\frac{2}{b}\left[(-1)^nJ_{4m}-J_{3m}\right]\\+D_x\frac{2}{a}\left[(-1)^{\frac{m-1}{2}}\left(\frac{\alpha_m^2}{4}+\mu_y\beta_n^2\right)I_{2n}-\frac{\alpha_m}{2}I_{3n}\right]\end{array}\right\} \quad m=1,3,5\cdots \quad (18)$$

$$\sum_{n=1}^{\infty}\beta_n(-1)^n A_{mn}\left\{\begin{array}{l} D_y\beta_n\frac{2}{b}\left[(-1)^n J_{4m}-J_{3m}\right] \\ +D_x\frac{2}{a}\left[(-1)^{\frac{m-1}{2}}\left(\frac{\alpha_m^2}{4}+\mu_y\beta_n^2\right)I_{2n}-\frac{\alpha_m}{2}I_{3n}\right] \end{array}\right\} \quad m=1,3,5\cdots \tag{19}$$

Through the above-mentioned derivation processes, we can only deal with the above systems of infinite linear algebra equations instead of solving complicated boundary value problems of free vibration governing PDE. Theoretically, we can only obtain an exact solution when n and m approach $+\infty$. Finite series terms can guarantee the precision of the present problem. In the present calculation process, the same terms, t, were selected for n and m, which implies that their upper limits are $N = t$ and $M = (2t-1)/2$, respectively. To obtain non-trivial solutions for plates' natural frequencies, the determinant matrix formed by Equations (16)–(19) should equal zero, by which non-zero solutions for constants I_{2n}, I_{3n}, J_{3m}, and J_{4m} are also determined. The successive substitution of the constants substituted into Equations (16)–(19) finally yield the corresponding vibration shape solutions.

3. Results for Frequency Parameters and Deformation Shapes of Plates

To confirm the capacity of the present two-dimensional modified Fourier series method in predicting clear free vibration behaviors of orthotropic thin plates under the mentioned boundary conditions, plates with different material properties and aspect ratios were examined. Due to the shortage of available analytic data, a comparison of the natural frequencies with the results offered by FEM was performed using Abaqus 6.13. The constituent materials considered in this paper are as follows: as for the orthotropic plates, the elastic constants adopted were $H = 0.5D_x$, $D_y = 0.5D_x$, $\mu_x = 0.6$ and $\mu_y = 0.3$; as for the isotropic thin plate, the Poisson's ratio $\mu_y = \mu_x = \mu = 0.3$. The length-to-width ratio b/a was assumed to range from 0.5 to 5.

4. Discussion

All the non-dimensional natural frequencies obtained by the present method and the finite element method are listed in Tables 1 and 2. Analysis of these data reveals a consistent trend wherein increasing aspect ratios lead to a decrease in natural frequencies across both isotropic and orthotropic materials. Notably, a minimum in natural frequency is evident at an aspect ratio of 0.5. Moreover, a rapid decline in natural frequency is observed as the aspect ratios transition from 0.5 to 1 and 1.5. Subsequent increases in aspect ratios, particularly from 1 to 5, exert a minimal impact on the natural frequency. Interestingly, the results emphasize that an aspect ratio of 0.5 employs a more pronounced influence on natural frequency compared with ratios ranging from 1 to 5, irrespective of the material type. Furthermore, the comparative analysis between isotropic and orthotropic materials for identical boundary conditions indicated that isotropic materials consistently exhibited higher natural frequencies. This disparity sheds light on the inherent mechanical differences between isotropic and orthotropic materials, emphasizing the importance of material selection in engineering applications to achieve desired performance characteristics. Through Tables 1 and 2, it is also evident that the percentage errors between the present solutions with the FEM data are no more than 1%. The corresponding deformation shapes for isotropic/orthotropic square plates are given in Figures 2 and 3. Through Figures 2 and 3, it is evident that the obtained plate deformation shapes strictly satisfy the edge conditions. Through the above comparison, it was found that all the given numerical and graphical solutions were very close to the FEM solutions, which provides sufficient evidence to exhibit the validity of the present approach and the precision of the analytical results acquired.

Table 1. Non-dimensional natural frequencies of the isotropic rectangular thin plate with one free edge and three clamped edges.

b/*a*	Method	Mode									
		1st	2nd	3rd	4th	5th	6th	7th	8th	9th	10th
0.5	Present	90.573	104.12	135.07	186.88	247.59	260.38	263.77	296.88	348.49	355.27
	FEM	90.528	104.07	135.01	187.03	247.49	260.31	263.66	296.75	348.33	355.16
1	Present	23.930	40.012	63.248	76.725	80.602	116.69	122.29	134.47	140.30	172.90
	FEM	23.918	39.991	63.216	76.704	80.562	116.64	122.23	134.43	140.23	172.83
1.5	Present	11.838	29.283	29.305	47.419	55.498	67.735	74.141	84.933	90.430	109.37
	FEM	11.832	29.269	29.292	47.395	55.470	67.721	74.104	84.907	90.385	109.32
2	Present	7.7778	17.544	25.860	32.231	36.036	51.210	51.835	64.926	71.104	74.341
	FEM	7.7748	17.536	26.232	32.215	36.018	51.184	51.809	64.915	71.069	74.322
2.5	Present	6.0112	12.179	21.526	24.386	30.850	34.042	40.666	49.708	53.519	63.697
	FEM	6.0094	12.173	21.516	24.375	30.835	34.025	40.646	49.682	53.493	63.688
3	Present	5.1190	9.3197	15.766	23.620	24.416	28.080	34.928	35.292	43.970	48.319
	FEM	5.1179	9.3158	15.759	23.609	24.404	28.066	34.911	35.275	43.949	48.294
3.5	Present	4.6193	7.6354	12.329	18.653	23.175	26.425	26.597	31.506	36.158	38.206
	FEM	4.6185	7.6326	12.324	18.643	23.165	26.413	26.584	31.491	36.140	38.188
4	Present	4.3164	6.5702	10.126	14.938	20.995	22.896	25.364	28.296	29.269	34.447
	FEM	4.3159	6.5681	10.121	14.931	20.985	22.886	25.352	28.282	29.255	34.431
4.5	Present	4.1210	5.8595	8.6357	12.412	17.176	22.708	22.923	24.646	27.735	29.656
	FEM	4.1207	5.8579	8.6323	12.406	17.167	22.698	22.911	24.635	27.722	29.641
5	Present	3.9884	5.3648	7.5855	10.621	14.460	19.098	22.575	24.135	24.533	26.643
	FEM	3.9881	5.3636	7.5827	10.616	14.453	19.089	22.565	24.124	24.521	26.630

Table 2. Non-dimensional natural frequencies of the orthotropic rectangular thin plate with one free edge and three clamped edges.

b/*a*	Method	Mode									
		1st	2nd	3rd	4th	5th	6th	7th	8th	9th	10th
0.5	Present	62.676	73.674	103.00	155.50	171.30	184.77	211.18	230.47	257.00	324.66
	FEM	62.642	73.634	102.96	155.43	171.22	184.68	211.08	230.40	256.86	324.50
1	Present	16.330	31.326	43.269	57.299	68.858	84.012	91.278	98.204	127.30	129.56
	FEM	16.322	31.310	43.246	57.269	68.843	83.968	91.244	98.152	127.26	129.50
1.5	Present	8.1418	19.810	25.375	35.630	37.770	52.846	61.836	64.447	73.038	76.747
	FEM	8.1384	19.800	25.363	35.612	37.749	52.819	61.803	64.434	73.018	76.707
2	Present	5.5800	11.783	21.728	23.704	28.900	35.171	37.919	50.794	52.058	63.138
	FEM	5.5784	11.777	21.717	23.693	28.886	35.153	37.900	50.767	52.031	63.126
2.5	Present	4.5790	8.2190	14.411	22.919	23.031	26.110	31.503	33.661	39.336	46.611
	FEM	4.5783	8.2156	14.403	22.907	23.020	26.098	31.487	33.644	39.315	46.586
3	Present	4.1296	6.4037	10.527	16.335	22.697	23.730	24.720	28.258	32.674	33.433
	FEM	4.1292	6.4015	10.522	16.327	22.686	23.718	24.709	28.244	32.657	33.416
3.5	Present	3.9037	5.3969	8.2637	12.426	17.793	22.508	23.935	24.318	26.419	30.054
	FEM	3.9035	5.3956	8.2603	12.421	17.784	22.497	23.924	24.305	26.407	30.039
4	Present	3.7789	4.8034	6.8588	9.9434	13.984	18.932	22.390	23.451	24.763	25.286
	FEM	3.7789	4.8025	6.8563	9.9390	13.977	18.922	22.380	23.440	24.750	25.274
4.5	Present	3.7043	4.4355	5.9467	8.2879	11.412	15.273	19.845	22.312	23.131	24.540
	FEM	3.7043	4.4349	5.9449	8.2846	11.407	15.266	19.835	22.302	23.121	24.529
5	Present	3.6569	4.1972	5.3335	7.1437	9.6074	12.686	16.354	20.592	22.258	22.909
	FEM	3.6569	4.1968	5.3322	7.1411	9.6031	12.680	16.345	20.582	22.248	22.899

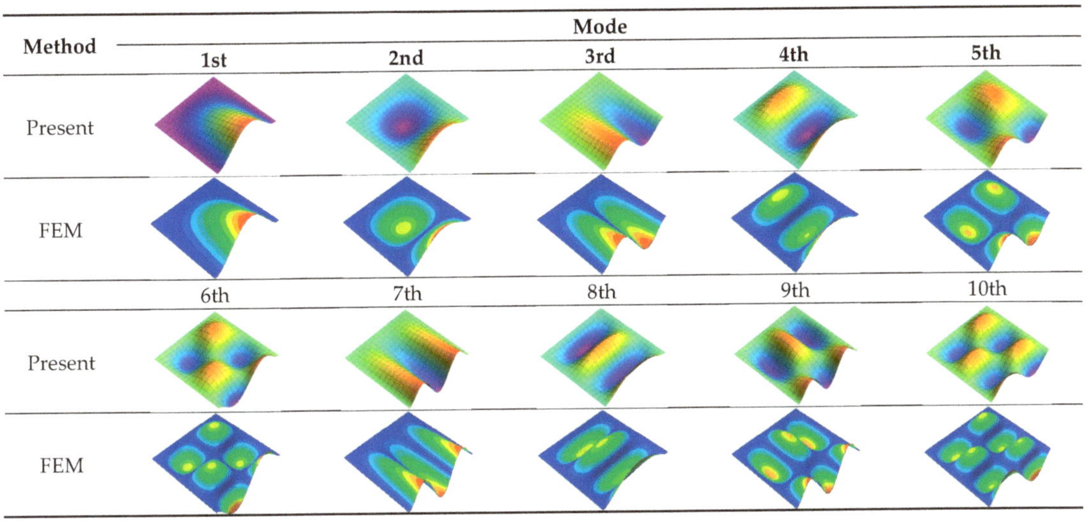

Figure 2. Mode shapes of an isotropic square thin plate with one edge free and three edges clamped.

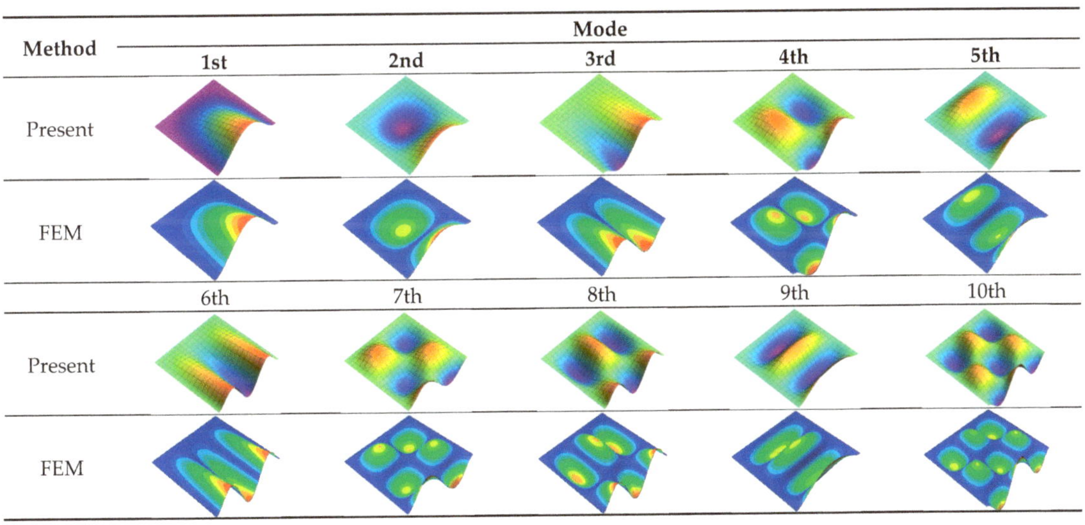

Figure 3. Mode shapes of an orthotropic square thin plate with one edge free and three edges clamped.

This study holds significant practical implications for engineering applications, particularly in structural design and material selection processes. The analysis of non-dimensional natural frequencies across various aspect ratios for both isotropic and orthotropic materials provides valuable insights into structural behavior. Engineers can utilize these findings to optimize the design of structures by adjusting aspect ratios to achieve desired natural frequencies, ensuring structural stability and performance. Moreover, the comparative analysis between isotropic and orthotropic materials highlights the importance of material selection in engineering applications, as isotropic materials consistently exhibit higher natural frequencies under identical boundary conditions. This understanding aids engineers in selecting the most suitable materials for specific applications, thereby enhancing the overall performance and durability of engineered systems. Additionally, the validation of analytical results against finite element method (FEM) data reinforces the accuracy and reliability of the analytical approach, providing engineers with confidence in utilizing these methods for structural analysis and design. Overall, this study offers practical guidance for engineers in optimizing structural designs, informing material selection processes, and improving engineering practices across various industries.

5. Conclusions

In the present study, we developed a new two-dimensional modified Fourier series method for studying the free vibration behavior of orthotropic plates with three edges clamped and one edge free. These solutions provide comprehensive information on the natural frequencies and vibration mode analysis, considering various aspect ratios. These solutions can be used as valuable reference data for evaluating other approximate/numerical approaches. The present approach is advantageous as it enables linear algebra equations to be solved instead of handling difficult boundary value problems of PDE, providing an easy-to-implement approach for the mechanical problems of plates. More importantly, further developments of this method are expected for analyzing problems of plates under other non-Levy edge conditions, employing different types of Fourier series.

Author Contributions: Conceptualization, writing—original draft preparation, methodology, formal analysis, and software, Z.W. and S.U.; funding acquisition, project administration, A.L.; methodology, validation, Y.W.; supervision, Z.Y. All authors have read and agreed to the published version of the manuscript.

Funding: This study was funded by Interaction Research Project between Hulin-Changchun Natural Gas Pipeline Project and Surrounding Seismic Stations (PC22-2023-005).

Data Availability Statement: Data are contained within the article.

Conflicts of Interest: Authors An Li and Zhiming Yin were employed by the company PipeChina Construction Project Management Company. Author Yu Wu was employed by the company Beijing Urban Construction Exploration & Surveying Design Research Institute Co., Ltd. The remaining authors declare that the research was conducted in the absence of any commercial or financial relationships that could be construed as a potential conflict of interest.

References

1. Chen, F.; Zhang, H.; Li, Z.; Luo, Y.; Xiao, X.; Liu, Y. Residual stresses effects on fatigue crack growth behavior of rib-to-deck double-sided welded joints in orthotropic steel decks. *Adv. Struct. Eng.* **2024**, *27*, 35–50. [CrossRef]
2. Luo, Y.; Liu, X.; Chen, F.; Zhang, H.; Xiao, X. Numerical simulation on crack–inclusion interaction for rib-to-deck welded joints in orthotropic steel deck. *Metals* **2023**, *13*, 1402. [CrossRef]
3. Shi, X.; Yang, Y.; Zhu, X.; Huang, Z. Stochastic dynamics analysis of the rocket shell coupling system with circular plate fasteners based on spectro-geometric method. *Compos. Struct.* **2024**, *329*, 117727. [CrossRef]
4. Zhang, C. The active rotary inertia driver system for flutter vibration control of bridges and various promising applications. *Sci. China Technol. Sci.* **2023**, *66*, 390–405. [CrossRef]
5. Lu, Z.; Yang, T.; Brennan, M.J.; Liu, Z.; Chen, L.-Q. Experimental investigation of a two-stage nonlinear vibration isolation system with high-static-low-dynamic stiffness. *J. Appl. Mech.* **2017**, *84*, 021001. [CrossRef]
6. Lu, Z.; Brennan, M.J.; Yang, T.; Li, X.; Liu, Z. An investigation of a two-stage nonlinear vibration isolation system. *J. Sound Vib.* **2013**, *332*, 1456–1464. [CrossRef]
7. Tran, V.-K.; Pham, Q.-H.; Nguyen-Thoi, T. A finite element formulation using four-unknown incorporating nonlocal theory for bending and free vibration analysis of functionally graded nanoplates resting on elastic medium foundations. *Eng. Comput.* **2022**, *38*, 1465–1490. [CrossRef]
8. Li, J.; Liu, Y.; Lin, G. Implementation of a coupled FEM-SBFEM for soil-structure interaction analysis of large-scale 3D base-isolated nuclear structures. *Comput. Geotech.* **2023**, *162*, 105669. [CrossRef]
9. Deng, E.-F.; Wang, Y.-H.; Zong, L.; Zhang, Z.; Zhang, J.-F. Seismic behavior of a novel liftable connection for modular steel buildings: Experimental and numerical studies. *Thin-Walled Struct.* **2024**, *197*, 111563. [CrossRef]
10. Sarrami-Foroushani, S.; Azhari, M. On the use of bubble complex finite strip method in the nonlocal buckling and vibration analysis of single-layered graphene sheets. *Int. J. Mech. Sci.* **2014**, *85*, 168–178. [CrossRef]
11. Civalek, Ö.; Avcar, M. Free vibration and buckling analyses of CNT reinforced laminated non-rectangular plates by discrete singular convolution method. *Eng. Comput.* **2022**, *38*, 489–521. [CrossRef]
12. Lai, S.K.; Xiang, Y. DSC analysis for buckling and vibration of rectangular plates with elastically restrained edges and linearly varying in-plane loading. *Int. J. Struct. Stab. Dyn.* **2009**, *9*, 511–531. [CrossRef]

13. Wu, W.X.; Shu, C.; Wang, C.M.; Xiang, Y. Free vibration and buckling analysis of highly skewed plates by least squares-based finite difference method. *Int. J. Struct. Stab. Dyn.* **2010**, *10*, 225–252. [CrossRef]
14. Albuquerque, E.L.; Sollero, P.; Fedelinski, P. Free vibration analysis of anisotropic material structures using the boundary element method. *Eng. Anal. Bound. Elem.* **2003**, *27*, 977–985. [CrossRef]
15. Fan, J.; Huang, J.; Ding, J.; Zhang, J. Free vibration of functionally graded carbon nanotube-reinforced conical panels integrated with piezoelectric layers subjected to elastically restrained boundary conditions. *Adv. Mech. Eng.* **2017**, *9*, 168781401771181. [CrossRef]
16. Motezaker, M.; Jamali, M.; Kolahchi, R. Application of differential cubature method for nonlocal vibration, buckling and bending response of annular nanoplates integrated by piezoelectric layers based on surface-higher order nonlocal-piezoelasticity theory. *J. Comput. Appl. Math.* **2020**, *369*, 112625. [CrossRef]
17. Civalek, Ö. Nonlinear dynamic response of laminated plates resting on nonlinear elastic foundations by the discrete singular convolution-differential quadrature coupled approaches. *Compos. Part B Eng.* **2013**, *50*, 171–179. [CrossRef]
18. Sharma, A. Free vibration of moderately thick antisymmetric laminated annular sector plates with elastic edge constraints. *Int. J. Mech. Sci.* **2014**, *83*, 124–132. [CrossRef]
19. Song, Z.; Li, W.; He, X.; Xie, D. Comparisons of matched interface and boundary (MIB) method and its interpolation formulation for free vibration analysis of stepped beams and plates. *Appl. Math. Comput.* **2021**, *394*, 125817. [CrossRef]
20. Papkov, S.O.; Banerjee, J.R. Dynamic stiffness formulation and free vibration analysis of specially orthotropic Mindlin plates with arbitrary boundary conditions. *J. Sound Vib.* **2019**, *458*, 522–543. [CrossRef]
21. Eftekhari, S.A.; Jafari, A.A. High accuracy mixed finite element-Ritz formulation for free vibration analysis of plates with general boundary conditions. *Appl. Math. Comput.* **2012**, *219*, 1312–1344. [CrossRef]
22. Xu, J.; Chang, L.; Chen, T.; Ren, T.; Zhang, Y.; Cai, Z. Study of the bending properties of variable stiffness chain mail fabrics. *Compos. Struct.* **2023**, *322*, 117369. [CrossRef]
23. Xu, J.; Zhang, Y.; Huang, Y.; Chang, L.; Chen, T.; Ren, T.; Cai, Z. Dynamic response of chain mail fabrics with variable stiffness. *Int. J. Mech. Sci.* **2024**, *264*, 108840. [CrossRef]
24. Zhang, W.; Kang, S.; Liu, X.; Lin, B.; Huang, Y. Experimental study of a composite beam externally bonded with a carbon fiber-reinforced plastic plate. *J. Build. Eng.* **2023**, *71*, 106522. [CrossRef]
25. Arefi, M.; Taghavian, S.H. Dynamic characteristics of composite micro lattice plates comprises of graphene nanoplatelets based on MCST theory. *Thin-Walled Struct.* **2022**, *175*, 109200. [CrossRef]
26. Arefi, M.; Firouzeh, S.; Mohammad-Rezaei Bidgoli, E.; Civalek, Ö. Analysis of porous micro-plates reinforced with FG-GNPs based on Reddy plate theory. *Compos. Struct.* **2020**, *247*, 112391. [CrossRef]
27. Ruocco, E.; Reddy, J.N. A closed-form solution for buckling analysis of orthotropic Reddy plates and prismatic plate structures. *Compos. Part B Eng.* **2019**, *169*, 258–273. [CrossRef]
28. Zenkour, A.M.; El-Shahrany, H.D. Hygrothermal forced vibration of a viscoelastic laminated plate with magnetostrictive actuators resting on viscoelastic foundations. *Int. J. Mech. Mater. Des.* **2021**, *17*, 301–320. [CrossRef]
29. Hosseini-Hashemi, S.; Fadaee, M.; Rokni Damavandi Taher, H. Exact solutions for free flexural vibration of Lévy-type rectangular thick plates via third-order shear deformation plate theory. *Appl. Math. Model.* **2011**, *35*, 708–727. [CrossRef]
30. Rezaei, A.S.; Saidi, A.R. Exact solution for free vibration of thick rectangular plates made of porous materials. *Compos. Struct.* **2015**, *134*, 1051–1060. [CrossRef]
31. Ray, M.C. Zeroth-Order Shear Deformation Theory for Laminated Composite Plates. *J. Appl. Mech.* **2003**, *70*, 374–380. [CrossRef]
32. Kobayashi, H.; Sonoda, K. Vibration and buckling of tapered rectangular plates with two opposite edges simply supported and the other two edges elastically restrained against rotation. *J. Sound Vib.* **1991**, *146*, 323–337. [CrossRef]
33. Cui, W.; Zhao, L.; Ge, Y.; Xu, K. A generalized van der Pol nonlinear model of vortex-induced vibrations of bridge decks with multistability. *Nonlinear Dyn.* **2024**, *112*, 259–272. [CrossRef]
34. Cui, W.; Caracoglia, L.; Zhao, L.; Ge, Y. Examination of occurrence probability of vortex-induced vibration of long-span bridge decks by Fokker–Planck–Kolmogorov equation. *Struct. Saf.* **2023**, *105*, 102369. [CrossRef]
35. Cui, W.; Zhao, L.; Ge, Y. Wind-Induced Buffeting Vibration of Long-Span Bridge Considering Geometric and Aerodynamic Nonlinearity Based on Reduced-Order Modeling. *J. Struct. Eng.* **2023**, *149*, 04023160. [CrossRef]
36. Zhang, J.; Zhou, C.; Ullah, S.; Zhong, Y.; Li, R. Two-dimensional generalized finite integral transform method for new analytic bending solutions of orthotropic rectangular thin foundation plates. *Appl. Math. Lett.* **2019**, *92*, 8–14. [CrossRef]
37. Zhang, J.; Guo, C.; Wang, K.; Zhang, C.; Jing, C.; Qi, W. On the finite integral transform approach for analytic thermal buckling solutions of orthotropic plates. *Acta Mech.* **2023**, *234*, 1901–1922. [CrossRef]
38. Zhang, J.; Zhao, Q.; Wang, X.; Ullah, S.; Zhao, D.; Civalek, Ö.; Xue, C.; Qi, W. New exact analytical thermal buckling solutions of composite thin plates with all edges rotationally-restrained. *Mech. Adv. Mater. Struct.* **2023**, 1–13. [CrossRef]
39. Zhang, J.; Ullah, S.; Zhong, Y. New analytical free vibration solutions of orthotropic rectangular thin plates using generalized integral transformation. *J. Comput. Appl. Math.* **2020**, *367*, 112439. [CrossRef]
40. Ullah, S.; Zhong, Y.; Zhang, J. Analytical buckling solutions of rectangular thin plates by straightforward generalized integral transform method. *Int. J. Mech. Sci.* **2019**, *152*, 535–544. [CrossRef]
41. Zhang, J.; Zhao, Q.; Ullah, S.; Zhao, D.; Qi, W.; Civalek, Ö. An Accurate Computational Method for Buckling of Orthotropic Composite Plate with Non-Classical Boundary Restraints. *Int. J. Struct. Stab. Dyn.* **2023**, *23*, 2350080. [CrossRef]

42. Zhang, J.; Zhao, Q.; Ullah, S.; Geng, L.; Civalek, Ö. A new analytical solution of vibration response of orthotropic composite plates with two adjacent edges rotationally-restrained and the others free. *Compos. Struct.* **2021**, *266*, 113882. [CrossRef]
43. Rahbar Ranji, A.; Rostami Hoseynabadi, H. A semi-analytical solution for forced vibrations response of rectangular orthotropic plates with various boundary conditions. *J. Mech. Sci. Technol.* **2010**, *24*, 357–364. [CrossRef]
44. Hu, Z.; Yang, Y.; Zhou, C.; Zheng, X.; Li, R. On the symplectic superposition method for new analytic free vibration solutions of side-cracked rectangular thin plates. *J. Sound Vib.* **2020**, *489*, 115695. [CrossRef]
45. Li, R.; Zhou, C.; Zheng, X. On New Analytic Free Vibration Solutions of Doubly Curved Shallow Shells by the Symplectic Superposition Method Within the Hamiltonian-System Framework. *J. Vib. Acoust.* **2021**, *143*, 011002. [CrossRef]
46. Hu, Z.; Zheng, X.; An, D.; Zhou, C.; Yang, Y.; Li, R. New analytic buckling solutions of side-cracked rectangular thin plates by the symplectic superposition method. *Int. J. Mech. Sci.* **2021**, *191*, 106051. [CrossRef]
47. Chen, G.; Zhou, J.; Yang, D. Benchmark solutions of stationary random vibration for rectangular thin plate based on discrete analytical method. *Probabilistic Eng. Mech.* **2017**, *50*, 17–24. [CrossRef]
48. Xing, Y.F.; Liu, B. New exact solutions for free vibrations of thin orthotropic rectangular plates. *Compos. Struct.* **2009**, *89*, 567–574. [CrossRef]
49. Zhang, M.; Jiang, X.; Arefi, M. Dynamic formulation of a sandwich microshell considering modified couple stress and thickness-stretching. *Eur. Phys. J. Plus* **2023**, *138*, 227. [CrossRef]
50. Yazdanpanah Moghadam, P.; Tahani, M.; Naserian-Nik, A.M. Analytical solution of piezolaminated rectangular plates with arbitrary clamped/simply-supported boundary conditions under thermo-electro-mechanical loadings. *Appl. Math. Model.* **2013**, *37*, 3228–3241. [CrossRef]
51. Gorman, D.J. Free vibration and buckling of in-plane loaded plates with rotational elastic edge support. *J. Sound Vib.* **2000**, *229*, 755–773. [CrossRef]
52. Kiani, Y.; Bagherizadeh, E.; Eslami, M.R. Thermal buckling of clamped thin rectangular FGM plates resting on Pasternak elastic foundation (Three approximate analytical solutions). *Z. Angew. Math. Mech.* **2011**, *91*, 581–593. [CrossRef]
53. Liew, K.M.; Hung, K.C.; Lim, M.K. Vibration of mindlin plates using boundary characteristic orthogonal polynomials. *J. Sound Vib.* **1995**, *182*, 77–90. [CrossRef]
54. Zhou, K.; Su, J.; Hua, H. Free and forced vibration analysis of moderately thick orthotropic plates in thermal environment and resting on elastic supports. *Arch. Appl. Mech.* **2018**, *88*, 855–873. [CrossRef]
55. Peng, X.; Zhong, Y.; Shi, J.; Shi, Z. Free flexural vibration analysis of composite sandwich plate with reentrant honeycomb cores using homogenized plate model. *J. Sound Vib.* **2022**, *529*, 116955. [CrossRef]
56. Rostami, H.; Rahbar Ranji, A.; Bakhtiari-Nejad, F. Free in-plane vibration analysis of rotating rectangular orthotropic cantilever plates. *Int. J. Mech. Sci.* **2016**, *115–116*, 438–456. [CrossRef]
57. Tang, X.; Guo, C.; Li, F.; Zhang, R.; Song, D.; Fu, P.; Liu, H. Thermal buckling analysis of rotationally-restrained orthotropic thin plates utilizing a two-dimensional improved Fourier series approach. *Meccanica* **2023**, *58*, 1443–1464. [CrossRef]
58. Tang, X.; Guo, C.; Wang, K.; Song, D.; Zhang, J.; Qi, W. New Fourier expansion for thermal buckling analysis of rectangular thin plates with various edge restraints. *Arch. Appl. Mech.* **2023**, *93*, 3411–3426. [CrossRef]
59. Green, A.E. Double Fourier series and boundary value problems. *Math. Proc. Camb. Philos. Soc.* **1944**, *40*, 222–228. [CrossRef]
60. Latifi, M.; Farhatnia, F.; Kadkhodaei, M. Buckling analysis of rectangular functionally graded plates under various edge conditions using Fourier series expansion. *Eur. J. Mech.-A/Solids* **2013**, *41*, 16–27. [CrossRef]

buildings

MDPI

Article

Clinker-Free Cement Manufactured with Metallurgical Slags

Marcel Demarco, Fernando Vernilli * and Sara Carvalho Zago

Department of Materials Engineering, Lorena School of Engineering, University of São Paulo—USP, São Paulo 12602-810, Brazil; marcel.demarco@usp.br (M.D.); saracarvalho@usp.br (S.C.Z.)

* Correspondence: fernando.vernilli@usp.br

Abstract: Steel slag is a significant environmental liability generated by pyrometallurgical processes. Residue generation, such as granulated blast furnace slag and basic oxygen slag (BOF), is intrinsic in steel production. Blast furnace slag, generated in the carbothermal reduction of iron ore, is almost entirely used as a supplementary cement material in Portland cement. BOF slag, produced in the conversion of pig iron into steel in a basic oxygen converter, is still not consolidated or valued for reuse. This research proposes the reuse and valorization of BOF slag combined with blast furnace slag in clinker-free cement production. Cement formulations were produced with different slag and gypsum contents, ranging from 80 to 90% blast furnace slag, 10 to 20% gypsum, and 10 to 15% BOF slag. All formulations were evaluated for compressive strength at ages of 3, 7, 14, 28, 91, and 180 days of curing. At the initial ages, the cement formulations exhibited high resistance. On the 3rd day, the cement formulations reached up to 10 MPa, and on the 7th day, 40 MPa. At late ages, the best-performing formulation, ECO2, showed, after 28 days of hydration, a compressive strength greater than 50 MPa, and at 180 days, a compressive strength greater than 80 MPa. It was possible to understand that BOF slag acts in cement alkaline activation with pH increase, more or less actively due to the presence of lime, portlandite, and calcite.

Keywords: BOF slag; granulated blast furnace slag; clinker-free cement; solid waste recovery

1. Introduction

Despite the relevant and negative environmental impacts related to the cement production chain, its consumption continues to soar, especially in developing nations, such as China, which represents 51% of global production, and India, the second largest producer in the world, in addition to countries in Southeast Asia, Latin America, and Africa [1].

The growing concern about the environmental impacts caused by the production of Portland cement, combined with possible technological and economic gains, has led to many changes in the cement industry. However, these changes were insufficient to significantly reduce the generated environmental problems, mostly related to the predatory extraction of minerals, mainly limestone and clays, and the consequent need for limestone decarbonization and clay dehydroxylation. Both calcination processes stand out for their high emission of greenhouse gases, mostly CO_2. In other words, the environmental problems are mainly related to the production of Portland clinker [1–3].

Alternative cement formulations using different materials and avoiding clinkerization to make the production chain less carbon-intensive are an important initiative to reduce emissions. Some technologies have been proposed without the conventional raw material use and with new technological routes. In some cases, the technologies start almost entirely from the reuse of waste, differing widely between them. Among these technologies, the production of alkali-activated cement, calcium aluminate cement (CAC), magnesium silicate cement (Novacem), and supersulfated cement (SSC) can be mentioned [1,4,5].

The production of these cements faces difficulties due to both the raw materials used and the understanding of their performance. Since the raw materials used may be of natural origin, as is the case with the use of bauxite (CAC) or magnesium silicate (Novacem), the limited supply of raw materials, either due to restricted availability in certain regions or due to competition with other production chains, can make the cement more expensive than Portland cement and limited to specific applications [4,5].

On the other hand, some formulations use high levels of industrial waste, as occurs in supersulfated cement. Its formulation uses up to 90% ground granulated blast furnace slag, 15% more than the maximum allowed by Brazilian standards [6] in the cement composition with the highest steel slag content (CPIII). The composition also includes 10–20% hydrated calcium sulfates but up to 5% of an alkaline activator, such as Portland cement or Portland clinker [4].

Given these formulations, the production of a clinker-free cement with low environmental impact and low greenhouse gas emissions from the exclusive use of steel waste, i.e., blast furnace slag (BFS) and basic oxygen furnace slag (BOF), combined with gypsum waste from construction and the ceramic industry, called eco-sustainable cement (ECO), was proposed. Eco-sustainable cement presents certain similarities to CSS regarding composition. However, it does not use either Portland clinker or Portland cement but uses BOF slag as an alkaline activator [7]. The mechanical and physical–chemical performance of ECO cement was similar to or superior to Brazilian blast furnace slag, Portland cement, and CSS [6–8].

In order to improve the mechanical performance of eco-sustainable cement in its final stages, this study was conducted. This study also aimed to test various cement formulations containing different amounts of ironmaking slags and gypsum waste, evaluate their mechanical performance, and understand the effect of raw materials on the cement hydration process, specifically in terms of chemical and mineralogical composition.

2. Materials and Methods

2.1. Materials

The raw materials used consisted of steelmaking slags coming from a blast furnace (blast furnace slag—BFS) and a Linz–Donawitz furnace (LD steel slag—BOF) obtained from Companhia Siderúrgica Nacional—CSN (Brazil)—and plaster residue from construction. As shown in Table 1, the same gypsum residue was used in the proposed formulations. However, three types of BOF slag and two types of blast furnace slag were used to evaluate the effect of different calcium oxides, aluminum, iron, and silicon levels in cement. After drying, the raw materials were fragmented to obtain a maximum particle size of 2.36 mm in diameter.

Table 1. Raw materials used for cement production.

Raw Materials	Abbreviation	Classification	Source
Blast furnace slag	BFS1 BFS2	Steelmaking slag	Steelmaking industry
Basic oxygen furnace slag	BOF1 BOF2 BOF3	Steelmaking slag	Steelmaking industry
Gypsum waste	GW	Recyclable wWaste	Waste treatment and recycling plant

2.2. Methods

The conditions of the chemical and mineralogical analyses of BFS, BOFS, and gypsum waste carried out using X-ray fluorescence (XRF) and X-ray diffraction (XRD) techniques are presented in Table 2. Rietveld Refinement was used to obtain quantitative results. An internal standard of 10% rutile was added to quantify the amorphous phase.

Table 2. Techniques and conditions for characterizing raw materials.

Analyses	Raw Materials	Analysis Conditions
XRF	BFS, BOF, GW	Lithium tetraborate and lithium metaborate fused pellets/panalytical spectrometer, model Axios
XRD	BFS, BOF, GW	Rigaku diffractometer, Windmax 1000 model, Cu Kα radiation with 40 KV—20 mA and scan speed of 2°/min

Ten cement formulations were proposed with different slag and gypsum contents, ranging from 80 to 90% BFS, 10 to 20% gypsum waste, and 10 to 15% BOF slag, as shown in Table 3. Due to the difference in the grindability of ironmaking slags, the cement grinding was carried out by fine grinding the BFS and GW mixture, with increasing replacements of (BFS + GW) with ground BOF slag to a Blaine fineness of 550 m^2/Kg.

Table 3. Composition of cementitious formulations.

Cementitious Formulations	Nomenclature	BOF	BFS	BFS [wt%]	GW [wt%]	BOF [wt%]
ECO1	ECO1-851510	BOF 1	BFS1	85	15	10
ECO2	ECO2-851510	BOF 2	BFS1	85	15	10
	ECO2-802010			80	20	10
	ECO2-802013			80	20	13
ECO3	ECO3-851510	BOF 3	BFS1	85	15	10
	ECO3-802010			80	20	10
	ECO3-802015			80	20	15
	ECO3-881213			88	12	13
ECO4	ECO4-802010	BOF 3	BFS2	80	20	10
	ECO4-901010			90	10	10

The cementitious formulations were evaluated for chemical composition, as shown in Table 2 (XFR), and alkalinity of the cement pastes. The pastes were prepared with a water/cement ratio of 0.31, which was determined based on the normal consistency of cement. The alkalinity measurements were taken using a peagameter, Dgimed model DM2.

The cement mortar specimens prepared for compressive strength tests, according to [9], were subjected to curing in a humid chamber (relative humidity of (95 ± 5)% and room temperature of (24 ± 2) °C) until the test ages of 3, 7, 28, 91, and 180 days. Compressive strength tests were carried out on a Forney compression machine, model F-25EX-F-CPILOT. The compression machine's working range of mechanical stress is from 20 to 1100 kN.

3. Results

3.1. Raw Material Characterization

The chemical composition of the BOF, BFS slags, and gypsum waste is shown in Table 4. The main oxides found for each raw material are different concerning their origin. BFS has high SiO_2, CaO, and Al_2O_3 content, essential for hydration product formation, such as aluminates and hydrated calcium silicates. In BOF slag, the oxides CaO, Fe_2O_3, and SiO_2 predominate, which help in the chemical activation of BFS and the formation of new hydration products, while the gypsum residue basically presents CaO and SO_3, essential in the formation of ettringite.

The gypsum waste from civil construction corresponds to the hydration residue of calcium sulfate hemihydrate. For this reason, its mineralogical composition corresponds mainly to gypsum; Table 5.

Table 4. Chemical composition of raw materials.

Chemical Composition	BOF1	BOF2	BOF3	BFS1	BFS2	GW
SiO_2	17.60	16.58	13.13	42.43	40.13	1.47
Al_2O_3	3.83	4.27	2.02	15.12	11.66	0.34
Fe_2O_3	29.60	27.77	32.08	0.28	0.36	0.28
CaO	37.62	41.46	41.34	38.30	37.68	41.34
MgO	7.28	5.82	5.20	5.19	6.52	0.66
K_2O	0.14	-	-	0.35	0.31	0.07
TiO_2	0.41	0.41	0.43	-	-	
P_2O_5	.....	......	1.86	-	-	0.20
MnO	2.87	2.88	3.31	0.58	0.32	
MgO	-	-	-	-	-	0.66
SO_3	-	-	-	-	-	37.90
LOI	0.44	0.28	0.34	0.38	0.31	-
Basicity Index	2.76	3.10	3.69	1.38	1.39	-

Table 5. Mineralogical composition of the gypsum waste and BOF slag.

Molecular Formula	Mineralogical Phase	GW %	BOF1 %	BOF2 %	BOF3 %
$CaSO_4.2H_2O$	Gypsum	92.79	-	-	-
$CaSO_4.0.5H_2O$	Hemihydrate	3.03	-	-	-
$CaSO_4$	Anhydrite	0.84	-	-	-
$CaMg(CO_3)_2$	Dolomite	1.4	-	-	-
FeO	Wustite	-	19.9	22.8	29.7
$CaCO_3$	Calcite	1.94	17.9	11.3	7.0
β-$2CaSiO_2$	Belite or Larnite	-	13.0	20.7	25.1
$Ca_2Fe_{1.4}Mg_{0.3}Si_{0.3}O_5$	Brownmillerite (Mg. Si-exchanged)	-	11.9	19.0	13.9
Fe_3O_4	Magnetite	-	10.9	7.1	5.8
Fe^0	Iron	-	2.1	1.4	0.5
SiO_2	Quartz	-	0.9	1.4	0.2
$Na_4(Si_8Al_4O_{24})\cdot 11H_2O$	Gmelinite-Na	-	0.3	0.2	0.2
$Ca_3Al_2(OH)_{12}$	Katoite	-	0.3	2.2	0.7
$Ca(OH)_2$	Portlandite	-	0.2	3.8	7.0
Amorphous Phase		-	22.6	10.1	9.9

The mineralogical composition of the BOF slag used (Table 5) demonstrates that despite the different percentages found, the majority of phases in the three samples correspond to wustite (FeO), calcite ($CaCO_3$), belite (β-$2CaSiO_2$), brownmillerite, and magnetite. Portlandite was also identified in all slags. However, portlandite content was significant for BOF2 and BOF3 slags.

BOF slag exerts a relevant influence on the reactivity of the reactional environment by the alkaline activator function. In this sense, BOF3 presented the highest portlandite content and had the highest basicity (3.7). $Ca(OH)_2$ has high solubility in water (1.6 g/L) [10], being easily solubilized and quickly raising the pH of the solution. On the other hand, BOF1 showed a high $CaCO_3$ content. Calcite can also change the pH of the solution by slowly releasing hydroxyl ions due to its low solubility in water (1 mg/L), as shown in the following equations [11]:

$$CaCO_3 \rightarrow Ca^{2+} + CO_3{}^{2-} \quad (1)$$

$$CO_3{}^{2-} + H_2O \rightarrow HCO^{3-} + OH^- \quad (2)$$

$$HCO^{3-} + H_2O \rightarrow H_2CO_3 + OH^- \quad (3)$$

In this way, both phases ($CaCO_3$ and $Ca(OH)_2$) can affect the basicity of the medium, but, depending on solubility, with different speeds.

Another factor relevant to reactivity is the percentage of the amorphous phase, which, due to the slow cooling of BOF slags, usually has a low crystallization energy level retained in its atomic structure. For this reason, BOF slags tend to be difficult to solubilize, given the high stability of the crystalline phases. In this sense, BOF2 and BOF3 slags presented similar contents of around 10%, while BOF1 presented twice the glass phase in its atomic structure, which may indicate greater reactivity and binding capacity [12,13].

In terms of hydraulic behavior, the most reactive phase present in BOF, in the initial ages, corresponds to brownmillerite, which appeared prominently in BOF2 (19%), as it begins hydration in the first 24 h to form hydrated calcium ferroaluminates or hydroxy compounds. At the final ages, belite is the phase responsible for the formation of hydrated calcium silicates that corroborate the gain of mechanical resistance in the cement and was identified in a higher percentage in BOF3 (25%) [13].

3.2. Cement Chemical Composition and Alkalinity

The evolution of the hydration process and the number of products formed in ECO cement are closely dependent on the chemical composition of the cement. Also, the development of mechanical resistance is mainly related to the precipitation of hydration products such as ettringite and hydrated calcium silicates (C-S-H). Table 6 shows the chemical composition of the cement.

Table 6. Chemical composition of cementitious formulations.

Chemical Composition	ECO1		ECO2			ECO3		ECO4	
	851510	802010	802013	851510	802010	802015	881213	802010	901013
SiO_2	34.59	32.63	32.21	34.29	32.32	31.49	34.71	30.65	33.6
Al_2O_3	12.08	11.45	11.26	12.12	11.24	10.84	12.05	8.73	9.55
Fe_2O_3	2.95	2.78	3.44	2.78	3.17	4.43	3.94	3.23	4.0
CaO	38.65	39.14	39.2	39	39.13	39.23	38.98	38.68	38.43
MgO	4.76	4.42	4.46	4.63	4.37	4.4	4.71	5.33	5.85
K_2O	0.28	0.27	0.26	0.28	0.27	0.26	0.28	0.24	0.25
Na_2O	-	0.01	0.01	-	0.01	0.01	-	0.01	-
SO_3	5.17	6.89	6.71	5.17	6.83	6.59	4.02	6.89	3.35
MnO	0.71	0.68	0.74	0.71	0.72	0.84	0.88	0.53	0.64
Alkalinity	12.3	12.2	12.6	12.3	12.3	13.1	12.7	12.3	12.8

By the time the anhydrous grains of the cement mixture come into contact with water, the dissolution of the blast furnace slag begins, but very slowly, which makes its use unfeasible. This is because the dissolution of the slag occurs by hydroxylic attack, that is, by OH^- ions. Thus, if the solution in contact with the grains is alkaline, dissolution will be faster as the solubility of the glassy structure of the silica that constitutes BFS is increased. In addition, the formation of hydrated silico-aluminous products on the surface of the slag grains is avoided, which would prevent the dissolution from continuing [14,15].

It is estimated that the initial pH of cement rich in blast furnace slag is around 11–12.5 and decreases as the hydration process develops [4,11]. The increase in pH in the solution is mainly related to the hydrated lime that makes up the BOF slag since calcium sulfate does not change the pH of the solution significantly.

This statement is confirmed by observing the alkalinity of the cements ECO3 802010 and 802015, which differ only in the BOF slag content, for which the alkalinity corresponds to 12.3 and 13.1, respectively. In addition to increasing the pH level, it is expected that lime introduces Ca^{2+} ions into the solution, causing the equilibrium of the solubility product to shift towards saturation, accelerating the hydration product precipitation. At the beginning of cement hydration, due to the high alkalinity, there are hydrates precipitated, such as ettringite, C-S-H, and C-A-H, ensuring the cement's high resistance at early ages. On the other hand, excessive alkalinity, as observed in ECO3 802015, can create instability in the products formed and can lead to covering the surface of anhydrous grains with precipitated products, harming the development of resistance at later ages as a consequence of earlier product precipitation.

For calcium sulfate, the dissolved SO_4^{2-} reacts with the aluminum released from BFS dissolution to form ettringite, one of the first products to be precipitated in this cement, which prevents the formation of low-permeability products on the surface of the slag particles. Therefore, the aluminum content is also a relevant factor for the initial strength gain.

The aluminum content in cement brings two relevant considerations: (i) the percentage of aluminum presented by the BFS, in which the higher the Al content, the higher the contribution to the increase in its dissolution speed; (ii) the aluminum content available in the mixture for the formation of ettringite.

Therefore, the dissolved aluminum content of the slag must be sufficient to react with the sulfate from the gypsum to appropriately form ettringite before the silicates. A low aluminum content and excess sulfate can impair the hydration of the BFS due to the rapid occurrence and growth of ettringite and monosulfate crystals on the surface of the BFS grain, causing its isolation and preventing hydration.

The inferences drawn from this study, together with the initial investigation for the ECO patent [7] and the relevant literature [4,5,12–15], have consistently demonstrated the points made in the previous observations and comments.

3.3. Compressive Strength of Cement Mortar Using ECO Formulations

Compressive strength results for cement mortar specimens with ECO1, ECO2, ECO3, and ECO4 cement are shown in Figures 1–4. Using analysis of variance (ANOVA), the effects of 'type of cement' and 'hydration age' were analyzed for all formulations. For all cement formulations, these effects are statistically significant variables to explain the different mechanical performances observed. In other words, within the same cement group, such as ECO2, the mechanical strength results of distinct formulations showed significant differences. The same was observed for ECO3 formulations.

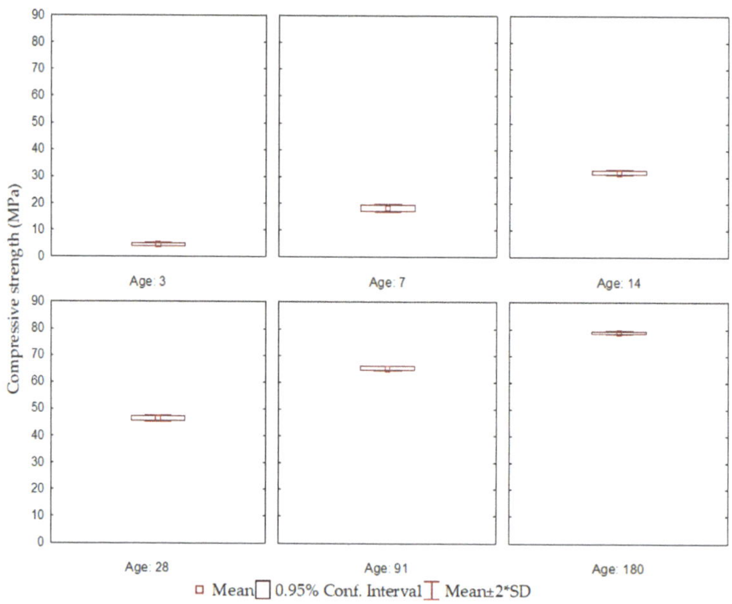

Figure 1. ECO1 cement compressive strength.

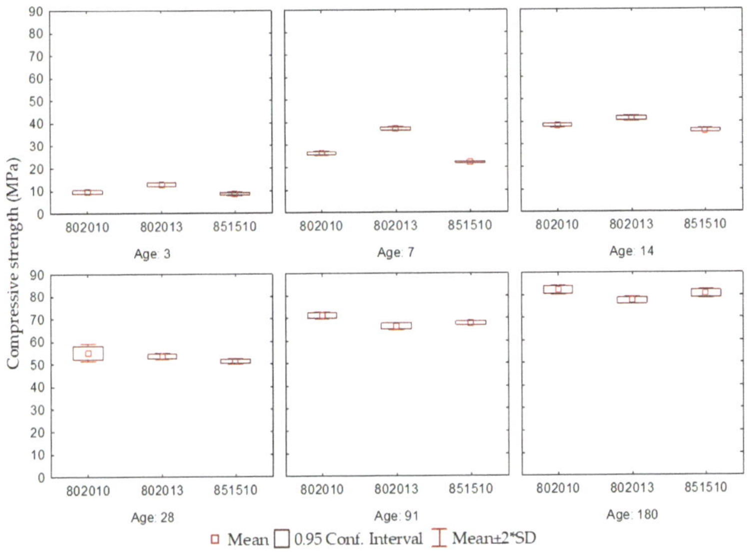

Figure 2. ECO2 cement compressive strength.

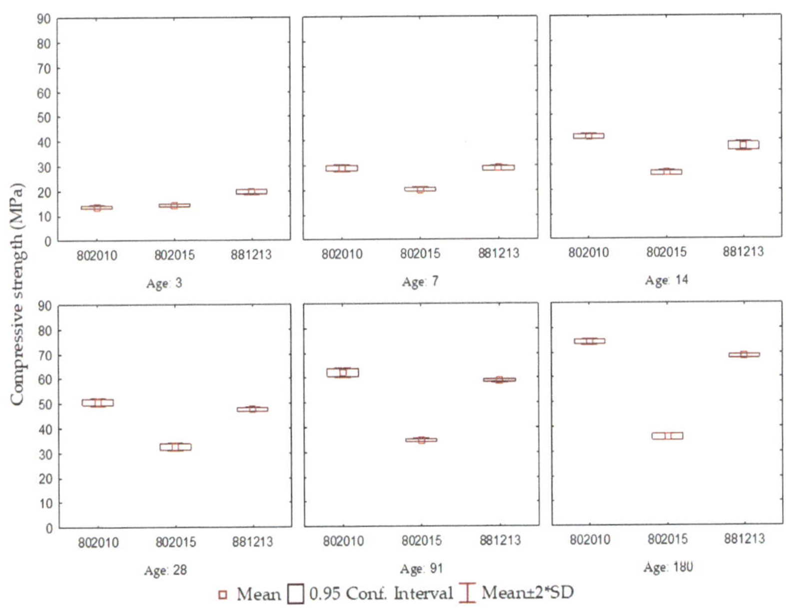

Figure 3. ECO3 cement compressive strength.

Figure 1 presents the results of the compressive strength of ECO1 cement, produced based on the initial formulation of ECO cement [7]. The cement showed a gain in resistance over the ages. However, the resistance at the initial ages was lower than the Brazilian normative limits [6]. This behavior is attributed to the BOF slag content used in the formulation, the lowest among all ten proposed cement formulations, and the basicity of the BOF1 slag (2.8). It is understood that both factors may not have favored the beginning of the hydration process. On the other hand, due to the blast furnace slag used (BFS1) and the high aluminum content present in its composition, a resistance gain was observed, even if more slowly.

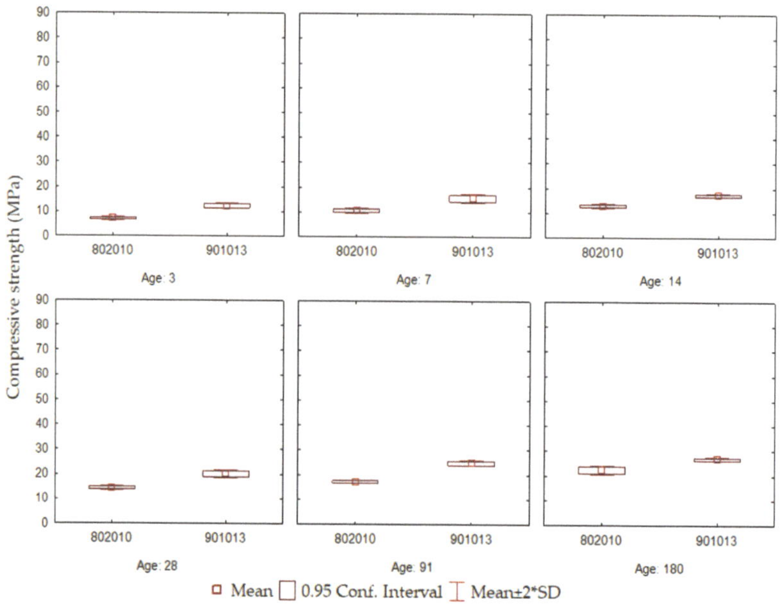

Figure 4. ECO4 cement compressive strength.

In the compressive strength results for the ECO2 cement, shown in Figure 2, it can be seen that the cement formulations showed a significant evolution in compressive strength over the ages.

At the initial ages, ECO2 cement exhibited high compressive strength. At 3 days, the compressive strength varied between 8 and 10 MPa, and at 7 days, from 20 to 40 MPa. At this last age (R7), the values approached the normative limits defined for most types of Portland cement at 28 days, as defined by [6]. The ECO2 cements were produced using BOF2, which presented high basicity (3.1) and the highest content of the brownmillerite phase, factors that may corroborate the development of initial resistance.

At early hydration ages, the ECO2-802013 formulation performed the best. It is noteworthy that this corresponds to the cement with the highest addition of BOF2 among the three formulations, which generated an environment of greater alkalinity, resulting in increased dissolution of blast furnace slag and accelerating the formation of hydration products.

At the later ages, the ECO2-802010 formulation demonstrated the best performance, with a compressive strength at 180 days greater than 80 MPa, corroborating the consistent strength growth throughout the hydration process. The ECO2-851510 formulation is attributed the worst performance due to the high BFS content and the reduction of gypsum, and consequently, the reduction in the contribution of calcium ions and sulfate ions, which compromised the availability of ions for the formation of hydration products.

For the ECO3 cement formulations, shown in Figure 3, the results demonstrate that the evolution of compressive strength over the ages did not occur uniformly for all cements. Compressive strength after 3 days of hydration reached values between 14 and 20 MPa, the highest among all the formulations studied. This behavior is understood through the basicity of the slag used, BOF3, which is the highest and equivalent to 3.7, responsible for accelerating the decomposition of blast furnace slag, given the alkalinity of the reaction environment. The best behavior is observed for the ECO3-802010 formulation, which maintains a constant evolution of compressive strength at all ages. It is seen that the ECO3-802015 cement had a compromised performance compared to the others, and this difference is more evident in the final ages. The mentioned formulation is composed of the highest BOF slag content, which allowed a rapid gain in resistance after the 3rd day, but from this age onwards, little evolution was observed (R7: 20.4 MPa to R180: 35.8 MPa).

The compressive strength results for the ECO4 formulation cements are shown in Figure 4 and demonstrate that they correspond to the lowest values observed among all formulations. Despite the development of initial resistance, there is no significant evolution over the ages, so between 3 and 180 days of curing, the difference was approximately 15 MPa. Among the formulations, the compound with the highest contents of BFS and BOF slag had slightly better results (ECO4-901013).

Figure 5 shows the average results for each group of cements. Observing the comparison of the evolution between them, it is seen that the cement mixtures of the ECO2 formulation, in addition to presenting a continuous gain in mechanical strength, showed less dispersion of the results, which demonstrates a more homogeneous behavior among them.

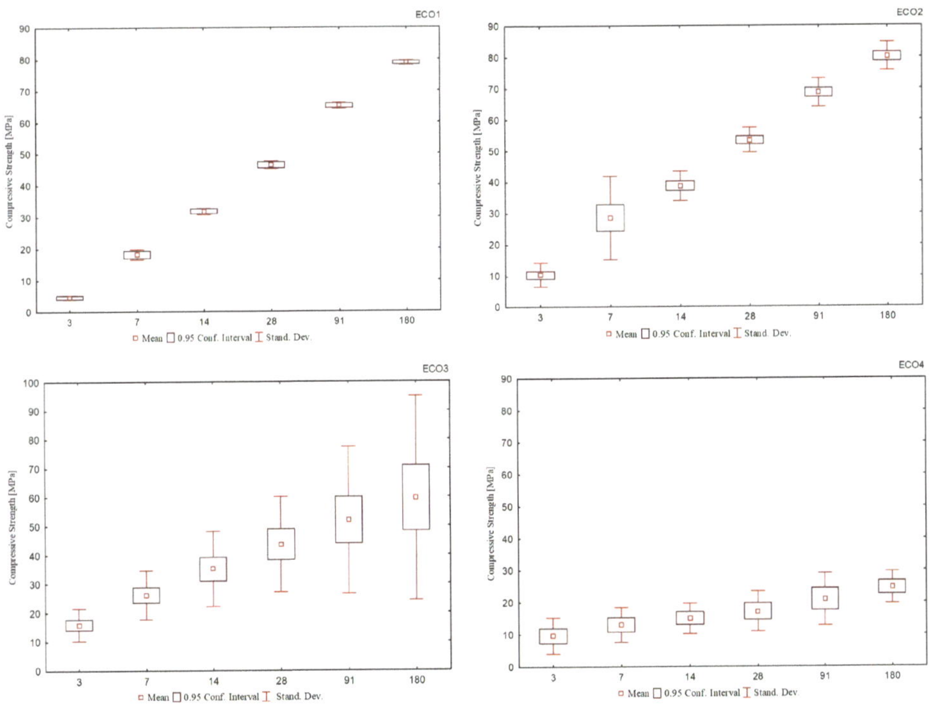

Figure 5. Average compressive strength of all cement formulations.

The ECO2 cement formulations were produced using BOF2 slag, with high basicity, the highest brownmillerite content, and a relevant dicalcium silicate content, corroborating the development at the initial and final ages. In addition, the BFS1 slag was used, which presented the highest aluminum content in its composition, supporting its solubilization and ettringite formation.

4. Conclusions

In this study, four different eco-sustainable types of cement (ECO1, ECO2, ECO3, and ECO4) were produced using iron-making slags and gypsum waste, varying the raw material proportions, ranging from 80 to 90% blast furnace slag, 10 to 20% gypsum, and 10 to 15% BOF slag.

The strength of ECO cement depends on the precipitation of ettringite, C-S-H, and C-A-H. This ensures that the cement gains high mechanical strength at an early age due to the dissolution of BFS by hydroxyl attack. On the 3rd day, the cement formulations reached up to 10 MPa, and on the 7th day, 40 MPa. The contribution of OH^- in the solution mainly comes from BOF slag, which provides an environment of high alkalinity from $Ca(OH)_2$ and $CaCO_3$ dissolution, as calcium sulfate does not have a significant effect on the pH level of the solution. BOF slag also takes part in the ECO cement hydration process through the hydration of brownmillerite.

Most ECO cement formulations showed a significantly high final strength, with the highest compressive strength values after 28 days of hydration, greater than 50 MPa, and at 180 days, greater than 80 MPa. This mechanical performance is believed to be influenced by the presence of BOF slag, which contains the belite phase commonly found in BOF slag and Portland cement. The belite phase is responsible for the gain in mechanical resistance after 28 days of curing due to its thermodynamic stability. During its hydration, C_2S generates C-S-H and releases $Ca(OH)_2$, which helps maintain an alkaline environment and allows the dissolution of BFS to continue progressing. However, excessive increases in alkalinity may favor the rapid dissolution of BFS and gain in initial strength, but they will also impede development in the final ages, due to covering the surface of anhydrous grains with precipitated products, harming the development of resistance at later ages.

This was observed in the ECO4 cement formulations. Despite the development of initial resistance, there is no significant evolution over the ages, so between 3 and 180 days of curing, the difference was approximately 15 MPa.

The ECO2 cement has demonstrated excellent mechanical performance in both the initial and final stages of the hydration process, with consistent strength growth throughout. This cement formulation was produced with BOF2 slag, which has a high basicity of 3.1, a significant brownmillerite content of 19%, and a relevant dicalcium silicate content of 21%, thus contributing to its development in the initial and final stages. Additionally, the BFS1 slag was used, which has the highest aluminum content (15%) in its composition, which supports its solubilization and ettringite formation.

5. Patents

Vernilli, F.; Oliveira, M. D. S.; Pereira, M. L. G.; Oliveira, L. M.; Zago, S.C. Cimento Ecossustentável sem clínquer à base de resíduos da siderurgia e da construção civil e uso do mesmo. 2022, Brasil. Número do registro: BR1020220227578, Instituição de registro: INPI—Instituto Nacional da Propriedade Industrial. Depósito: 8 November 2022.

Author Contributions: Conceptualization, S.C.Z., F.V., and M.D.; methodology, S.C.Z., F.V., and M.D.; validation, S.C.Z. and M.D.; formal analysis, M.D.; investigation, S.C.Z. and M.D.; resources, S.C.Z., F.V., and M.D.; data curation, S.C.Z.; writing—original draft preparation, S.C.Z.; writing—review and editing, S.C.Z., F.V., and M.D.; visualization, S.C.Z. and M.D.; supervision, F.V.; project administration, M.D. All authors have read and agreed to the published version of the manuscript.

Funding: This research received no external funding.

Data Availability Statement: The original contributions presented in the study are included in the article, further inquiries can be directed to the corresponding authors.

Conflicts of Interest: The authors declare no conflicts of interest.

References

1. IEA. Global Cement Production in the Net Zero Scenario, 2010–2030, IEA, Paris. IEA. Licence: CC BY 4.0. Available online: https://www.iea.org/data-and-statistics/charts/global-cement-production-in-the-net-zero-scenario-2010-2030-5260 (accessed on 20 January 2024).
2. Capmas, A. Concreto e desenvolvimento sustentável. In *Durabilidade do Concreto*; Geraldo, C.I., Translator; Ibracon: São Paulo, Brazil, 2014; pp. 3–13.

3. *ROADMAP Tecnológico do Cimento: Potencial de Redução das Emissões de Carbono da Indústria do Cimento Brasileira Até 2050*; SNIC: Rio de Janeiro, Brazil, 2019; 64p.
4. Juenger, M.C.G.; Winnefeld, F.; Provis, J.L.; Ideker, J.H. Advances in alternative cementitious binders. *Cem. Concr. Res.* **2011**, *41*, 1232–1243. [CrossRef]
5. Imbabi, M.S.; Carrigan, C.; McKenna, S. Trends and developments in green cement and concrete technology. *Int. J. Sustain. Built Environ.* **2012**, *1*, 194–216. [CrossRef]
6. *NBR 16697*; Cimento Portland—Requisitos. Associação Brasileira de Normas Técnicas: Rio de Janeiro, Brazil, 2018.
7. Oliveira, M.D.S. Estudo da Obtenção de Cimento sem Clínquer a Partir de Misturas de Escórias Siderúrgicas. Master's Thesis, Universidade de São Paulo, São Paulo, Brazil, 2021.
8. *EN 15743:2010*; Supersulfated Cement—Composition, Specifications and Conformity Criteria. Comité Européen de Normalisation-CEN: Brussels, Belgium, 2010.
9. Associação Brasileira de Normas Técnicas. *NBR 7215. Cimento Portland—Determinação da Resistência à Compressão*; ABNT: Rio de Janeiro, Brazil, 2019.
10. Nonat, A. *A Hidratação dos Cimentos*; Alba Cincotto, M., Translator; Ibracon: São Paulo, Brazil, 2014.
11. Baird, C.; Cann, N. *Environmental Chemistry*, 5th ed.; W.H. Freeman and Company: New York, NY, USA, 2012.
12. Kaja, A.M.; Melzer, S.; Brouwers, H.J.H.; Yu, Q. On the optimization of BOF slag hydration kinetics. *Cem. Concr. Compos.* **2021**, *124*, 104262. [CrossRef]
13. Zago, S.C.; Vernilli, F.; Cascudo, O. The Reuse of Basic Oxygen Furnace Slag as Concrete Aggregate to Achieve Sustainable Development: Characteristics and Limitations. *Buildings* **2023**, *13*, 1193. [CrossRef]
14. Wu, Q.; Xue, Q.; Ye, Z. Research status of super sulfate cement. *J. Clean. Prod.* **2021**, *294*, 126228. [CrossRef]
15. Liu, Z.; Ni, W.; Li, Y.; Ba, H.; Li, N.; Ju, Y.; Zhao, B.; Jia, G.; Hu, W. The mechanism of hydration reaction of granulated blast furnace slag-steel slag-refining slag-desulfurization gypsum-based clinker-free cementitious materials. *J. Build. Eng.* **2021**, *44*, 103289. [CrossRef]

buildings

Article

Time-Dependent Behavior of Ultra-High Performance Concrete Beams under Long-Term Bending Loads

Jiayue Li [1], Yankai Lu [1], Xiaorui Jia [1], Bo Liu [1,*], Juannong Chen [1] and Qingjuan Meng [2]

1 College of Civil and Architectural Engineering, North China University of Science and Technology, Tangshan 063210, China; lijiayue@ncst.edu.cn (J.L.); luyankai1999@outlook.com (Y.L.); jxiaorui0116@outlook.com (X.J.); chenjuannong@ncst.edu.cn (J.C.)
2 School of Civil Engineering, Tangshan University, Tangshan 063000, China; mqj27@outlook.com
* Correspondence: liubo19840311@ncst.edu.cn

Abstract: In the past, scholars have studied the creep of UHPC, mainly in compression and tension but not bending creep. In this research, 20 ultra-high performance concrete (UHPC) beams were tested for bending creep under long-term loading, and the changes of beam deflection, temperature, and humidity with time were obtained for 445 days of continuous loading. The deflection patterns of UHPC beams with time were analyzed for different steel fiber content, curing systems, water/binder ratio, sand/binder ratio, and stress levels. The results showed that steel fiber had an obvious inhibition effect on initial deflection, but a dosage of steel fiber too high would offset part of the inhibition effect of steel fiber on creep. The use of heat treatment had a better inhibition of creep in the later stage of UHPC, but heat treatment must be matched with necessary moisture content, and hot water maintenance was the most efficient. Both a high water/binder ratio and high stress level increased the bending creep of the specimen. Bending creep increased with the increase in the sand/binder ratio. Therefore, attention should be paid to the total amount and ratio of cementitious materials and fine aggregates in UHPC.

Keywords: UHPC; steel fiber; bending creep; heat treatment; water/binder ratio

1. Introduction

All concrete structures experience time-dependent deformations known as shrinkage and creep. Shrinkage is a reduction in volume due to the evaporation of water or a chemical reaction within the concrete, independent of external loading. Creep is the increasing deformation of concrete under sustained stress in the direction of the applied load. Shrinkage and creep are inherent properties of concrete, and both significantly affect the long-term performance of structures, especially in large structures. Therefore, it is of great engineering significance to understand the pattern of change of shrinkage and creep of concrete materials.

In order to assess tensile and bending creep, Ranaivomanana et al. [1] created a test setup. They compared basic creep at the three stress levels with various loading modes and provided findings from experiments that were subjected to sustained stresses of 30%, 40%, and 50% of tensile or compressive strength. Babafemi et al. [2] reported delayed cracking of cracked concrete incorporated with short discrete synthetic fibers under 8 months of service conditions. The tensile creep properties of early age concrete were studied by Liang et al. [3], and they developed a method for calculating incremental tensile creep and enhanced the Kelvin model based on the degree of hydration. In order to evaluate the difference between the creep response of cracked plastic fiber concrete beams and steel fiber concrete beams under bending loads, Pujadas et al. [4] discussed the influence of crack cracking and environmental conditions on the long-term deformation behavior of beams. Jahami et al. [5] investigated the mechanical properties of low-cost, high-strength concrete by partially replacing fine aggregates with waste glass sand. Manjunatha et al. [6]

investigated the freshness, strength properties, microstructure analysis, and environmental impact assessment of an M60 grade self-compacting concrete prepared with silica fumes, ground granulated blast furnace slag, and different proportions of PVC waste powder, and they conducted a full life cycle assessment. Many scholars have also studied the different types of creep of the same type of concrete [7–10] and fiber-reinforced concrete [11–15].

Ultra-high performance concrete (UHPC) is a new cement-based composite material, and it has a dense matrix, a low water/binder ratio, and excellent tensile and compressive strength as well as ductility and durability. Moreover, it has outstanding low permeability, strong resistance to corrosion and carbonation, and strong freeze–thaw stability. In addition, the high volume-doped fibers reinforce the UHPC matrix, resulting in a high tensile capacity even after cracking of the UHPC. Due to its superior mechanical characteristics and longevity, UHPC is being utilized more frequently in pre-stressed bridge building. UHPC provides larger spans and excellent durability for pre-tensioned pre-stressed girders. However, creep and shrinkage deformation are particularly important in pre-stressed beams. Creep and shrinkage can lead to a gradual loss of pre-stress, thereby affecting the load-bearing capacity of components and potentially causing usability issues in the structure. For this reason, accurately estimating the pre-stress loss caused by long-term deformations such as shrinkage and creep is crucial for the design of pre-tensioned UHPC girders.

In recent years, with the wide application of UHPC, many scholars have also conducted a lot of research on the creep properties of UHPC. Fiber optic grating sensors were employed by Yazdizadeh et al. [16] to assess the creep and shrinkage of regular concrete, high-performance concrete, and UHPC. There was a strong link between the creep and shrinkage test findings. Yang et al. [17] conducted an experimental study on the creep performance of NC-UHPC composite columns. The results showed that the creep coefficients of the NC-UHPC composite columns were significantly lower than those of the NC columns. Zhu et al. [18] developed an ABAQUS user subroutine using the recursion of adjacent stress increments in the time history algorithm to simulate the creep shrinkage of plain concrete and UHPC. The long-term performance of UHPC beams, including bending and compression creep, was examined by Llano et al. [19]. Xu et al.'s [20] study examined the compression creep behavior of specimens with water/binder ratios of 0.16 and 0.22 and steel fiber volume levels of 0%, 1%, and 2%. The findings demonstrated that the creep coefficients of 1% and 2% ultrafine steel fibers dropped dramatically by 25.4% and 13.4% after loading for 180 days, respectively, in comparison to the unloaded ones. The creep behavior of UHPC was adversely affected by an increase in the water/cement ratio. The effects of the fiber type and admixture, water-to-cement ratio, and cementitious material content on UHPC shrinkage and creep were examined by Chen et al. [21]. Zhang et al. [22,23] investigated the creep behavior of UHPC creep damage under high uniaxial compressive stresses. Mohebbi et al. [24] measured the compressive creep properties of various UHPC materials, assessed the impact of various environments (such as high, low, and hermetic conditions) on the unconfined shrinkage and compressive creep of various UHPC materials, and created prediction equations.

Many scholars have also studied the creep of UHPC under different heat treatment conditions. Garas [25] studied the effect of fiber content on the compressive creep of UHPC under different heat treatment conditions. The results indicated that heat treatment can improve the creep deformation resistance of steel fibers by increasing the interfacial strength between fibers and the matrix. Garas et al. [26] considered three curing temperatures (23 °C, 60 °C, and 90 °C). The results indicate that the creep of UHPC was mainly determined by the temperature level, rather than the total heat input. Cui [27] designed an experimental program to study the creep behavior of UHPC under various curing schemes, and the results showed that under the combined curing scheme, the creep deformation of UHPC was significantly reduced. Abid et al. [28] investigated the steady-state creep behavior of UHPC at high temperatures. The results indicated that the creep of UHPC at room temperature was comparable and that the steady-state creep increases with the increase in the load level. The above scholars have considered the effects of various heat treatments on the creep of UHPC, but the types of heat treatments are still limited.

In the past, scholars have studied the creep of UHPC mainly in compression and tension, with limited reports on the bending creep of UHPC. The problem of excessive mid-span deflections exists in bridge engineering, and these excessive deflections and the resulting cracks may lead to poor bridge service quality and a series of durability problems. UHPC has excellent compressive and tensile strength, as well as significant durability, and is increasingly being used in bridge engineering. However, creep and shrinkage have a significant impact on the long-term performance of UHPC. Thus, for the application of UHPC in bridge engineering, it is crucial to comprehend the bending creep features of UHPC.

To study the flexural creep performance of UHPC, an experimental study of the deformation performance of 20 UHPC beams under long-term loading was carried out. The temperature, humidity, and deflection changes of the beams were obtained over a period of 445 days of continuous loading, and the changes in deflection of UHPC beams were analyzed for various steel fiber content, curing systems, water/binder ratio, sand/binder ratio, and stress levels. The results of the experiments can serve as a reference for the computation of UHPC beams' long-term deformation. The test findings can be used as a guide to determine how much UHPC beams will deform over time.

2. Experimental Program

2.1. Test Materials

P·II 52.5R Portland cement specific surface area is 375 m^2/kg. Fly ash 45 μm square hole screening ratio is 9.6%. The SiO_2 content of the silica fume is 94%, and the ignition loss at 950 °C is 1.15%. Mineral powder specific surface area is 419 m^2/kg. The diameter of quartz sand is 0.85–1.7 mm. Superplasticizer was added to obtain appropriate workability. Two types of copper-plated steel fibers (RS65/8) and end-hooked steel fibers (RS60/13) were incorporated into UHPC, with a volume ratio of 1:2 between the two. Steel fiber mechanical properties are shown in Table 1.

Table 1. Steel fiber mechanical properties.

Type	Elastic Modulus/GPa	Tensile Strength/MPa	Diameter/mm	Length/mm	Aspect Ratio	Density/(kg/m^3)
RS65/8	210	2850	0.12	8	65	7800
RS60/13	210	2850	0.22	13	60	7800

The volume mixing rate of steel fibers was 2.0%, the water/binder ratio of UHPC utilized in the reference specimen RS was 0.16, the sand/binder ratio was 1.0, standard maintenance was applied, and the mixing ratios are displayed in Table 2. The reference mix proportion (specimen RS) in this experiment was a mix proportion independently tested and used by our research group for a long time, and its physical properties met the requirements of use. The fitment ratios of the remaining specimens were similar to those of the UHPC used in specimen RS, except that the relevant adjustments were made according to the test variables of the group, as detailed in Table 3.

Table 2. Mix proportions of reference specimen RS (kg/m^3).

Coagulation Material				Quartz Sand	Water	Superplasticizer	Steel Fiber	
Cement	Silica Powder	Fly Ash	Mineral Powder				RS65/8	RS60/13
646	215	108	107	1076	172	14	52	104

Table 3. Specimen details.

Group	Specimen Number	Steel Fiber Content/%	Water/Binder Ratio	Sand Binder Ratio	Curing Condition	Stress Level	f_f/MPa	f_{cu}/MPa
RS	RS	2.0	0.16	1.0	SC	0.3	17.40	129.80
SF	SF-0 SF-1.0 SF-1.5 SF-2.5	0 1.0 1.5 2.5	0.16	1.0	SC	0.3	10.85 16.07 19.02 20.67	81.83 128.06 140.35 145.63
CUR	NC HW2 250DA3 HW2-250DA3	2.0	0.16	1.0	NC HW2 250DA3 HW2-250DA3	0.3	18.50 15.03 15.71 20.32	120.30 140.52 136.20 156.52
WBR	WBR-0.14 WBR-0.18 WBR-0.20	2.0	0.14 0.18 0.20	1.0	SC	0.3	15.03 19.22 14.67	130.41 137.26 123.40
SBR	SBR-0.9 SBR-1.1 SBR-1.2	2.0	0.16	0.9 1.1 1.2	SC	0.3	20.02 19.41 11.03	143.23 148.75 86.20
SL	RS/0.2 NC/0.2 SBR-0.9/0.2 SBR-1.1/0.2 SBR-1.2/0.2	2.0	0.16	1.0	SC	0.2	17.40 18.50 20.02 19.41 11.03	129.80 120.30 143.23 148.75 86.20

To determine UHPC's cubic compressive strength (f_{cu}) and flexural strength (f_f) for each specimen, three cubic specimens (100 × 100 × 100 mm) and three flexural specimens (100 × 100 × 400 mm) were cast simultaneously. The flexural strength (f_f) provided a reference for loading the specimen at the appropriate stress level.

2.2. Design of Specimen

The research methodology followed for the present study is presented in Figure 1 with the help of a flow chart. A total of 20 UHPC small beams were designed, with dimensions of 100 × 100 × 400 mm and a clear span of 300 mm. Based on the test variables, six groups of specimens were created.

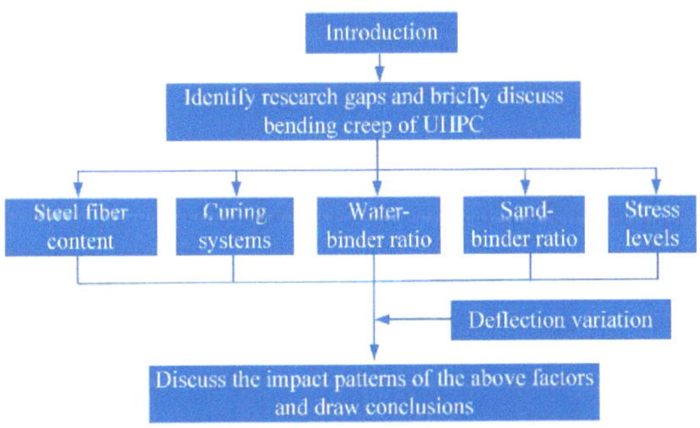

Figure 1. The research methodology followed in the present study.

The reference specimens, designated as Group 1 (RS) specimens, comprised a single specimen bearing the specimen named RS. Group 2's (SF) test variable was steel fiber content and the group contained 4 specimens. The specimens were named SF-0, SF-1,

SF-1.5, and SF-2.5, respectively, and steel fiber content was 0, 1%, 1.5%, and 2.5%. Group 3's (CUR) test variable was the curing system, and the group contained 4 specimens. The following four curing systems were established: (1) natural curing, (2) hot water curing (two days of hot water curing at 90 °C; then, placed under natural environment to the desired age after completion), (3) dry heat curing (three days of dry heat curing at 250 °C; then, placed under natural environment to the desired age after completion), and (4) hot water and dry heat combined curing (two days of hot water curing at 90 °C and then three days of dry heat curing at 250 °C, followed by being placed under natural environment to the desired age after completion). The specimen numbers NC, HW2, 250DA3, HW2-250DA3 corresponded to the four distinct curing regimens mentioned above. Group 4's (WBR) test variable was the water/binder ratio, which contained three specimens with water/binder ratio ratios of 0.14, 0.18, and 0.20, with specimens named WBR-0.14, WBR-0.18, and WBR-0.20, in this order. The test variable for Group 5 (SBR) was the sand/binder ratio, which consisted of three specimens with sand/binder ratios of 0.9, 1.1, and 1.2, and the specimens were named SBR-0.9, SBR-1.1, and SBR-1.2, respectively. The stress level of the specimens for the above five groups was 0.3. The sixth group of test variables comprised stress level (SL), and all stress levels were 0.2, containing five specimens. The specimens were named RS/0.2, NC/0.2, SBR-0.9/0.2, SBR-1.1/0.2, and SBR-1.2/0.2, in this order.

Except for the Group 3 (CUR) specimens, all specimens were cured using standard curing (SC), which means they were immediately placed in a standard curing room with a temperature of 20 ± 2 °C and a relative humidity of over 95% after demolding. Details of the test specimens are shown in Table 3.

2.3. Loading and Measurement Scheme

The UHPC bending creep test used a spring loading device designed according to Hooke's law, as shown in Figure 2. The device applies a load to a specimen by compressing the spring, ordering the spring with a pre-given spring stiffness, and controlling the amount of stress by controlling spring compression deformation. The small size of the device and the negligible temperature-induced error satisfied the need for large-volume durability testing in a short period of time.

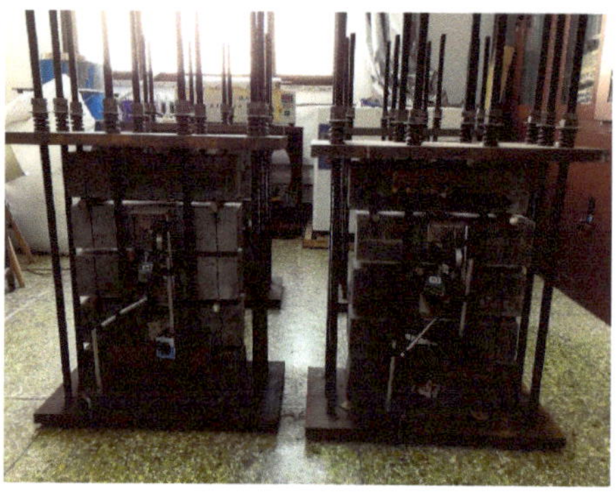

Figure 2. Test loading device.

Before loading, the flexural strength of different specimens was tested. Every specimen had a clear span of 300 mm and was only supported at both ends. The micrometer's magnetic table holder was positioned appropriately, and the deflection value of the beam in the span was measured using the device, whose configuration is depicted in Figure 3. Additionally, a temperature and humidity recorder were employed to document the variations in temperature and humidity at the loading site over time.

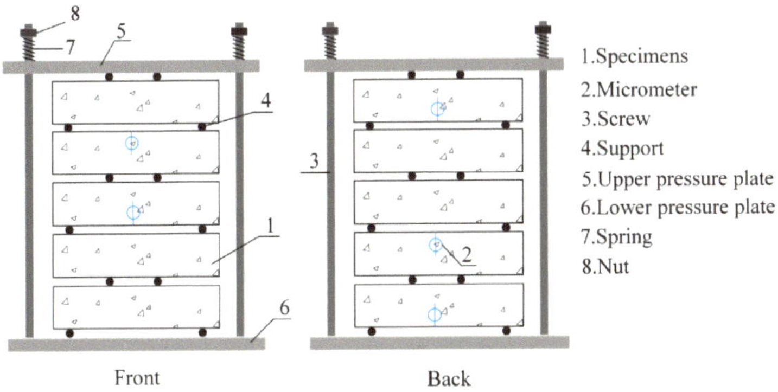

Figure 3. Dial indicator arrangement.

3. Test Results

After all specimens were cured for 28 days, a bending creep test was carried out for 445 days. Temperature and humidity recorders were used to record the change rule of temperature and humidity with time at the loading site, as shown in Figure 4. The test had an average temperature of 20.4 °C and an average humidity of 33.4%. A micrometer was used to record the variation rule of the mid-span deflection of the UHPC beam specimen with time. The results are displayed in Table 4.

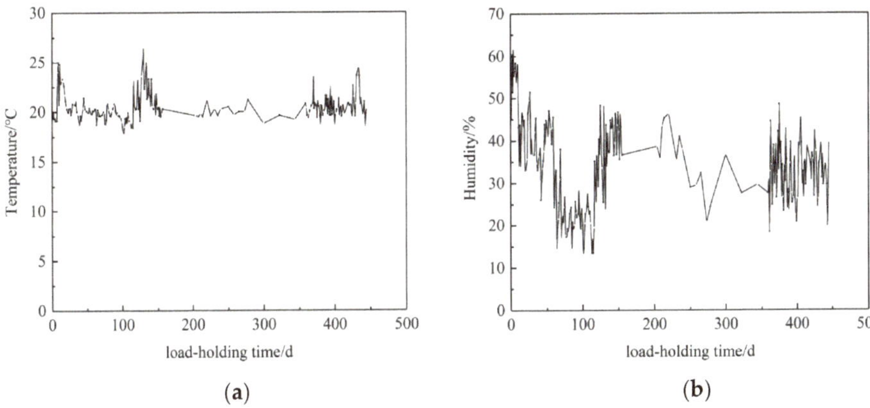

Figure 4. Curves of temperature and humidity. (**a**) Temperature variation curve. (**b**) Humidity change curve.

The deflection creep coefficient θ was defined to characterize the effect brought about by the specimens' creep.

$$\theta = f_c / f_0 \quad (1)$$

$$f = f_0 + f_c \quad (2)$$

where f_0 represents the initial deflection after loading, f_c represents the creep deflection resulting from long-term load bearing, and f represents the total deflection, which is the sum of the initial and creep deflections.

Table 4. Measured deflection of the specimen under 445 days loading.

Group	Specimen Number	f_0/mm	f_c/mm	f/mm	θ	Completion Days/d	
						50% θ	90% θ
RS	RS	0.039	0.276	0.315	7.077	300	414
SF	SF-0	0.072	0.221	0.293	3.069	142	231
	SF-1.0	0.047	0.199	0.246	4.234	265	410
	SF-1.5	0.022	0.273	0.295	12.409	273	388
	SF-2.5	0.059	0.374	0.433	6.339	232	366
CUR	NC	0.053	0.538	0.591	10.151	204	415
	HW2	0.047	0.311	0.358	6.617	250	400
	250DA3	0.121	0.501	0.622	4.140	181	415
	HW2-250DA3	0.034	0.357	0.391	10.500	305	403
WBR	WBR-0.14	0.037	0.243	0.280	6.568	300	401
	WBR-0.18	0.056	0.429	0.485	7.661	204	395
	WBR-0.20	0.108	0.504	0.612	4.667	153	413
SBR	SBR-0.9	0.038	0.454	0.492	11.947	310	398
	SBR-1.1	0.054	0.638	0.692	11.815	315	419
	SBR-1.2	0.161	0.538	0.699	3.342	189	405
SL	RS/0.2	0.033	0.215	0.248	6.515	322	419
	NC/0.2	0.058	0.458	0.516	7.897	157	399
	SBR-0.9/0.2	0.030	0.207	0.237	6.900	312	409
	SBR-1.1/0.2	0.077	0.414	0.491	5.377	290	382
	SBR-1.2/0.2	0.069	0.490	0.559	7.101	306	403

4. Analysis of Influencing Factors

4.1. Steel Fiber Content

The effect of different steel fiber doping rates on the flexural creep of UHPC is shown in Figure 5. Among them, Figure 5a shows the deflection time course curves of specimen deflection development with time for different steel fiber volume doping rates, and Figure 5b shows the deflection development ratio for different specimens.

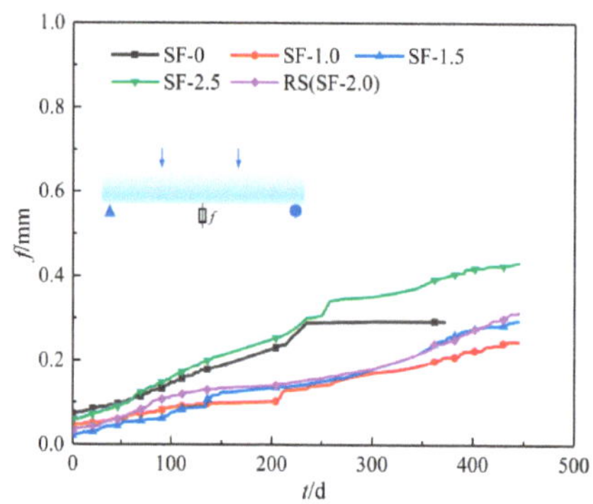

(a)

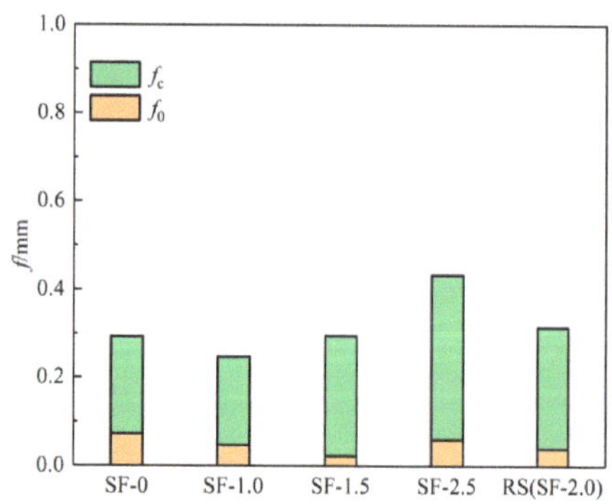

(b)

Figure 5. Influence of steel fiber content on bending creep. (**a**) Deflection time course curve. (**b**) Deflection development ratio.

The initial deflection of SF-1.0, SF-1.5, RS (2%, steel fiber content), and SF-2.5 decreased by 34.72%, 69.44%, 45.83%, and 18.05%, respectively, when compared to specimen SF-0, as shown in Figure 5. Creep deflection increased by −9.95%, 23.53%, 24.89%, and 69.23%, respectively. The specimens' initial deflection dropped, their creep deflection increased, and their total deflection first decreased and subsequently increased when the steel fiber doping rate increased. As a result, the specimens' initial deflection was visibly inhibited by the steel fiber. Remarkably, SF-0, devoid of steel fibers, exhibits the greatest initial deflection and the quickest rate of deflection growth; in total, 50% of the overall creep process (445 days) was completed in 142 days, and the fracture happened at 300 day of loading age. The biggest initial and creep deflections were found in SF-2.5, suggesting that an excess of steel fibers may lessen their ability to limit the creep of UHPC.

Steel fibers with a high modulus of elasticity and high tensile strength had good interfacial bonding with UHPC, which can significantly improve the connection, deformation, and cracking resistance of the hardened slurry. The hardened matrix of UHPC was prone to shrinkage and creep under load. By causing deformation and bonding slip, steel fibers added to UHPC can absorb energy, reallocate stress within the microstructure, and prevent UHPC from creeping or shrinking. Excessive steel fiber integration, though, may lessen this capability. This was due to the low UHPC water/binder ratio and the fact that adding more steel fiber dose decreased the fluidity of newly mixed UHPC. This led to a weaker interfacial transition zone between the steel fibers and the matrix and more new defects in the UHPC, which partially offset the creep inhibition effect of the steel fibers. Nevertheless, the mechanical characteristics of UHPC were diminished when the volume doping rate of steel fibers was less than 1%, since the steel fibers were unable to effectively form a mesh to enhance the matrix microstructure. As a result, UHPC's steel fiber doping level has to fall within a suitable range. In conjunction with the test findings, 1–2% steel fiber content in UHPC was recommended.

4.2. Maintenance System Curing Systems

The effect of different maintenance regimes on the flexural creep of UHPC is shown in Figure 6, wherein Figure 6a shows the deflection time course curves of the specimen deflection development with time for different maintenance regimes, and Figure 6b shows the proportion of deflection development for different specimens.

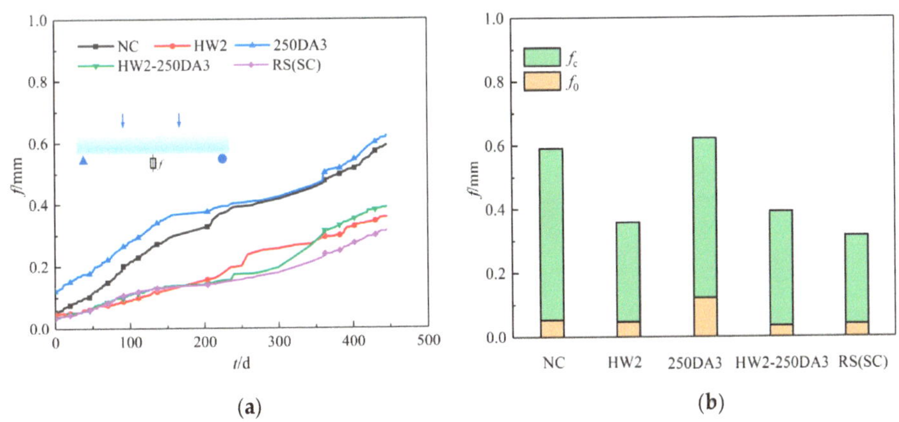

Figure 6. Influence of curing system on bending creep. (**a**) Deflection time course curve. (**b**) Deflection development ratio.

As can be seen from Figure 6, compared with specimen NC, the initial deflections of HW-2, 250DA3, HW2-250DA3, and RS were reduced by 11.32%, −128.30%, 35.85%, and 26.42%, respectively; the creep deflections were reduced by 42.19%, 6.88%, 33.64%, and 48.70%; the total deflections were sequentially reduced by 39.42%, −5.25%, 33.84%, and 46.70%; and the deflection creep coefficient was reduced by 34.81%, 59.21%, −3.44%, and 30.28%. It can be seen that the initial deflection of HW2-250DA3 was the smallest, RS's creep deflection was the smallest, the initial deflection and creep deflection of NC and

250DA3 were the highest, and the creep development rate was faster. It only took 204 days and 181 days, respectively, to complete 50% of the total creep process (445 days).

Heat treatment during the curing stage could effectively reduce the shrinkage of the concrete material in the later stage, while the concrete would continue to shrink in the later stage after the completion of natural curing. Heat treatment was used to speed up hydration and modify the concrete matrix's microstructure during the curing stage. This microstructure refinement was most noticeable near the fibers. The fiber–matrix interface's improved structure and characteristics had a higher ability to prevent UHPC shrinkage and creep in later phases. Without a heat treatment of UHPC, the casting process may form a water film around the fibers, leading to a higher local water/binder ratio. Heat treatment could promote a further reaction of the cement paste, leading to a reduction in porosity around the fibers and an improvement in fiber–matrix interface defects.

In addition to the binding water found in the material, a significant amount of water was needed for the rehydration of concrete, and this water needed to originate from the surrounding environment. Even though the heat treatment could accelerate the hydration reaction, if the UHPC hydration response was insufficient, a shortage of water during the curing process could also lead to an increase in creep. For instance, NC and 250DA3 did not have access to a water environment during the curing, and they exhibited high initial and creep deflections as well as a rapid rate of creep development. By using hot water at 90 °C for just two days, HW2 was able to achieve results that were nearly identical to RS (normal curing for 28 days). This resulted in a significant reduction in curing time and increased labor efficiency, and it may find widespread use in the assembly of components.

4.3. Water/Binder Ratio

The effect of different water/binder ratios on the bending creep of UHPC is shown in Figure 7, wherein Figure 7a shows the deflection time course curves of the deflection development with time for the specimens with different water/binder ratios, and Figure 7b shows the percentage of deflection development for different specimens.

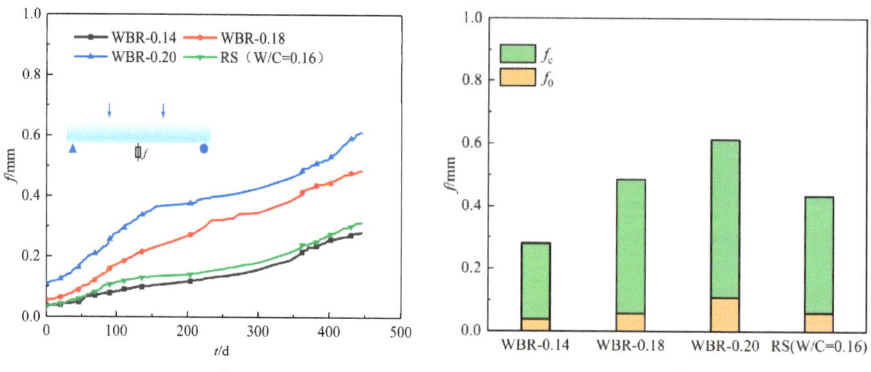

(a) (b)

Figure 7. Influence of water/binder ratio on bending creep. (**a**) Deflection time course curve. (**b**) Deflection development ratio.

From Figure 7, it can be seen that compared with specimen WBR-0.14, the initial deflection of RS, WBR-0.18, and WBR-0.20 increased by 5.41%, 51.35%, and 191.89%; the creep deflection increased by 13.58%, 76.54%, and 107.41%; the total deflection increased by 12.50%, 73.21%, and 118.57%; and the deflection creep coefficient increased by 7.75%, 16.63%, −28.95%, respectively. It was evident that the specimens' initial deflection, creep deflection, and total deflection all greatly increased as the water/binder ratios grew. The creep deflection of WBR-0.18 and WBR-0.20 developed quickly; in total, 50% of the whole creep process (445 days) was completed in 204 days and 153 days, respectively.

The type and nature of hydration products, porosity, and microstructure can all be strongly impacted by the water/binder ratio. Because more water reacts with cementitious material and produces hydration products, the chemical self-shrinkage of UHPC increases as the water/binder ratio rises. Concurrently, there was a higher potential for creep because of how readily a substantial quantity of free water in UHPC can evaporate. The effect of the water/binder ratio on the creep of UHPC is significant. This study pointed out that the movement of water is one of the most important factors leading to the creep. Moreover, the larger the water/binder ratio, the more free the water remains after the hydration of cement, the greater the evaporation of water from the hardened concrete, the higher the internal porosity, and the greater the creep of UHPC. It can be seen that the water/binder ratio of UHPC should be controlled within a reasonable range, and it is recommended that it should generally not exceed 0.20.

4.4. Sand/Binder Ratio

The effect of different sand/binder ratios on the flexural creep of UHPC is shown in Figure 8, wherein Figure 8a shows the deflection time course curves of the specimen deflection development with time for different sand/binder ratios, and Figure 8b shows the percentage of deflection development for different specimens.

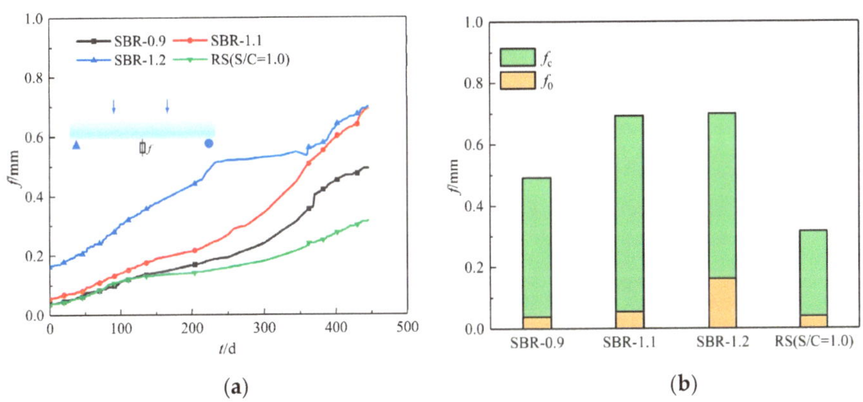

Figure 8. Influence of sand/binder ratio on bending creep. (**a**) Deflection time course curve. (**b**) Deflection development ratio.

As observed in Figure 8, the initial deflection of RS, SBR-1.1, and SBR-1.2 increased by 2.63%, 42.11%, and 323.68%, respectively, when compared to specimen SBR-0.9; the creep deflection increased by −39.21%, 40.53%, and 18.50%; the total deflection increased by −35.98%, 40.65%, and 42.07%; and the deflection creep factor decreased by 40.76%, 1.11%, and 72.03%, respectively. It was evident that as the sand/binder ratio rose, the specimens' initial deflection rose along with their creep deflection and total deflection, which first dropped and then increased. SBR-1.2's creep deflection developed at the quickest pace; in total, 50% of the whole creep process (445 d) was completed in just 189 days. It can be seen that the appropriate sand/binder ratio had a certain inhibitory effect on the creep.

In general, the harder the aggregate, the higher the modulus of elasticity. Further, the larger the volume proportion occupied by the aggregate, the smaller the deflection induced by the pressure transferred from the gel flow to the aggregate. Nonetheless, based on test results, the initial deflection and creep deflection increase as the sand/binder ratio increases, with the exception of RS (sand/binder ratios of 1.0). Specimens SBR-0.9, RS, SBR-1.1, and SBR-1.2 maintained the same capacity, and the proportion of cementitious material became smaller and smaller as the sand/binder ratio increased. The calculated cement dosage of specimens SBR-0.9, RS, SBR-1.1, and SBR-1.2 was 679 kg/m^3, 646 kg/m^3, 614 kg/m^3, and 587 kg/m^3, respectively. Additionally, as the cement dosage was decreasing, the hydration was not sufficient, and the creep increased. This showed that the total amount of cementitious materials and fine aggregates in UHPC and the ratio of the two should be within a reasonable range.

4.5. Stress Levels

The effect of different stress levels on the flexural creep of UHPC is shown in Figure 9, wherein Figure 9a shows the deflection time course curves of the specimen deflection development with time for different stress levels, and Figure 9b shows the percentage of deflection development for different specimens.

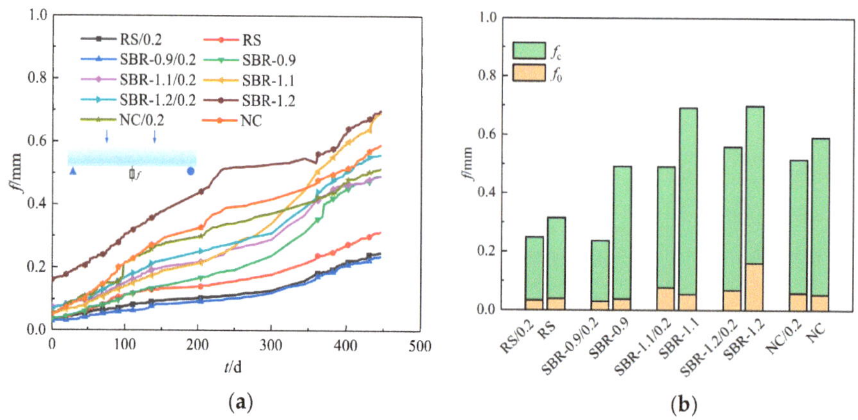

Figure 9. Influence of stress level on bending creep. (**a**) Deflection time course curve. (**b**) Deflection development ratio.

From Figure 9, it can be seen that the initial deflections of specimens RS, SBR-0.9, SBR-1.1, SBR-1.2, and NC decreased by 15.38%, 21.05%, −29.87%, 57.14%, and −8.62%, respectively. When the stress levels of specimens RS, SBR-0.9, SBR-1.1, SBR-1.2, and NC were reduced from 0.3 to 0.2, the creep deflections decreased by 22.10%, 54.41%, 35.11%, 8.92%, 14.87%. Consequently, there was a 21.27%, 51.83%, 29.05%, 20.03%, and 12.69% reduction in total deflection, and a 7.94%, 42.25%, 54.49%, −52.94%, 22.20% reduction in the deflection creep coefficient, in this order. It was evident that the specimens' initial deflection, creep deflection, and total deflection all generally increased with the stress level. The rate at which creep developed was also strongly influenced by the stress level. For example, specimens SBR-1.2/0.2 and SBR-1.2 took 306 days and 189 days, respectively, to complete 50% of the total creep process (445 days), whereas specimens NC/0.2 and NC took 157 days and 204 days, respectively, to complete 50% of the total creep process (445 days).

Concrete's creep was directly correlated with its stress level: the higher the stress level, the higher the creep. The gel flowed more quickly, and the pace of creep development became faster as the stress level increased. As a result, selecting a suitable range of pre-stress is essential when employing UHPC for pre-stressing tasks.

5. Conclusions

The deformation properties of 20 UHPC beams under long-term loading were studied in this research study to determine the changes in the beams' deflection patterns for 445 days of continuous loading. The effects of steel fiber content, curing systems, water/binder ratio, sand/binder ratio, and stress level on the deflection of UHPC beams over time were investigated. The following main conclusions were obtained:

(1) With the increase in steel fiber content, the initial deflection of the specimens decreased, the creep deflection increased, and the steel fiber had an obvious inhibiting

effect on the initial deflection of the specimen. However, a dosage of steel fiber too high led to a relatively weak interfacial transition zone between the steel fiber and matrix, which would offset part of the inhibitory effect of the steel fiber on creep, and it was recommended that the dosage rate of the steel fiber in UHPC should be 1~2%.

(2) At the maintenance stage, heat treatment can hasten the hydration effect, leading to improved UHPC shrinkage and creep inhibition later on. NC's and 250DA3's maintenance periods were not provided with a water environment, the initial deflection and creep deflection were very large, and the rate of creep development was fast. Therefore, heat treatment must be coupled with necessary moisture. HW2's curing time was short and efficient, and it can be popularized in the fabrication of assembly components.

(3) The larger the water/binder ratio, the more free the water remaining after cement hydration, the greater the evaporation of water from the hardened concrete, the higher the internal porosity, the greater the creep of UHPC. The water/binder ratio of UHPC should be controlled within a reasonable range, and it is recommended that it should not exceed 0.20 in general.

(4) Both initial and creep deflections increased with an increasing sand/binder ratio, except for RS (sand/binder ratio of 1.0). The total amount of cementitious materials and fine aggregates as well as the ratio of the two should be taken care of in UHPC.

(5) The creep of UHPC had a close relationship with the stress level: the greater the stress level, the greater the creep. Increasing the stress level accelerated the flow of gel and the development rate of creep. Therefore, when UHPC is used in pre-stressing works, a reasonable range of pre-stress should be selected.

Finally, for future research, the authors recommend a comparative study of the variation patterns of compressive creep and bending creep in UHPC under the same size and conditions to be carried out. In addition, it is worth studying the long-term effects of bending creep on the structural integrity of UHPC elements.

Author Contributions: Conceptualization, J.L.; methodology, J.L.; software, Y.L. and X.J.; formal analysis, B.L.; investigation, J.C.; resources, J.L. and B.L.; data curation, Q.M.; writing—original draft preparation, J.L.; writing—review and editing, J.L. and B.L.; visualization, B.L.; supervision, J.L. and B.L. All authors have read and agreed to the published version of the manuscript.

Funding: This research received no external funding.

Data Availability Statement: The data that support the findings of this study are available upon reasonable request from author Jiayue Li.

Conflicts of Interest: The authors declare no conflicts of interest.

References

1. Ranaivomanana, N.; Multon, S.; Turatsinze, A. Tensile, compressive and flexural basic creep of concrete at different stress levels. *Cem. Concr. Res.* **2013**, *52*, 1–10. [CrossRef]
2. Babafemi, A.J.; Boshoff, W.P. Testing and modelling the creep of cracked macro-synthetic fiber reinforced concrete (MSFRC) under flexural loading. *Mater. Struct.* **2016**, *49*, 4389–4400. [CrossRef]
3. Siming, L.; Ya, W. Research on tensile creep model based on degree of hydration for early-age concrete. *Eng. Mech.* **2016**, *33*, 171–177.
4. Pujadas, P.; Blanco, A.; Cavalaro, S.H.P.; De La Fuente, A.; Aguado, A. The need to consider flexural post-cracking creep behavior of macro-synthetic fiber reinforced concrete. *Constr. Build. Mater.* **2017**, *149*, 790–800. [CrossRef]
5. Jahami, A.; Khatib, J.; Raydan, R. Production of low-cost, high-strength concrete with waste glass as fine aggregates replacement. *Buildings* **2022**, *12*, 2168. [CrossRef]
6. Manjunath, M.; Seth, D.; Balaji, K.; Roy, S.; Tangadagi, R.B. Utilization of industrial-based PVC waste powder in self-compacting concrete: A sustainable building material. *J. Clean. Prod.* **2023**, *428*, 139428. [CrossRef]
7. Tailhan, J.; Boulay, C.; Rossi, P.; Le Maou, F.; Martin, E. Compressive, tensile and bending basic creep behaviours related to the same concrete. *Struct. Concr.* **2013**, *14*, 124–130. [CrossRef]
8. Kim, S.G.; Park, Y.S.; Lee, Y.H. Comparison of concrete creep in compression, tension, and bending under drying condition. *Materials* **2019**, *12*, 3357. [CrossRef]
9. Farah, M.; Grondin, F.; Alam, S.; Loukili, A. Experimental approach to investigate creep-damage bilateral effects in concrete at early age. *Cem. Concr. Res.* **2019**, *96*, 128–137. [CrossRef]

10. Berger, J.; Gericke, O.; Feix, J.; Sobek, W. Experimental investigations on actively bent concrete shells. *Struct. Concr.* **2020**, *21*, 2268–2281. [CrossRef]
11. Ding, Y.; Fang, Y.; Jin, W.; Zhang, J.; Li, B.; Mao, J. Numerical method for creep analysis of strengthened fatigue-damaged concrete beams. *Buildings* **2023**, *13*, 968. [CrossRef]
12. Buratti, N.; Mazzotti, C. Experimental tests on the effect of temperature on the long-term behaviour of macrosynthetic fibre reinforced concretes. *Constr. Build. Mater.* **2015**, *95*, 133–142. [CrossRef]
13. Buratti, N.; Ferracuti, B.; Savoia, M. Concrete crack reduction in tunnel linings by steel fibre-reinforced concretes. *Constr. Build. Mater.* **2013**, *44*, 249–259. [CrossRef]
14. Taengua, E.; Arango, S.; Vargas, M. Flexural creep of steel fiber reinforced concrete in the cracked state. *Constr. Build. Mater.* **2014**, *65*, 321–329. [CrossRef]
15. Vrijdaghs, R.; Prisco, M.D.; Vandewalle, L. Sectional analysis of the flexural creep of cracked fiber reinforced concrete. *Struct. Concr.* **2021**, *22*, 1817–1830. [CrossRef]
16. Yazdizadeh, Z.; Marzouk, H.; Hadianfard, M.A. Monitoring of concrete shrinkage and creep using fiber bragg grating sensors. *Constr. Build. Mater.* **2017**, *137*, 505–512. [CrossRef]
17. Zhang, Y.; Zhu, P.; Zhu, Y.; Bao, C.; Shao, X.; Shi, J. NC-UHPC composite structure for long-term creep-induced deflection control in continuous box-girder bridges. *J. Bridge Eng.* **2018**, *23*, 04018034. [CrossRef]
18. Zhu, L.; Wang, J.-J.; Li, X.; Zhao, G.-Y.; Huo, X.-J. Experimental and numerical study on creep and shrinkage effects of ultra high-performance concrete beam. *Compos. Part B* **2020**, *184*, 107713. [CrossRef]
19. Llano, T.A.; Jose Rocio Martí-Vargas Serna, P. Flexural and compressive creep behavior of UHPFRC specimens. *Constr. Build. Mater.* **2020**, *244*, 118254. [CrossRef]
20. Xu, Y.; Liu, J.; Liu, J.; Zhang, P.; Zhang, Q.; Jiang, L. Experimental studies and modeling of creep of UHPC. *Constr. Build. Mater.* **2018**, *175*, 643–652. [CrossRef]
21. Chen, Y.; Liu, P.; Sha, F.; Yu, Z.; He, S.; Xu, W.; Lv, M. Effects of type and content of fibers, water-to-cement ratio, and cementitious materials on the shrinkage and creep of ultra-high performance concrete. *Polymers* **2022**, *14*, 1956. [CrossRef] [PubMed]
22. Zhang, Z.; Xu, T.; Deng, K.; Tong, T.; Zhou, H. Experimental study on creep failure of non-steam-cured ultrahigh-performance concrete under high uniaxial compressive stress. *J. Mater. Civ. Eng.* **2022**, *34*, 04022105. [CrossRef]
23. Zhang, Y.; Zhu, Y.; Xu, Z.; Shao, X. Long-term creep behavior of NC filled UHPC tube composite column. *Eng. Struct.* **2022**, *259*, 114214. [CrossRef]
24. Mohebbi, A.; Graybeal, B.; Haber, Z. Time-dependent properties of ultrahigh-performance concrete: Compressive creep and shrinkage. *J. Mater. Civ. Eng.* **2022**, *34*, 04022096. [CrossRef]
25. Garas, V.Y. Multi-Scale Investigation of Tensile Creep of Ultra-High Performance Concrete for Bridge Applications. Ph.D. Thesis, Georgia Institute of Technology, Atlanta, GA, USA, 2009.
26. Garas, V.Y.; Kurtis, K.E.; Kahn, L.F. Creep of UHPC in tension and compression: Effect of thermal treatment. *Cem. Concr. Compos.* **2012**, *34*, 493–502. [CrossRef]
27. Cui, C. Influence of Curing Regime on Shrinkage, Creep and Basic Mechanical Proper-Ties of Ultra-High Performance Concrete. Master's Thesis, Beijing Jiaotong University, Beijing, China, 2018.
28. Abid, M.; Hou, X.; Zheng, W.; Hussain, R.R.; Cao, S.; Lv, Z. Creep behavior of steel fiber reinforced reactive powder concrete at high temperature. *Constr. Build. Mater.* **2019**, *205*, 321–331. [CrossRef]

buildings

MDPI

Article

Study on the Vibration Isolation Performance of Sliding–Rolling Friction Composite Vibration Isolation Bearing

Yankai Lu [1], Jiayue Li [1], Bo Liu [1,*], Juannong Chen [1], Wanying Zhang [1] and Qingjuan Meng [2]

[1] School of Civil Architectural Engineering, North China University of Science and Technology, Tangshan 063000, China; luyankai1999@outlook.com (Y.L.); lijiayue@ncst.edu.cn (J.L.); chenjuannong@163.com (J.C.); zwy_sep03@163.com (W.Z.)
[2] School of Civil Engineering, Tangshan University, Tangshan 063000, China; mqjmqj2728@126.com
* Correspondence: liubo19840311@ncst.edu.cn

Abstract: This study focuses on investigating the newly proposed sliding–rolling friction composite seismic isolation bearing. It begins by establishing the dynamic equilibrium equation for the structure. Subsequently, this paper proposes a calculation model for the sliding–rolling friction composite seismic isolation bearing, integrating fundamental theories of structural dynamic response analysis and numerical solution methods. Utilizing finite element analysis software ABAQUS (2021), the mechanical properties of the seismic isolation bearing are comprehensively assessed. Through this evaluation, the optimal parameters of the seismic isolation bearing are determined. The findings reveal that the optimal parameters include a friction coefficient (μ) of 0.04, four U-type dampers at 45° angles, a width of 60 mm, five balls, and two shims.

Keywords: sliding–rolling friction composite seismic isolation bearing; U-shaped damper; hysteresis curve; skeleton curve

1. Introduction

China, positioned at the convergence of several seismic zones, experiences active crustal movements and frequent earthquakes, notably in regions such as Sichuan, Yunnan, and Inner Mongolia. Consequently, the advancement of seismic isolation technology is imperative to mitigate earthquake-related challenges. Notably, seismic isolation techniques have historical precedents, albeit lacking a comprehensive theoretical framework. For instance, during the construction of the Forbidden City in Beijing, glutinous rice was mixed into the foundation material due to its favorable flexibility and integrity. This incorporation facilitated uniform deformation during earthquakes, yielding favorable seismic effects. Similarly, the Small Wild Goose Pagoda in Xi'an features a tower body and foundation arranged in an arc, exhibiting a "non-tilting" structure akin to contemporary friction pendulum support systems [1].

The formal conceptualization of seismic isolation emerged in 1881 through the work of Kozo Kawai in Japan. Since then, extensive research endeavors have been undertaken worldwide to explore the mechanical properties of seismic isolation bearings through experimentation, numerical simulations, and the application of novel materials. Moreover, the development of new models has been pursued both domestically and internationally [2–7].

Seismic isolation bearings represent a crucial component of structural isolation technology, serving to enhance the seismic resilience of building structures. These seismic isolation bearings not only have excellent damping performance, but also have a wide variety of characteristics. Zayas, V.A. et al. [8] analyzed the effect of friction pendulum bearing (FPS) for isolating torsional motions of eccentric and irregular structures in buildings, and the results demonstrated that the reduction in seismic loads can be as much as eight times greater with the correct design. Quaglini, V. et al. [9] analyzed the effect of friction pendulum bearings (FPS) for isolating torsional motions in buildings by changing the pad material or lubrication conditions to provide different equivalent damping ratios for the seismic isolation system. Modifying the coefficient of friction of the bearing by altering the pad material or lubrication conditions yields disparate equivalent damping ratios for the seismic isolation system. Fenz, D.M. et al. [10] validated the theoretical force–displacement relationship by characterizing bearings with sliding surfaces exhibiting the same radius of curvature and coefficient of friction. The outcomes demonstrate that the property is predominantly a rigid bilinear hysteresis, which collapses to a rigid linear hysteresis for equal coefficients of friction.

Composite seismic isolation bearings have been extensively utilized to address the limitations of traditional seismic isolation bearings by amalgamating various seismic isolation materials and techniques, thereby enhancing the seismic isolation performance of structures [11,12]. In this study, a novel sliding–rolling friction composite isolation bearing is introduced, which combines the features of sliding and rolling isolation bearings while incorporating a U-shaped damper for reset. Utilizing ABAQUS software, the mechanical properties of the sliding–rolling friction composite seismic isolation bearing were simulated and analyzed. The optimal parameters of the seismic isolation bearing were identified, offering valuable data references for engineering applications.

2. Establishment of Structural Dynamic Equations

The use of sliding–rolling friction composite isolation bearings for foundation isolation results in two states of relative static and relative motion for the superstructure and foundation under seismic action. The state of relative motion depends on whether the horizontal seismic force on the new composite isolation bearings reaches the critical value. To accurately analyze the actual force situation of the building structure under seismic action, this paper selects the "tandem mass system" model according to the characteristics of structural discretization and vibration models. The model assumes that all the mass of the structure is centrally distributed at the key points where the translational displacements need to be calculated. The total mass at any node is equal to the sum of the masses assigned to that node by the segments connected to it.

2.1. Relative Stationarity

When the seismic action generates a base shear force that is less than the maximum static friction of the bearing, indicated by $\left|\sum_{i=0}^{n} m_i \ddot{X}_g\right| < -\mu \sum_{i=1}^{i=n} m_i g$, the structure remains relatively stationary. At this point, the maximum static friction of the seismic isolation layer is sufficient to balance the generated shear force. The seismic isolation layer and the superstructure as a whole remain in a seismic state, allowing the structure to dissipate energy. The superstructure's mass, stiffness, and damping matrices are as follows, and the structural system has n degrees of freedom:

$$M_S = \begin{bmatrix} m_1 & \dots & 0 \\ \vdots & \ddots & \vdots \\ 0 & \dots & m_n \end{bmatrix} \tag{1}$$

$$K_S = \begin{bmatrix} k_1 & -k_1 & & \\ -k_1 & k_1 + k_2 & -k_3 & \\ & & & \vdots \\ & & -k_n & k_n \end{bmatrix} \tag{2}$$

$$C_S = \begin{bmatrix} a_0 \sum_1^n m_i + a_1 k_1 & \cdots & -a_0 m_n \\ \vdots & \ddots & \vdots \\ & \cdots & a_0 m_n + a_1 k_n \end{bmatrix} \tag{3}$$

Style:

$m_1, m_2, \cdots, m_n$—Mass at level i of the structural system;
k_i—Shear stiffness of structural system layer i.
The Rayleigh damping Equation (4) is as follows

$$C = a_0 M + a_1 K \quad (4)$$

where a_0, a_1 are solved by (5) and (6) below.

$$a_0 + a_1 w_1^2 = 2\xi_1 w_1 \quad (5)$$

$$a_0 + a_1 w_2^2 = 2\xi_2 w_2 \quad (6)$$

Style:
a_0, a_1—Scale factor;
w_1, w_2—First and second modes of vibration of structural systems;
ξ_1, ξ_2—First and second damping ratios for structural systems, reinforced concrete structure ξ_1 = 0.05, ξ_2 = 0.07; Steel structure ξ_1 = 0.02, ξ_2 = 0.03.
Its corresponding equation of motion is:

$$M_S \ddot{X} + C_S \dot{X} + K_S X = -M_S I \ddot{X}_g \quad (7)$$

Style:
$X, \dot{X}, \ddot{X}$—Lateral displacement, velocity and acceleration vectors for each mass of the superstructure;
$\ddot{X}_g$—earthquake acceleration vector.

2.2. Relative State of Motion

When the earthquake's base shear force exceeds the maximum static friction of the bearing, indicated by $\left|\sum_{i=0}^{n} \ddot{X}_{gG} m_i\right| > -\mu \sum_{i=0}^{i=n} m_i g$, the structure enters a state of relative sliding. Even after offsetting the maximum static friction of the seismic isolation layer, the shear force remains high, and the seismic isolation bearing and the superstructure work together to dissipate energy.

In this case, the seismic isolation layer is an additional layer in the structural system, which increases the number of degrees of freedom of the seismic isolation structure to n+1. The mass matrix, stiffness matrix, and damping matrix of the seismic isolation structure can be introduced based on the matrix construction of the superstructure.

$$M_G = \begin{bmatrix} m_0 & \cdots & 0 \\ \vdots & \ddots & \vdots \\ 0 & \cdots & m_n \end{bmatrix} \quad (8)$$

$$K_G = \begin{bmatrix} K_0 + k_1 & -k_1 & & \\ -k_1 & k_1 + k_2 & -k_3 & \\ & & & \vdots \\ & & -k_n & k_n \end{bmatrix} \quad (9)$$

$$C_G = \begin{bmatrix} C_0 + a_0 \sum_1^n m_i + a_1 k_1 & \cdots & -a_0 m_n \\ \vdots & \ddots & \vdots \\ & \cdots & a_0 m_n + a_1 k_n \end{bmatrix} \quad (10)$$

Style:
m_0—The total mass of the seismic isolation layer, denoted as $m_0 = \sum m_s$, m_s is the mass of a single seismic isolation bearing;

K_0—The horizontal stiffness of the seismic isolation layer, denoted as $K_0 = \sum K_s$, K_s is the horizontal stiffness of a single seismic isolation bearing;

C_0—The equivalent damping ratio of the seismic isolation layer, denoted as $C_0 = 2\sum m_s\omega_0\zeta_{eq}$, ω_0 is the horizontal stiffness of a single seismic isolation bearing, and ζ_{eq} is the equivalent damping ratio of the seismic isolation layer.

Its corresponding equation of motion is:

$$M_G\ddot{X}_G + C_G\dot{X}_G + K_GX_G = -M_GI\ddot{X}_g \tag{11}$$

Style:

$X_G, \dot{X}_G, \ddot{X}_G$-Lateral displacement, velocity, and acceleration vectors for each mass of the seismically isolated structure;

$\ddot{X}_g$—Seismic acceleration vectors.

3. ABAQUS Finite Element Analysis of Seismic Isolation Bearings

3.1. Support Structure

The sliding–rolling friction composite seismic isolation bearing is composed of a number of components, including upper and lower connection plates, an intermediate column, a spring, a ball, a friction plate, and other components. Additionally, a U-shaped damper is set around the bearing to assist in energy consumption. The connecting plate is connected to the intermediate column, U-shaped damper, and friction plate via bolts, facilitating ease of installation and dismantling. The lower connecting plate is coated with a layer of PTFE, a white wax-like substance with semi-transparency, heat resistance, cold resistance, acid and alkali resistance, insolubility in other solvents, and a low coefficient of friction. This coating provides an ideal lubricating surface for sliding friction. The design of sliding–rolling friction composite seismic isolation bearings is based on the principles of energy dissipation through sliding and rolling friction, as well as the synergistic effect of springs and U-shaped dampers. The spring compression is adjusted by increasing or decreasing the number of shims, and the number of balls in the grooves is changed, thus proportionally distributing the loads applied from the upper part to the sliding surfaces and the ball group. This reduces the seismic transmission to the superstructure through the deformation of energy dissipation.

3.2. Material Intrinsic Relationship

The sliding–rolling friction composite seismic isolation bearing consists of upper and lower connecting plates, U-shaped dampers, springs, and ball rollers, all made of steel. The material properties are defined using the bifold principal model for all principal relationships of steel. The stress–strain curves are shown in Figure 1. The decision to use the bifold model, rather than more complex models such as the triple-fold model, is based on several factors. Firstly, the bifold model has been widely applied in engineering and has been practically validated. Additionally, it can succinctly and efficiently describe the stress–strain relationship of steel before and after yielding. Secondly, this model offers high computational efficiency and stability while maintaining computational accuracy [13]. It is suitable for simulating and analyzing sliding–rolling friction composite seismic isolation bearings. The model assumes a constant slope of the stress–strain relationship after yielding, which is expressed by Equation (12).

$$\begin{cases} \delta = E_s\varepsilon_s & \varepsilon_s \le \varepsilon_y \\ \delta = \delta_y + E_s'(\varepsilon_s - \varepsilon_y) & \varepsilon_y < \varepsilon_s \le \varepsilon_{cu} \end{cases} \tag{12}$$

Style:

E_s—Modulus of elasticity of steel;

E_s'—Slope of the hardened section of the steel;

σ_y—Yield strength of steel;

ε—Strain in steel;

ε_y—Yield strain of steel;

ε_{cu}—The peak strain corresponding to the time when the steel reaches its ultimate tensile strength.

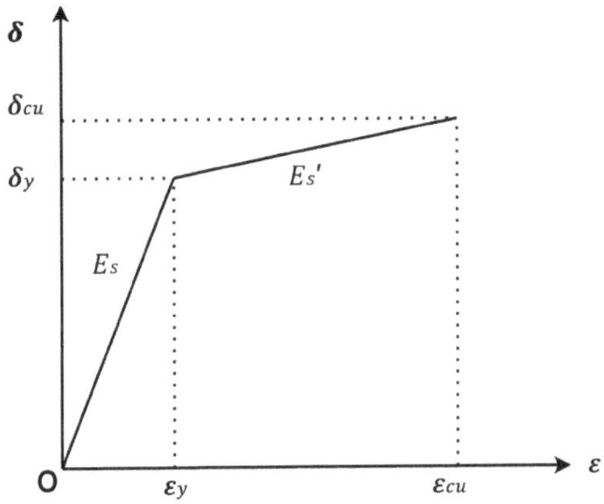

Figure 1. Steel bifold intrinsic model.

The basic parameters of the various types of materials used in the support are shown in Table 1.

Table 1. Table of material properties.

Makings	Modulus of Elasticity (MPa)	Poisson's Ratio	Yield Stress (N/mm^2)	Mass Density (kg/m^3)
45#steel	2.11 × 1011	0.269	430	7890
65 Mn	2.09 × 1011	0.288	355	7820
GCr15	2.06 × 1011	0.3	1800	7810
PTFE	2.8 × 1011	0.35	0	2320
Q345	2.11 × 1011	0.3	345	7890

3.3. Model Simplification Processing

During the ABAQUS finite element modeling process, simplification of the physical model is necessary to improve computational efficiency and highlight key features. This simplification aids in mesh delineation and improves computational speed, ultimately facilitating model convergence.

This paper presents a model of a sliding–rolling friction composite seismic isolation bearing, which consists of a superstructure, U-shaped damper, PTFE coating, ball, and friction plate. The connection relationship between the upper connection plate and the intermediate column is simplified using the merge method in a Boolean operation, replacing the complex bolt connection with an overall modeling approach to construct a more simplified superstructure. This simplification improves the calculation speed and enhances the convergence of the model. This paper simplifies the bolted relationship between the U-shaped damper and the support into a binding connection. The main mechanical properties of the U-shaped damper are retained while effectively simplifying the model's structure and improving analysis efficiency. Figure 2 displays the simplified components and three-dimensional model of the sliding–rolling friction composite seismic isolation bearing.

To assess the effectiveness of the simplified treatment, we compared computational time and convergence. The simplified model significantly reduced the total time required for a full analysis by one-third compared to the pre-simplified model. Additionally, the simplified model showed faster convergence in the iterative solving process, requiring fewer iterations and reducing computation time per iteration.

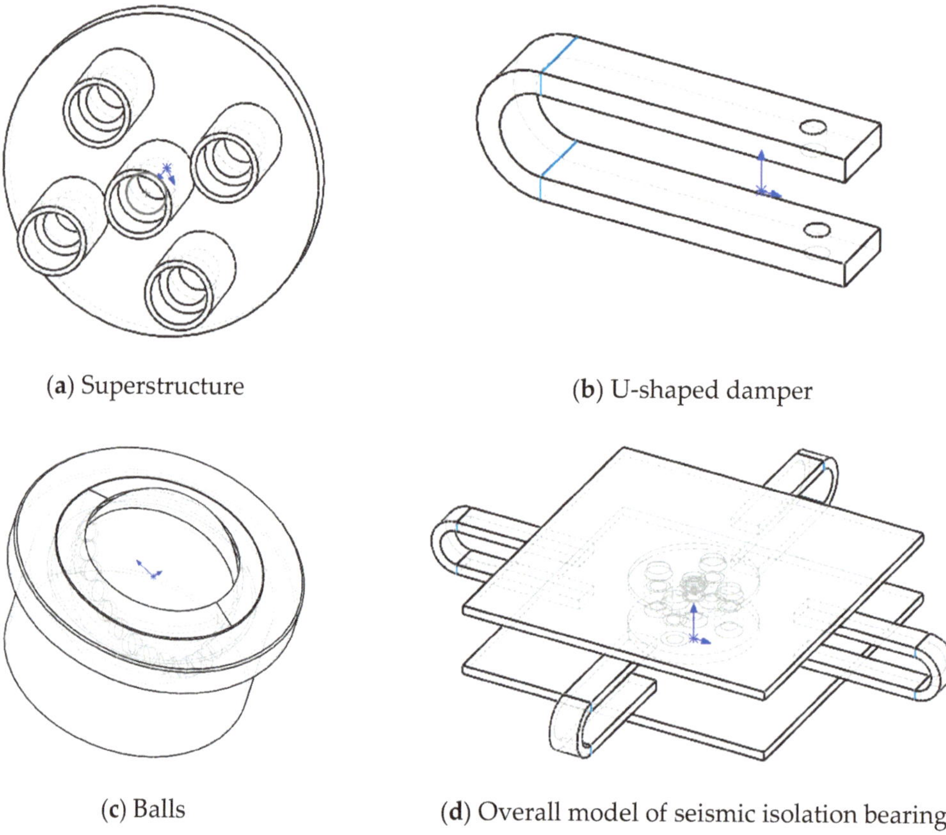

Figure 2. Sliding–rolling friction composite seismic isolation bearing components and overall modeling.

3.4. *Definition of Exposure*

This paper meticulously defines and sets parameters for the mechanical behavior of sliding–rolling friction composite seismic isolation bearings. Firstly, the connection relationship between the U-shaped damper and the upper and lower friction plates is considered, whose main functions are fixation and force transmission. To ensure a solid connection between the two and almost no slip in the simulation [14], the binding constraint (Tie) is chosen in this paper. Secondly, the spring regulates the load distribution between the ball and the sliding surface in the seismic isolation bearing. To define the spring connecting the ball and the intermediate column, the Connector Element is used. This not only saves computational resources but also ensures model accuracy. Finally, the contact relationship between the ball and other components is crucial as it is a key component in the seismic isolation bearing. This paper adopts a face-to-face approach to more realistically simulate the contact behavior between the ball and the ball base, the ball and the friction plate, and the PTFE coating and the friction plate. The contact method considers the geometry and relative motion of the contact surfaces, resulting in simulation outcomes that are closer to the actual situation. The contact surfaces are characterized by 'hard contact' for normal contact behavior. For tangential contact behavior, the Cullen friction model is used to define the Pentaly function, which simulates the friction between the contact surfaces by setting the friction coefficient.

The ultimate shear stress expression [14] in the slip state using the small slip formulation between the faces is as follows:

$$\tau_{\text{crit}} = \mu p \quad (13)$$

Style:
μ—Coefficient of friction.
p—Contact pressure between contact surfaces.

3.5. Boundary Conditions and Load Step Treatment

This study focuses on the analysis of a sliding–rolling friction composite seismic isolation bearing, with boundary conditions set according to the initial constraints of the bearing. The lower section of the friction plate is immobile, thus restricting the degrees of freedom in the X, Y, and Z directions to ensure stable initial boundary conditions. In the preliminary analysis, a reference point RP3 is established on the upper friction plate. Subsequently, the upper surface of the plate is linked with RP3, and axial pressure of 200 Kn along with gravity is applied to the upper part of RP3, resulting in surface loading on the top of the upper friction plate. In the subsequent phase of the analysis, the model is subjected to a loading regime involving horizontal displacement in the direction of U1 to investigate its mechanical response. The objective is to comprehend the behavior of the model when subjected to horizontal displacement.

For the load step treatment, this paper employs a cyclic loading regime controlled by displacement loading. Displacement loading control is preferred because it directly controls the bearing's displacement variable, more accurately simulating the specific working conditions in the actual project. The study aimed to investigate the mechanical behavior of seismic isolation bearings under different horizontal displacements. The amplitude of displacement loading was increased by 15 mm in each cycle. The loading regime was cycled five times.

3.6. Grid Division

To ensure efficient, stable, and fast computation in finite element analysis, the number of meshes must be determined by weighing the following three aspects: 1. selecting a reasonable cell type; 2. ensuring good cell shape; and 3. strictly controlling mesh density based on size [15].

To regulate mesh density, this paper employs a strategy that combines splitting component entities and arranging seeds. This approach ensures that the mesh arrangement meets both computational accuracy requirements and efficiency considerations. Secondly, to ensure a smooth transition between meshes, we have adopted the mesh transition technique. This technique effectively avoids errors that may occur due to sudden changes in meshes and improves the accuracy of the analysis.

Figure 3 shows that detailed meshing was performed for critical areas of the model, such as the stress concentration area near the bend of the U-shaped damper and the contact portion of the lower connecting plate with the ball. This fine meshing helps to accurately analyze the model's behavior in these critical regions and predict its performance more accurately. For non-core regions, the mesh size was appropriately increased to improve computational efficiency. This strategy ensures computational accuracy and analytical efficiency, providing a solid foundation for comprehensive evaluation of the performance of sliding–rolling friction composite seismic isolation bearings.

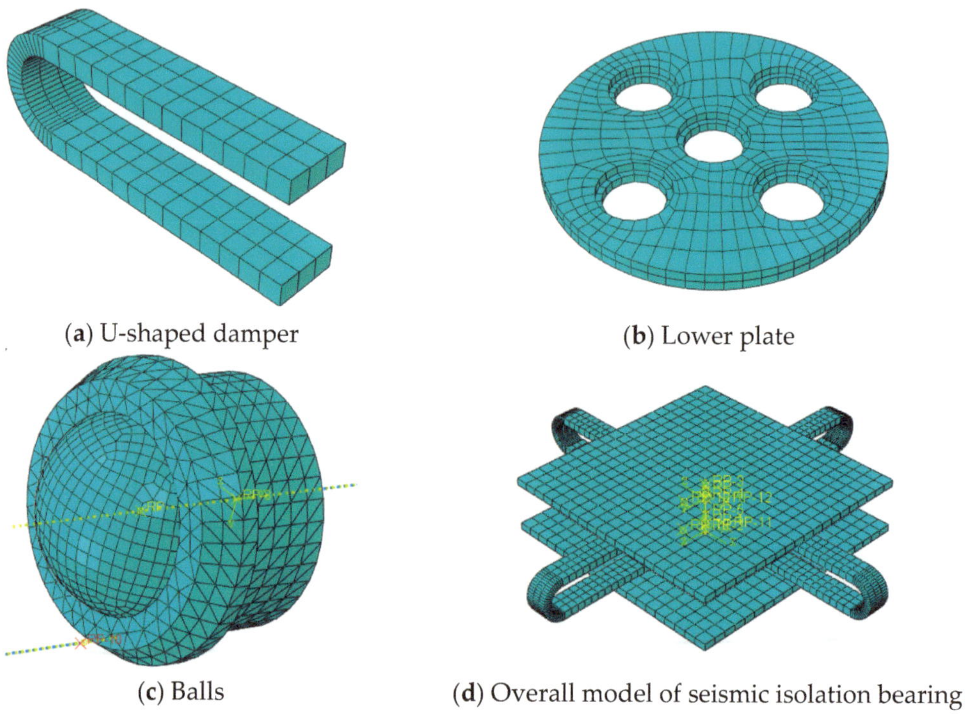

Figure 3. Mesh delineation of seismic isolation bearing.

4. Hysteresis Curve Analysis of Sliding–Rolling Friction Composite Seismic Isolation Bearings

4.1. Effect of Friction Coefficient on Hysteresis Curve

The hysteresis curve characterizes the energy dissipation generated by the elastic–plastic deformation of a structure or component. The size of the hysteresis loop area enclosed by the cyclic motion in one cycle is used as the evaluation criterion. The fuller the shape of the curve and the larger the area, the stronger the energy dissipation capacity and the better the seismic performance of the structure or component. To investigate the effect of friction coefficient on the seismic isolation performance of sliding–rolling friction composite isolation bearings, numerical simulations were conducted. The bearing was set to have zero balls and shims, and four U-shaped dampers with a width of 40 mm (at an angle of 90°) were arranged around it. Hysteresis curves were obtained for the seismic isolation bearing with friction coefficients of 0.04, 0.05, and 0.06, respectively. Figure 4 illustrates the energy dissipation capacity performance of the seismic isolation bearing at varying friction coefficients.

Based on the hysteresis curves in Figure 4, it is evident that the sliding–rolling friction composite seismic isolation bearings exhibit a complete shuttle shape, regardless of the variation in friction coefficient. This aligns with the elastic–plastic energy dissipation model. Furthermore, after reaching the yield point. the hysteresis curves remain almost parallel due to the small differences between the analyzed friction coefficients.

When the friction coefficient is increased from 0.04 to 0.06, the maximum damping force of the seismic isolation bearings changes from 201.34 kN to 201.45 kN. This indicates that the increase in friction coefficient does not significantly affect the maximum damping force.

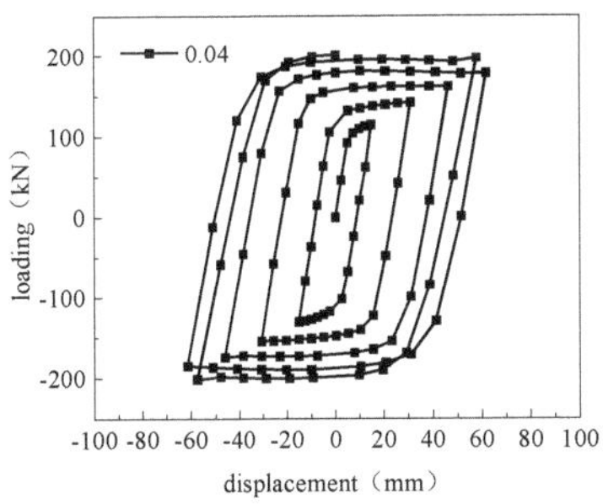

(**a**) Friction coefficient 0.04

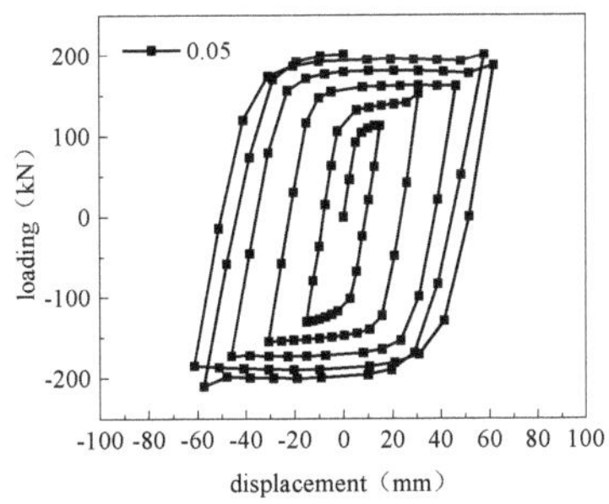

(**b**) Friction coefficient 0.05

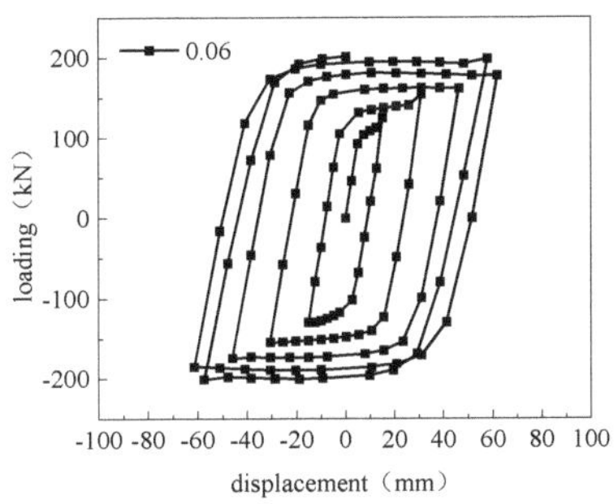

(**c**) Friction coefficient 0.06

Figure 4. Hysteresis curves under different friction coefficients.

Based on the hysteresis curve data presented in Table 2, it is evident that an increase in the friction coefficient from 0.04 to 0.05 results in a decrease of 0.16% and 0.24% in the hysteresis loop area and equivalent damping ratio, respectively. Similarly, an increase in the friction coefficient from 0.05 to 0.06 leads to a decrease of 0.12% and 0.24% in the hysteresis loop area and equivalent damping ratio, respectively. This indicates that the change of the friction coefficient has a very limited effect on the energy dissipation capacity of the seismic isolation bearings and further confirms that the change of the friction coefficient does not have a significant effect on the improvement of the performance of the bearings.

Table 2. Statistics of hysteresis curves under different friction coefficients.

Coefficient of Friction	Hysteresis Loop Area (J)	Maximum Value of Displacement in the Cycle (mm)	Maximum Value of the Load during the Cycle (kN)	Equivalent Damping Ratio
0.04	32,114	61.86	201.34	0.411
0.05	32,060.9	61.85	201.29	0.41
0.06	32,020	61.86	201.45	0.409

After comprehensive consideration, a friction coefficient of 0.04 was selected to ensure that the seismic isolation bearing maintains its energy-consuming performance while effectively realizing the seismic isolation effect.

4.2. Effect of the Number of U-Dampers on the Hysteresis Curve

The U-shaped damper is arranged based on the angle between it and the horizontal displacement loading direction of the sliding–rolling friction composite seismic isolation bearing: '0°' when the two directions are the same, '45°' at an angle of 45°, and '90°'

vertically. The arrangement options are that the '90°' arrangement is used when the two directions are the same. Figure 5 displays the number and arrangement of dampers considered in the simulation.

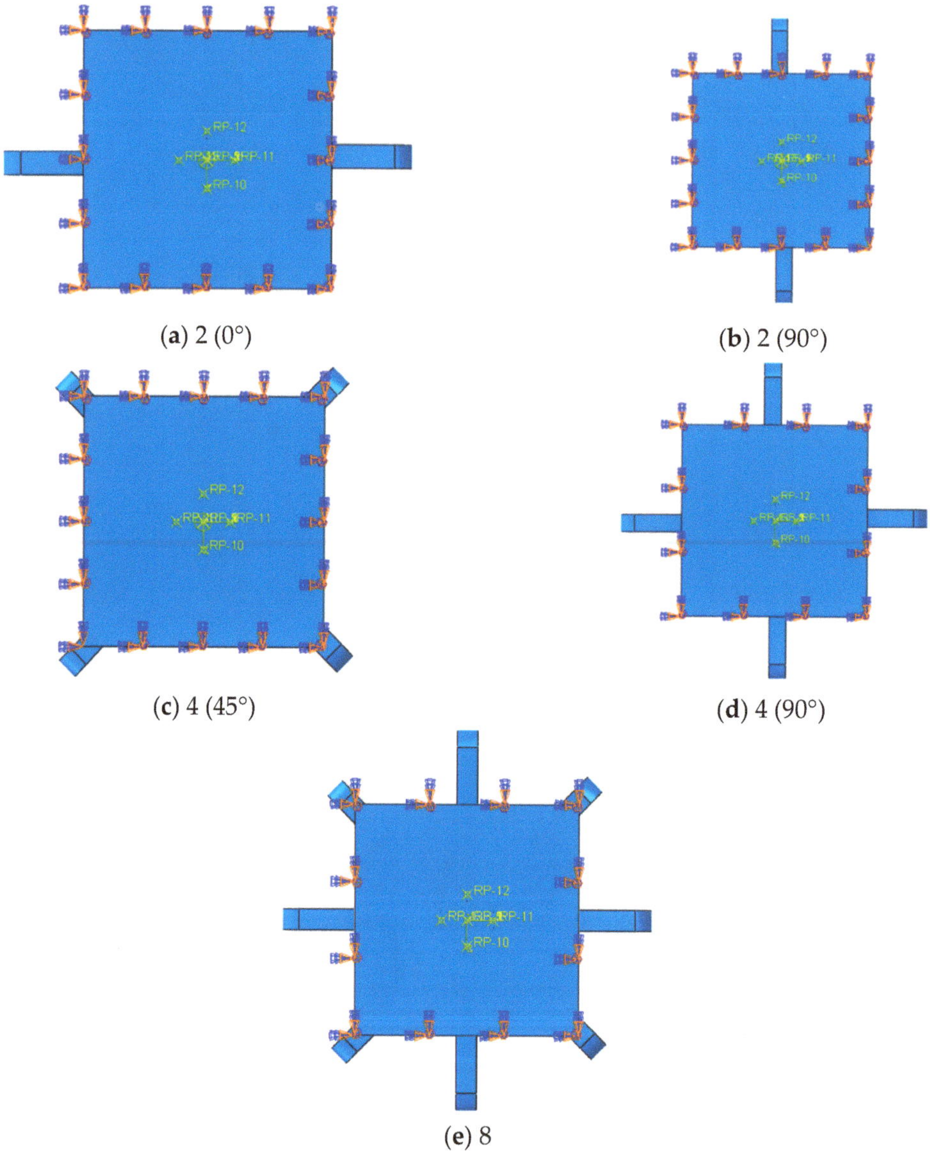

Figure 5. Arrangement of U-dampers.

To investigate the influence of the number of U-dampers on the seismic isolation performance of the bearing, numerical simulations were conducted. The experimental conditions maintained a consistent number of shims and balls, a friction coefficient of 0.05, and a U-damper width of 60 mm. The seismic isolation bearing configurations included zero, two, four, and eight U-dampers, and hysteresis curves were generated under different

U-damper quantities. Figure 6 illustrates the hysteresis curves corresponding to various numbers of U-dampers.

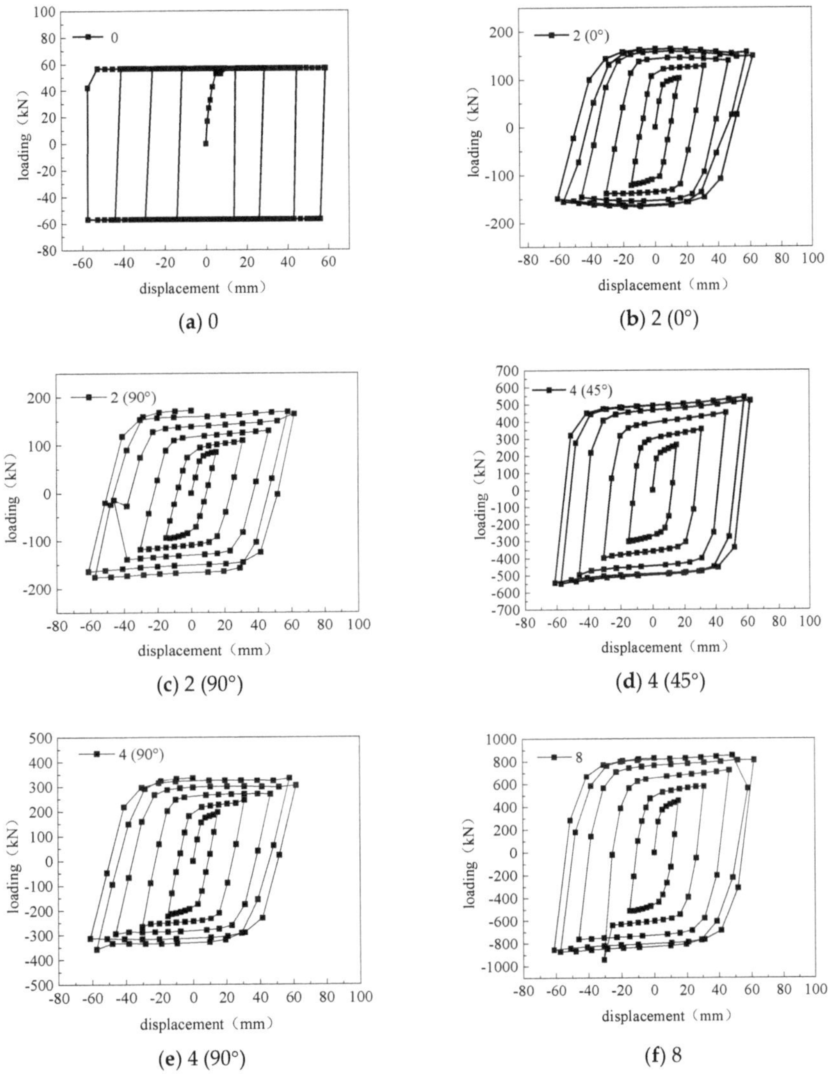

Figure 6. Hysteresis curves under the action of different numbers of U-dampers.

The hysteresis curve in Figure 6 shows that the support experiences significant slip during the stressing process when there is no U-shaped damper in action, as evidenced by the clear rectangular shape of the curve. The bearing provides almost no resistance during the loading phase, allowing slip to accumulate rapidly and potentially impacting the structural stability. During the unloading stage, residual deformation significantly impacted the overall performance of the structure due to incomplete recovery from slip-induced deformation. The addition of a U-shaped damper improved the energy dissipation capacity and stability of the support, as evidenced by the hysteresis curve changing from a rectangular to a full shuttle shape. The hysteresis curve of the bearing has a shuttle shape, which bends noticeably during both the loading and unloading phases. This indicates that the bearing can effectively absorb and dissipate energy during the stressing process, thereby enhancing the seismic performance and stability of the structure.

From a quantitative perspective, the maximum damping force exhibits a notable increase from 61.11 kN to 172.237 kN when the number of U-dampers is augmented from zero to two. This is attributed to the fact that the enhancement in stiffness resulting from the increase in the number of U-dampers implies the introduction of more energy-consuming units for energy dissipation. Subsequently, increasing the number of U-dampers from two to four leads to a further increase in the maximum damping force, from 164.545 kN to 543.278 kN. Moreover, expanding the number of dampers from four to eight yields a maximum damping force of 855.845 kN. These findings illustrate a notable upward trend in the maximum damping force of the seismic isolation bearing with an increase in the number of U-dampers. The inclusion of U-shaped dampers augments the overall energy dissipation capacity and stability of the structure by absorbing and dissipating energy under external forces, thereby enhancing the maximum damping force. This approach proves effective and pragmatic in achieving these objectives.

The maximum damping force increases from 164.545 kN to 172.237 kN when there are two dampers, indicating a slight influence of the arrangement mode on the damping force. However, with four dampers, the maximum damping force varies significantly depending on the arrangement. When distributed at a 45° angle, the maximum damping force reaches 543.278 kN, while at a 90° angle, it decreases to 336.369 kN. This suggests that a well-planned arrangement can distribute U-shaped dampers more evenly in space, reducing stress concentration and facilitating a uniform dispersion of external force among the dampers. This, in turn, enhances the efficiency of each damper, improving the stability and energy consumption capacity of the entire structure.

Based on the hysteresis curves presented in Table 3, it is evident that the quantity and arrangement of U-dampers have a substantial impact on both the hysteresis loop area and the equivalent damping ratio.

Table 3. Presents the statistics of the hysteresis curve data when subjected to varying numbers of U-dampers.

Number of Dampers	Hysteresis Loop Area (J)	Maximum Value of Displacement in the Cycle (mm)	Maximum Value of the Load during the Cycle (KN)	Equivalent Damping Ratio
0	10,019.85	58.852	61.110	0.404
2 (0°)	25,887.50	61.871	164.545	0.405
2 (90°)	28,606.36	61.872	172.237	0.427
4 (45°)	96,009.74	61.840	543.278	0.455
4 (90°)	54,508.73	61.840	336.369	0.417
8	150,495.98	61.808	855.845	0.453

Regarding the change in quantity, as the number of dampers increased from zero to two, the hysteresis loop area and equivalent damping ratio increased by 185.52% and 5.69%, respectively. Similarly, when the number of dampers increased from two to four, the hysteresis loop area and equivalent damping ratio increased by 235.62% and 6.56%, respectively. However, when the number of dampers increased from four to eight, the hysteresis loop area increased by 176.1%, but the equivalent damping ratio decreased by −0.44%. The results demonstrate that the hysteresis loop area, which is surrounded by force and displacement, shows a clear increasing trend with the addition of U-shaped dampers. This verifies that increasing the number of U-shaped dampers can effectively enhance the energy dissipation capacity of seismic isolation bearings. However, increasing the number of U-shaped dampers beyond a certain point does not increase the equivalent damping ratio. This may be due to the uneven distribution of energy dissipation caused by too many dampers, resulting in some dampers failing to fully play their role in energy dissipation.

Regarding the arrangement, when there are two U-type dampers arranged from 0° to 90°, the hysteresis loop area decreases by 9.11%, and the equivalent damping ratio increases by 9.54%. When there are four U-type dampers arranged from 45° to 90°, the hysteresis loop area decreases by 0.9%, and the equivalent damping ratio increases by 4.19%. This demonstrates that when the number of dampers is fixed, the arrangement has a relatively minor impact on the hysteresis loop area, but a more noticeable effect on the equivalent damping ratio.

Therefore, when selecting the number of U-dampers, it is important to consider not only the enhancement of the energy dissipation capacity of the seismic isolation bearing but also the influence of its arrangement on the equivalent damping ratio. This will help achieve the optimal balance between seismic isolation performance and cost. Taken together, the arrangement of four U-dampers at a 45° angle has the most outstanding performance in improving the energy dissipation and damping characteristics of the seismic isolation bearing. Therefore, it is the optimal choice for efficient energy dissipation.

4.3. *Effect of U-Damper Width on Hysteresis Curve*

Numerical simulations were conducted to investigate the impact of U-shaped damper width on the seismic isolation performance of the bearing. The U-shaped damper widths of 40 mm, 50 mm, and 60 mm were tested while keeping the number of shims and balls constant and maintaining a coefficient of friction of 0. Figure 7 shows the hysteresis curves of the vibration isolation bearings with four U-shaped dampers arranged at 90° and different widths. The figure also demonstrates the energy dissipation performance of the bearings under the action of different U-shaped damper widths.

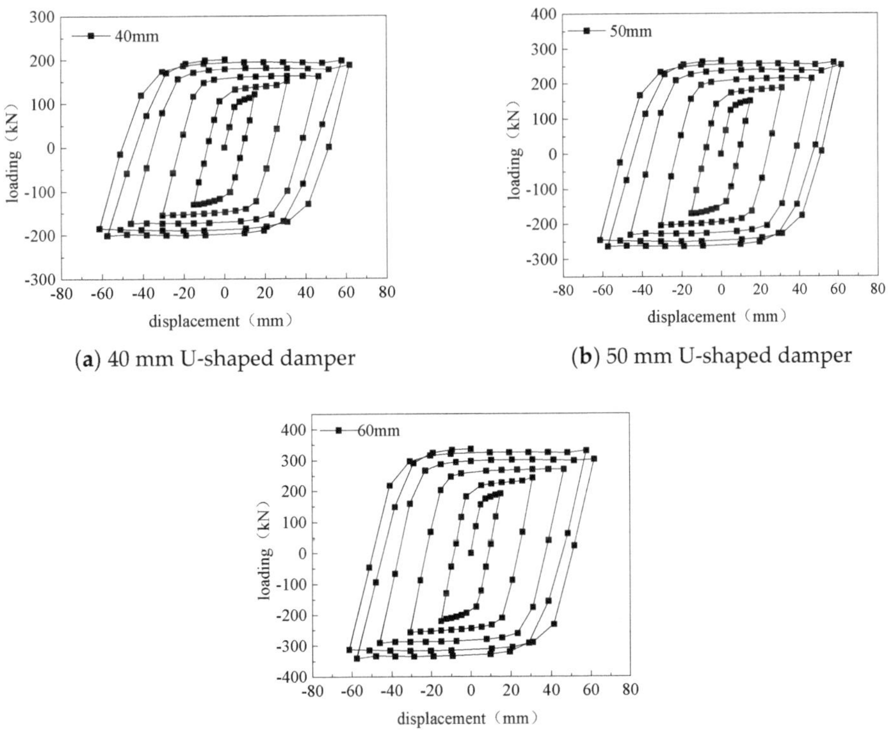

(**a**) 40 mm U-shaped damper (**b**) 50 mm U-shaped damper

(**c**) 60 mm U-shaped damper

Figure 7. Hysteresis curves under the action of different U-damper widths.

Based on the hysteresis curve in Figure 7, it is evident that the full shuttle shape is maintained regardless of the width of the U-shaped damper. This aligns with the characteristics of the elastic-plastic energy dissipation model. Increasing the width of the damper from 40 mm to 50 mm results in an increase of the maximum damping force of the seismic isolation bearing from 201.289 kN to 265.743 kN. Similarly, increasing the width from 50 mm to 60 mm results in a further increase of the maximum damping force from 265.743 kN to 336.369 kN. With an increase in damper width, the maximum damping force of the seismic isolation bearing shows a clear upward trend. This is due to the wider U-shaped damper providing a larger contact area, resulting in more material involved in the deformation and energy dissipation process, thus generating a greater damping force. Furthermore, as the damper width increases, its internal stress distribution becomes more uniform, reducing the occurrence of stress concentration, and ultimately enhancing the damper's load-carrying capacity and energy dissipation performance.

Based on the hysteresis curve data presented in Table 4, it is evident that the energy dissipation performance of the seismic isolation bearing increases significantly with the widening of the U-shaped damper. Increasing the width of the damper from 40 mm to 50 mm significantly increases the hysteresis loop area and equivalent damping ratio by 26.08% and 24.07%, respectively. This suggests that widening the damper can effectively enhance the energy dissipation capacity of the seismic isolation bearing. When the width was increased from 50 mm to 60 mm, the hysteresis loop area and equivalent damping ratio increased by 20.43% and −0.69%, respectively. This suggests that increasing the width has a positive effect on energy dissipation, but the enhancement of damping performance may gradually weaken as the width continues to increase.

Table 4. Presents the statistics of the hysteresis curve data when subjected to various U-damper widths.

Damper Width (mm)	Hysteresis Loop Area (J)	Maximum Value of Displacement in the Cycle (mm)	Maximum Value of the Load during the Cycle (KN)	Equivalent Damping Ratio
40	32,060.9	61.853	201.289	0.41
50	43,370.7	61.853	265.743	0.42
60	54,508.7	61.84	336.369	0.417

Increasing the width of the U-shaped damper is an effective strategy for enhancing the energy dissipation capacity and stability of seismic isolation bearings. After considering all factors, a width of 60 mm is recommended for the U-shaped damper. This width ensures good stability while maintaining a high energy dissipation capacity for the seismic isolation bearing.

4.4. *Effect of Number of Balls on Hysteresis Curve*

To examine the impact of the number of balls on the seismic isolation performance of the bearing, we utilized the control variable method to investigate how changes in the number of balls affect the bearing's performance. The mechanical behavior of isolation bearings with different numbers of balls was simulated in ABAQUS. Hysteresis curves were obtained to visualize the energy dissipation performance of the bearings under the action of different balls, as shown in Figure 8.

Based on the hysteresis curves in Figure 8, it is evident that the curves exhibit a complete shuttle shape when subjected to different balls, consistent with the characteristics of the elastic–plastic energy dissipation model. When the number of balls increases from zero to one, the maximum damping force decreases from 304.69 kN to 266.942 kN. This is mainly due to the intervention of the balls, which changes the contact state of the support. As a result, it becomes easier for the support to undergo relative displacement when subjected to external force, thus reducing the friction damping force. When the number of balls increases from one to four, the maximum damping force increases from 266.942 kN to

336.48 kN. This is due to the interaction between the balls, which restricts the displacement of the bearing and improves the damping force. When the number of balls increases from four to five, the maximum damping force only slightly increases from 336.48 kN to 337.794 kN. This suggests that as the number of balls increases, the enhancement of the maximum damping force gradually decreases and may even reach saturation. This is because having too many balls can complicate the transfer of energy between them, leading to the dissipation of energy in the form of heat. This can also hinder the increase of the damping force.

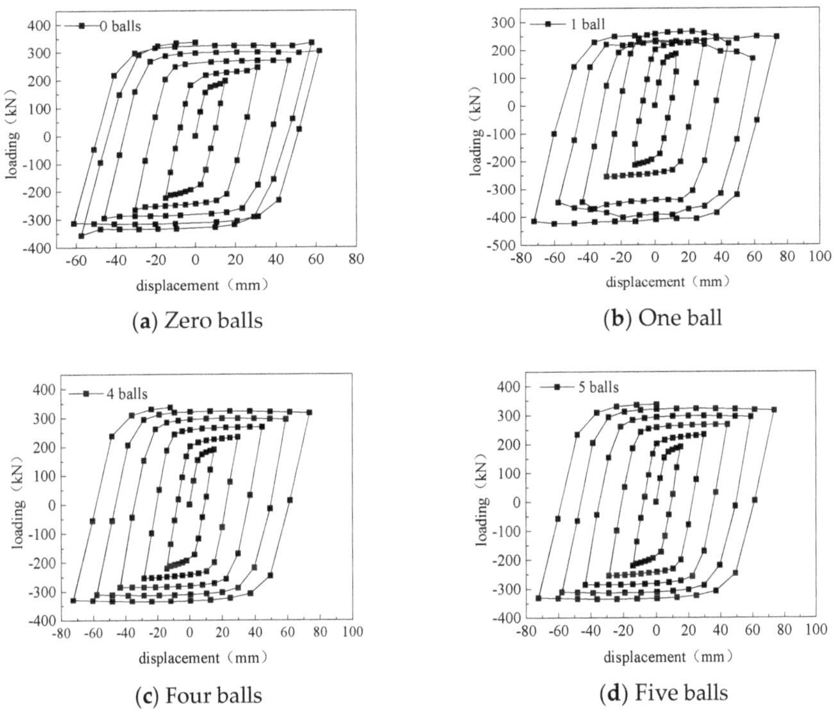

Figure 8. Hysteresis curves for different numbers of balls.

Based on the hysteresis curve data presented in Table 5, it is evident that the hysteresis loop area enclosed by force and displacement and the equivalent damping ratio exhibit an increasing-then-decreasing trend with the increase in the number of balls. When the number of balls increases from zero to one, the hysteresis loop area and equivalent damping ratio increase by 8.22% and 15.34%, respectively. This indicates that the addition of balls has a positive effect on the energy dissipation capacity of the seismic isolation bearing, which in turn effectively enhances the seismic performance of the structure. When the number of balls increased from one to four, the hysteresis loop area and equivalent damping ratio increased by 30.75% and 4.44%, respectively. This suggests that the growth rate of energy dissipation efficiency was slowing down while maintaining the energy dissipation capacity of the bearing. The interaction of the balls resulted in an increase in the loss of energy in the process of energy transfer and dissipation, which in turn lowered the energy dissipation efficiency of the bearing. When the number of balls increased from four to five, the hysteresis loop area increased by 0.46%, while the equivalent damping ratio remained almost unchanged. This suggests that after a certain number of balls, additional balls have a limited effect on the energy dissipation capacity and efficiency of the support.

Table 5. Presents the statistics of hysteresis curves obtained with varying numbers of balls.

Number of Balls	Hysteresis Loop Area (J)	Maximum Value of Displacement in the Cycle (mm)	Maximum Value of the Load during the Cycle (KN)	Equivalent Damping Ratio
0	51,284.7	61.84	304.69	0.39
1	55,499.6	73.57	266.942	0.45
4	72,567.1	73.62	336.48	0.47
5	72,900.1	73.62	337.794	0.47

When designing seismic isolation bearings, it is important to balance the number of balls with energy consumption and efficiency to achieve optimal performance. Therefore, selecting four balls is a more reasonable choice.

4.5. Effect of Number of Shims on Hysteresis Curve

According to the shape of the hysteresis curve in Figure 9 and the hysteresis curve data in Table 6, it is evident that the curve maintains a full pike shape regardless of the number of shims used. This is consistent with the characteristics of the elastic-plastic energy dissipation model. When the number of shims increases from zero to two, the maximum damping force increases from 307.794 kN to 338.599 kN. This is because the increase in the number of shims enhances the spring pre-stress, causing the ball group to share more loads and form a more effective synergistic effect with the sliding surface. When the number of shims increases from two to four, the maximum damping force decreases from 338.599 kN to 337.618 kN. Further increasing the number of shims to six results in a decrease in the maximum damping force to 337.44 kN. This decrease is due to excessive shims, which cause excessive spring prestressing. As a result, the ball group shares too much load, and the energy dissipation of the sliding surface decreases.

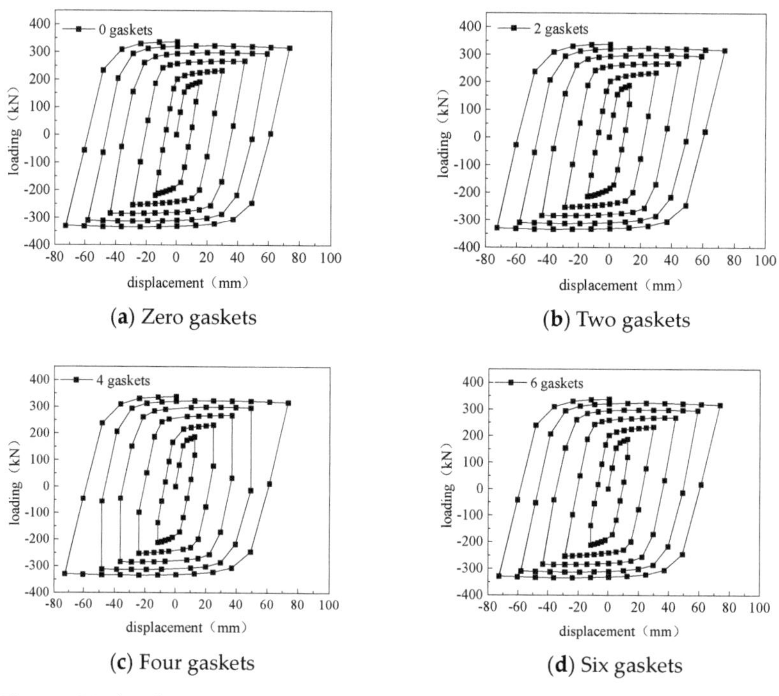

(a) Zero gaskets (b) Two gaskets

(c) Four gaskets (d) Six gaskets

Figure 9. Displays hysteresis curves for various numbers of shims.

Table 6. Statistics of hysteresis curves under different number of shims.

Number of Gaskets	Hysteresis Loop Area (J)	Maximum Value of Displacement in the Cycle (mm)	Maximum Value of the Load during the Cycle (kN)	Equivalent Damping Ratio
0	72,900.1	73.6209	307.794	0.467
2	76,806.7	73.5153	338.599	0.493
4	76,648.5	73.5101	337.618	0.492
6	76,632.2	73.5146	337.44	0.492

5. Skeleton Curve Analysis of Sliding–Rolling Friction Composite Seismic Isolation Bearings

5.1. Analysis Curves for Different Parts of the Skeleton

After analyzing the hysteresis curve data in Section 3, we plotted the variation of the skeleton curve of the isolation bearing under different parameters in Figure 10.

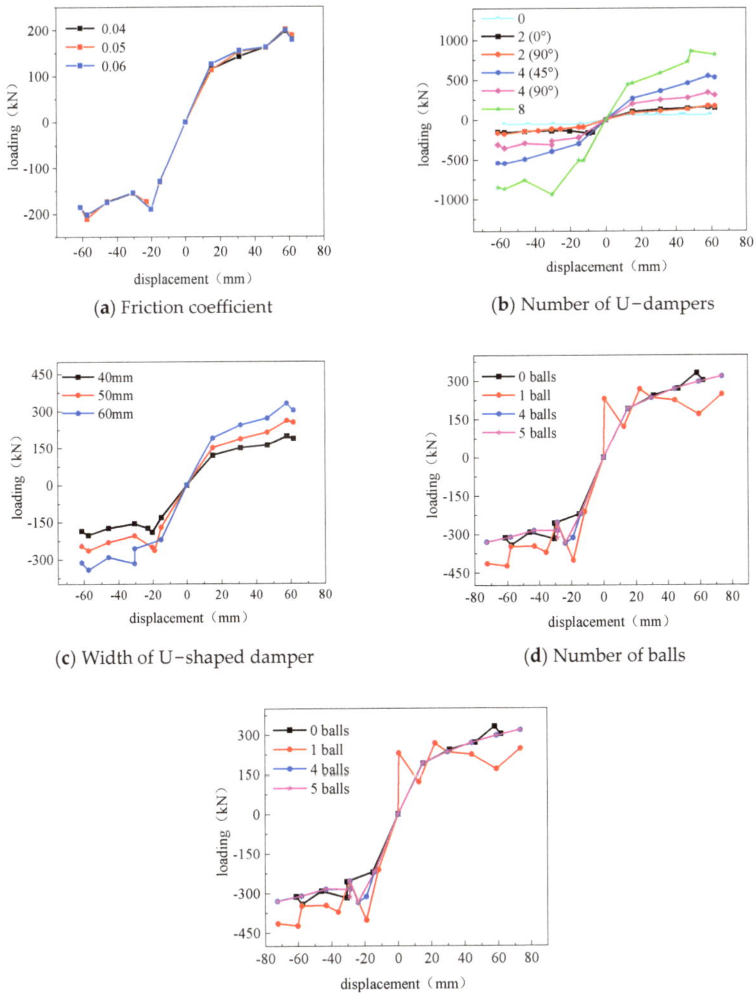

(**a**) Friction coefficient (**b**) Number of U−dampers

(**c**) Width of U−shaped damper (**d**) Number of balls

(**e**) Number of gaskets

Figure 10. Skeleton curves under different parameters.

Based on the skeleton curve presented in Figure 10, it is evident that the width and number of U-dampers, as well as the number of balls, have a more significant impact on the bearing compared to changes in the coefficient of friction and the number of shims. Therefore, when designing seismic isolation bearings, it is crucial to prioritize the width, number of U-dampers, and number of balls.

Therefore, the next step is to analyze the skeleton curve formed by the width and number of U-shaped dampers and the number of ball rollers. Then, the optimal design parameters of the seismic isolation bearing can be determined by analyzing key data indexes such as the ductility coefficient, yielding load, yielding displacement, and ultimate load under different parameters.

5.2. Analysis of the Characteristic Parameters of the Skeleton Curve

The key performance data were statistically derived from the skeleton curves provided above.

Table 7 shows the performance indexes of the bearing parameters. The ultimate load, yield load, and ductility of the seismic isolation bearings are significantly affected by the number and arrangement method of U-type dampers. In terms of quantity, the yield load, ultimate load, and ductility coefficient increased by approximately 81.89%, 119.62%, and 32.52%, respectively, when the number of dampers increased from zero to two. Similarly, when the number of dampers increased from two to four, the yield load, ultimate load, and ductility coefficient increased by approximately 156.01%, 244.08%, and 11.74%. The yield load and ductility coefficient increased by 156.01% and 244.08%, respectively, when the number was increased from four to eight. Similarly, increasing the number from four to seven significantly affected the yield load and ductility coefficients. Further increasing the number to eight increased by about 66.4% in yield load, 57.5% in ultimate load, and 9.2% in ductility coefficient. Increasing the number of dampers can effectively improve the bearing capacity and ductility of seismic isolation bearings. Regarding the arrangement, if there are two dampers, changing the arrangement can increase the yield load, ultimate load, and ductility coefficient by 20.46%, 7.52%, and 34.8%, respectively. If there are four dampers, changing the arrangement will decrease the yield load and ultimate load by 25.23% and 38.4%, respectively, but increase the ductility coefficient by 3.93%.

Table 7. Shows the performance indexes of the support's skeleton curve parameters under different numbers of U-dampers.

Number of U-Dampers	Yield Load (kN)	Ultimate Load (kN)	Yield Displacement (mm)	Limit Displacement (mm)	Ductility Factor
0	56.81	61.11	14.18	58.87	2.06
2 (0°)	103.33	134.21	15.04	46.48	2.73
2 (90°)	85.78	144.3	15.04	51.54	3.68
4 (45°)	264.54	461.8	16.33	47.5	3.05
4 (90°)	197.8	284.48	15.03	47.03	3.17
4 (45°)	440.47	727.47	15.02	46.49	3.33

To ensure stability and safety, the seismic isolation bearing must withstand and disperse horizontal seismic forces during earthquakes. It is necessary to balance the bearing capacity and deformation capacity. Based on the analysis, four U-shaped dampers arranged at 45° are the optimal parameters that meet the performance requirements and ensure the structure's safety and stability.

Based on the performance indexes of the bearing parameters presented in Table 8, it is evident that the yield load and ultimate load exhibit a significant growth trend with an increase in the width of the U-type damper. Specifically, when the damper width increases from 40 mm to 50 mm, the yield load and ultimate load increase by 24.4% and 31.5%, respectively. Similarly, when the damper width increases from 50 mm to 60 mm, the yield load and ultimate load increase by 31.3% and 28.4%, respectively.

Table 8. Shows the performance indexes of the support's skeleton curve parameters under different widths of U-dampers.

Width of U-Dampers	Yield Load (kN)	Ultimate Load (kN)	Yield Displacement (mm)	Limit Displacement (mm)	Ductility Factor
40	120.93	168.38	15.03	47.04	3.08
50	150.48	221.49	15.03	46.92	3.07
60	197.80	284.48	15.03	47.03	3.17

Increasing the damper width improves the ductility performance of seismic isolation bearings, as shown by the overall increasing trend of the ductility coefficient. It is important to note that this evaluation is objective and based solely on the data presented.

Based on the bearing and deformation capacity, the optimal choice is the U-type damper with a width of 60 mm. This damper not only enhances the seismic isolation bearing's load-bearing capacity but also maintains excellent ductility performance.

Table 9 shows the performance indexes of the bearing parameters. The number of balls has a significant impact on the yield load and ultimate load. As the number of balls increases, the ultimate load and yield load initially decrease and then increase. When the number of balls increased from zero to one, the yield and ultimate load decreased by 39.0% and 26.3%, respectively. This was due to the addition of balls, which altered the original contact state and resulted in a temporary decrease in the load-carrying capacity. When the number of balls was increased from one to four, the yield load and ultimate load increased by 57.5% and 28.5%, respectively. This indicates that the structural load-carrying capacity was effectively enhanced with the further increase in the number of balls. When increasing the number of balls from four to five, the yield load and ultimate load increased only slightly. This suggests that the load-carrying capacity is gradually weakened by increasing the number of balls to a certain extent.

Table 9. Shows the performance indexes of the support's skeleton curve parameters under different number of balls.

Number of Balls	Yield Load (kN)	Ultimate Load (kN)	Yield Displacement (mm)	Limit Displacement (mm)	Ductility Factor
0	197.80	284.48	15.03	47.03	3.17
1	120.88	209.49	12.63	43.56	4.16
4	190.83	269.25	15.07	44.35	3.00
5	192.04	269.31	15.07	44.41	3.00

The ductility coefficient shows an increasing and then decreasing effect with the increase in the number of balls. Specifically, from zero to one ball, the ductility coefficient increased by 14.5%, indicating a positive effect of adding a ball. However, when the number of balls increased from one to four, the ductility coefficient decreased by 5.36%, suggesting that a further increase in the number of balls may not always be favorable to the ductility coefficient. Notably, there is almost no difference in the ductility coefficient when the number of balls is four and five.

Based on the comprehensive performance index, the optimal parameter for the number of balls is four. This maintains a high load-carrying capacity while also allowing for good deformation ability.

To ensure a comprehensive analysis, this paper suggests designing the optimal parameters of the sliding–rolling friction composite isolation bearing as follows: a friction coefficient of 0.04, four U-shaped dampers arranged at 45° with a width of 60 mm, four ball rollers, and two shims.

6. Conclusions

According to the concept of performance-based seismic engineering, the seismic loss analysis of eccentrically braced steel frame structures is of great significance for the selection of structural layout. In this paper, different forms of eccentrically braced steel frame structures are designed, which are K-shaped, V-shaped, and D-shaped, respectively, and the vulnerability of the structure and earthquake loss are studied. The main conclusions are as follows.

This study established a model for a sliding–rolling friction composite seismic isolation bearing using ABAQUS software. The model was optimized and analyzed for parameters such as friction coefficient, width of U-dampers, number of U-dampers, number of balls, and number of shims using the method of control variables. After comparing performance indexes, such as hysteresis loop shape, area, and equivalent damping ratio, it is concluded that the width and number of U-dampers, as well as the number of balls, are the key factors that affect the performance of seismic isolation bearings.

The study analyzes the effects of the number of U-shaped dampers, width, and number of balls on the performance of seismic isolation bearings. The characteristic parameters in the skeleton curves are extracted, and key performance indexes such as yield load, ultimate load, and ductility coefficient are compared. This analysis aims to determine the optimal design parameters of the seismic isolation bearings. The recommended parameters for this system are a friction coefficient of 0.04, four U-shaped dampers with a width of 60 mm arranged at a 45° angle, four balls, and two shims.

Author Contributions: Conceptualization, Y.L.; Methodology, J.L.; Software, B.L.; Validation, J.C.; Formal analysis, W.Z.; Investigation, Q.M.; Resources, Q.M.; Writing—original draft, Y.L.; Writing—review & editing, J.L. and B.L. All authors have read and agreed to the published version of the manuscript.

Funding: This research received no external funding.

Data Availability Statement: Data is contained within the article.

Conflicts of Interest: The authors declare that they have no known competing financial interests or personal relationships that could have appeared to influence the work reported in this paper.

References

1. Lin, X. Seismic Performance Analysis of Frame Structures Using Seismic Isolation Technology. Master's Thesis, Southeast University, Nanjing, China, 2019.
2. Liu, W.; Zhou, F.; Zhong, X.; Bai, Y. Study on various related properties and long-term performance of lead-core laminated rubber seismic isolation pads. *J. South China Constr. Inst.* **1999**, 12–20.
3. Yang, L.; Liu, Y.; Chang, Y.; Cheng, C.; Sun, F. Global patent analysis of seismic isolation bearing technology. *Eng. Seism. Reinf. Retrofit.* **2018**, *40*, 7–12.
4. Yang, L.; Sun, F.; Chang, Y.; Cheng, C. Study on the patent status of building seismic isolation bearing in China. *Eng. Seism. Reinf. Retrofit.* **2018**, *40*, 1–6.
5. Li, J. Comparison of Seismic Response Analysis of Frame Structures with Different Isolation Schemes. Master's Thesis, Shandong University of Architecture, Jinan, China, 2020.
6. Jin, J.; Huang, X.; Zhong, X.; Shen, Z. Study on the value of stiffness before yielding of lead core rubber bearing (LRB) in seismic isolation design. *J. Guangzhou Univ. (Nat. Sci. Ed.)* **2006**, 63–67.
7. Wang, B.; Tan, P.; Xu, K.; Zhou, F.; Ning, L. Experimental study on mechanical properties of new fiber reinforced engineering plastic plate sandwich rubber isolation bearing. *J. Civ. Eng.* **2012**, *45*, 187–191.
8. Zayas, V.A.; Low, S.S.; Mahin, S.A. A Simple Pendulum Technique for Achieving Seismic Isolation. *Earthq. Spectra* **1990**, *6*, 317–333. [CrossRef]
9. Quaglini, V.; Gandelli, E.; Dubini, P. Experimental investigation of the re-centring capability of curved surface sliders. *Struct. Control. Health Monit.* **2017**, *24*, e1870. [CrossRef]
10. Fenz, D.M.; Constantinou, M.C. Behaviour of the double concave Friction Pendulum bearing. *Earthq. Eng. Struct. Dyn.* **2006**, *35*, 1403–1424. [CrossRef]

11. Wang, Q.T. Analysis of Vibration Damping Performance of Lead-Core Steel Pipe Seismic Isolation Bearing with Stiffening Ring. Master's Thesis, Jilin University of Architecture, Changchun, China, 2022.
12. Harvey, P.S.; Wiebe, R.; Gavin, H.P. On the chaotic response of a nonlinear rolling isolation system. *Phys. D Nonlinear Phenom.* **2013**, *256–257*, 36–42. [CrossRef]
13. Zhang, J.; Jia, J. Research on the seismic isolation effect of the ring spring–friction pendulum bearing in the dakai underground subway station. *Appl. Sci.* **2023**, *13*, 7093. [CrossRef]
14. Sheng, T.; Liu, G.B.; Bian, X.C.; Shi, W.X.; Chen, Y. Development of a three-directional vibration isolator for buildings subject to metro and earthquake-induced vibrations. *Eng. Struct.* **2022**, *252*, 113576. [CrossRef]
15. Han, J.; Guo, Z.; Li, M.; Li, L.; Hou, B.; Du, X. Nonlinear seismic response of free-field soil under longitudinal non-uniform seismic excitations. *Rock Soil Mech.* **2019**, *40*, 2581–2592.

buildings

MDPI

Article

Study on Seismic Behavior of Different Forms of Eccentrically Braced Steel Frames

Bo Liu [1,*], Yankai Lu [1], Weitao Li [1], Jiayue Li [1], Jingchen Zhao [2,*], Shuhe Wang [2], Guowei Ni [1] and Qingjuan Meng [3]

[1] College of Civil and Architectural Engineering, North China University of Science and Technology, Tangshan 063000, China; luyankai1999@outlook.com (Y.L.); lwt1999123@outlook.com (W.L.); lijiayue@ncst.edu.cn (J.L.); tjngw@126.com (G.N.)
[2] School of Civil and Resource Engineering, University of Science and Technology Beijing, Beijing 100083, China; wangshuhe2001@163.com
[3] School of Civil Engineering, Tangshan University, Tangshan 063000, China; mqjmqj2728@126.com
* Correspondence: liubo203@outlook.com (B.L.); liubo19840311@ncst.edu.cn (J.Z.)

Abstract: The arrangement of eccentric bracing has a significant impact on the seismic performance of structures. However, there is no further stipulation on different forms of eccentric bracing in the current Chinese code. At the same time, there is a lack of research on the seismic loss of eccentrically braced structures by Chinese domestic scholars. Therefore, this paper designs different forms of eccentrically braced frames and analyzes them according to the concept of seismic engineering based on performance, which provides some reference for the selection of the eccentrically braced steel frame structure layout in future engineering practice. In this paper, K-shaped, V-shaped, and D-shaped eccentrically braced steel frame structures with 3, 5, and 8 floors are designed, and the finite element analysis model is used for static napping and dynamic time history analysis. The results show that the K-shaped eccentrically braced structure has the best performance in bearing capacity and stiffness and has good seismic and collapse resistance performance. In the FEMA P-58 seismic assessment and vulnerability assessment, it is found that the V-shaped eccentrically braced structure has the smallest loss. However, it is necessary to fully consider the acceleration sensitivity of the non-structural components in the design. In general, the seismic performance of the eccentrically braced structure is improved by the energy dissipation beam yielding to consume energy, which provides a useful reference for structural design.

Keywords: eccentric braces; vulnerability; structural response; seismic loss

1. Introduction

With the rapid development of China's economy, the sharp increase in steel production capacity has played an important role in driving China's domestic GDP, which has made structural steel popular as a sustainable construction material. The steel structure system is widely used in high-rise and super high-rise buildings, including the bending steel frame, central braced steel frame, eccentrically braced steel frame, etc. The eccentrically braced structure can provide good ductility and seismic resistance and is considered an economical and effective choice for a wide range of applications. Eccentrically braced steel frame structures combine the advantages of pure steel frames to provide good ductility and sufficient energy dissipation capacity with the advantage of the high stiffness of centrally braced steel frames [1–3], sing the controllable energy dissipation beam yield to achieve seismic energy consumption [4]. In order to achieve good seismic performance of eccentrically braced structures, it is necessary to reasonably set up the form of eccentrically braced structures according to the characteristics of the structural system. In this regard, scholars at home and abroad have carried out a series of studies (Yu Anlin et al. [5]; Qian Jiaru et al. [6]; Bosco and Rossi et al. [7]; Wang Feng et al. [8]; Tian Xiaohong et al. [9,10]; Li Shen et al. [11]). Yasin O. Ozkılıc et al. [12–16] conducted a series of studies on the shear links of eccentrically supported frame structures. They performed a comprehensive numerical analysis and experimental exploration of shear links. The drift ability and service life of the shear links are improved, and the performance of the eccentric frame structure is optimized. These studies have deepened the understanding of the energy dissipation characteristics of different forms of eccentrically braced structures.

At the same time, in seismic design codes across various countries, the traditional design standard of "minor earthquakes do not cause damage, moderate earthquakes are reparable, and major earthquakes do not cause collapse" is widely adopted, showcasing a hierarchical approach to seismic design. For example, the "Code for Seismic Design of buildings" GB50011-2010 [17] and the American "International Building Code" IBC [18] are all based on this concept. Buildings designed according to the above approach can effectively mitigate overall structural collapse. They also minimize casualties during severe earthquakes within the building. However, it is powerless to the direct or indirect economic loss caused by the earthquake disaster. In recent years, several destructive earthquakes have revealed the limitations of conventional seismic design methods. Performance-based earthquake engineering (PBEE) has emerged in our field as a response to these challenges. Aslani et al. [19] took many factors as random variables and considered the influence of non-structural members on earthquake loss. Mitrani-Reiser et al. [20] and Ye Shanshan et al. [21] studied the seismic performance of the structure from the perspective of direct and indirect economic loss caused by the earthquake. Zareian et al. [22] and Ramirez et al. [23] all put forward a single building loss assessment method from the floor level. Gobbo et al. [24], Zeng Xiang et al. [25], Zhu Hanbo et al. [26], and Yandeng et al. [27] used the FEMA P-58 assessment method to assess the loss of different forms of structures.

The arrangement of eccentric bracing has a significant impact on the seismic performance of structures. However, there are no further regulations on different forms of eccentric bracing in current Chinese specifications [17,28,29]. Therefore, discussing the arrangement forms of eccentric bracing is necessary; it helps in finding more reasonable layouts, aiming to reduce the structural response and enhance the seismic performance of structures. At the same time, the research on the earthquake loss of eccentrically braced structures is also lacking. Therefore, different forms of eccentrically braced steel frames are designed in this paper. According to the concept of seismic engineering based on performance, a seismic loss analysis is carried out, which provides some reference for the selection of eccentrically braced steel frame structure layouts in future engineering practice.

2. Structural Design Modeling

2.1. Results of Structural Design

The seismic performance of eccentrically braced structures is investigated in this study, adhering strictly to the provisions outlined in Code for Seismic Design of buildings [17] and Steel structure Design Standard [28]. Three sets of examples are designed, consisting of buildings with three floors, five floors, and eight stories, respectively. Each group of examples includes K-shaped, V-shaped, and D-shaped eccentrically braced structures, for a total of nine structural models. It is assumed that all the structural models studied in this paper are office buildings.

In each group of examples, the plane layout of the three eccentrically braced frames is the same, as shown in Figure 1. The structure name and elevation layout are shown in Figure 2 (taking the elevation layout of three types of models 3K, 5V, and 8D as an example, the different elevations of the same type of model are similar). The structural calculation example is classified as Class B for seismic fortification, with an importance factor of 1.1 and a design life of 50 years. It is fortified against an intensity of 8 degrees, with a design acceleration of 0.2 g, falling under Seismic Grade II and Site Soil Category II. The system incorporates a damping ratio of 0.04 and a period reduction coefficient of 0.85, categorized within the second seismic design group with a characteristic period of 0.4 s. Frame columns and frame beams are made of Q345 low-alloy steel. The energy dissipation beam section and the support section are made of Q235 low-alloy steel. The floor and roof panels are C30 concrete. According to building structure load code GB 50009-2012 [30], the permanent and live loads for roof and floor surface stories are both 5 kN/m^2 and 2 kN/m^2, respectively. Considering door and window openings and infill walls, the load on the beam is taken as 6 kN/m. The permanent and live loads are converted to loads on the beam, which are 36 kN/m and 14.4 kN/m, respectively. The floor is an ordinary concrete floor with a thickness of 120 mm. The uniform load on the beam is converted to 21 KN/m. The rough category of the site is Class B. The basic wind pressure is 0.45 KN/m^2. The section dimensions of each component are shown in Tables 1–3.

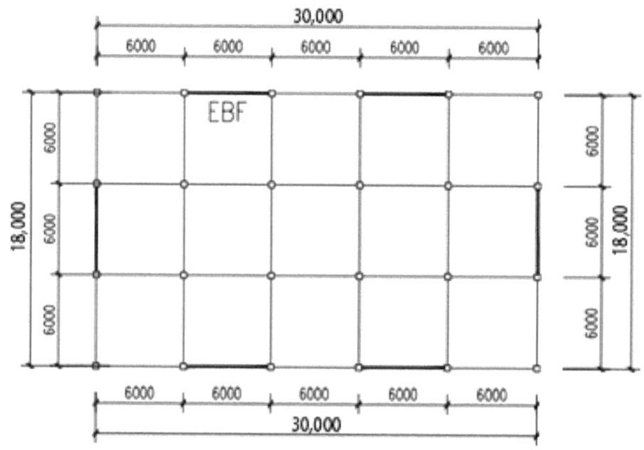

Figure 1. Structural layout plan (unit: mm).

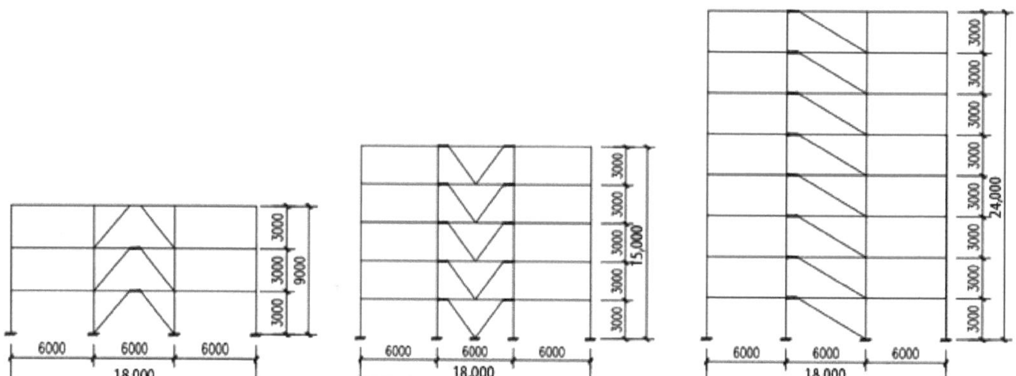

Model-3K Model-5V Model-8D

Figure 2. Elevation layout of example structure (unit: mm).

Table 1. Section size (mm) of each member of a 3-story example.

Floor	Frame Column	Frame Beam	Energy Dissipation Beam Section	Braced	$\rho = e/k$
3	300 × 300 × 18	H380 × 180 × 10 × 16	H380 × 180 × 10 × 16	H220 × 220 × 10 × 16	1.20
2	320 × 320 × 20	H400 × 200 × 10 × 16	H400 × 180 × 10 × 16	H220 × 220 × 10 × 16	1.18
1	320 × 320 × 20	H400 × 200 × 10 × 16	H400 × 180 × 10 × 16	H220 × 220 × 10 × 16	1.18

Table 2. Section size (mm) of each member of a 5-story example.

Floor	Frame Column	Frame Beam	Energy Dissipation Beam Section	Braced	$\rho = e/k$
5	300 × 300 × 18	H400 × 180 × 10 × 16	H400 × 180 × 10 × 16	H220 × 220 × 8 × 12	1.18
4	300 × 300 × 18	H400 × 180 × 10 × 16	H400 × 180 × 10 × 16	H220 × 220 × 8 × 12	1.18
3	400 × 400 × 20	H470 × 200 × 10 × 16	H420 × 180 × 10 × 16	H250 × 250 × 10 × 16	1.17
2	400 × 400 × 20	H470 × 200 × 10 × 16	H470 × 180 × 10 × 16	H250 × 250 × 10 × 16	1.06
1	400 × 400 × 20	H470 × 200 × 10 × 16	H470 × 180 × 10 × 16	H250 × 250 × 10 × 16	1.06

Table 3. Section size (mm) of each member of an 8-story example.

Floor	Frame Column	Frame Beam	Energy Dissipation Beam Section	Braced	$\rho = e/k$
8	450 × 450 × 20	H400 × 200 × 10 × 16	H400 × 180 × 10 × 16	H220 × 220 × 8 × 12	1.18
7	450 × 450 × 20	H400 × 200 × 10 × 16	H400 × 180 × 10 × 16	H220 × 220 × 8 × 12	1.18
6	500 × 500 × 20	H450 × 200 × 10 × 16	H450 × 180 × 10 × 16	H250 × 250 × 10 × 16	1.07
5	500 × 500 × 20	H450 × 200 × 10 × 16	H450 × 180 × 10 × 16	H250 × 250 × 10 × 16	1.07
4	500 × 500 × 20	H450 × 200 × 10 × 16	H450 × 180 × 10 × 16	H250 × 250 × 10 × 16	1.07
3	550 × 550 × 20	H550 × 240 × 10 × 16	H500 × 200 × 10 × 16	H280 × 280 × 12 × 18	1.03
2	550 × 550 × 20	H550 × 240 × 10 × 16	H500 × 200 × 10 × 16	H280 × 280 × 12 × 18	1.03
1	550 × 550 × 20	H550 × 240 × 10 × 16	H500 × 200 × 10 × 16	H280 × 280 × 12 × 18	1.03

2.2. Establishment of SAP2000 Finite Element Model

The model of the example structure is established according to reference [31] in the finite element program SAP2000. When modeling, the beam and column are selected for beam unit simulation. As reported by FEMA 356 [32], for the frame column, considering the coupling between the axial force and the bending moment, the default P-M2-M3 hinge is adopted. Because the plastic area of the beam and column is mainly concentrated at the end of the member, the plastic hinges are arranged at 0.1 L and 0.9 L (L is the length of the beam and column member). For the braced, the default Axial-P hinge is defined in this paper, which is arranged at 0.5 L (L is the length of the inclined bar) at the midpoint of the inclined bar. When setting the specific parameters of the shear hinge in SAP2000, the yield strength is the shear yield strength of the material, the shear ultimate strength is 1.6 times the yield strength, and the corresponding plastic strain-strengthening section length is 18 times the yield displacement. Tables 4–8 present the initial three modal characteristics of Model-3K, Model-5K, Model-5V, Model-5D, and Model-8K.

Table 4. Model-3K modal characteristics.

Mode No.	Period (s)	Angle	Translational Coefficient	Torsion Coefficient
1	0.4474	90.00	1.00	0.00
2	0.3491	0.00	1.00	0.00
3	0.2813	0.00	0.00	1.00

Table 5. Model-5K modal characteristics.

Mode No.	Period (s)	Angle	Translational Coefficient	Torsion Coefficient
1	0.6534	90.00	1.00	0.00
2	0.5122	0.00	1.00	0.00
3	0.4135	0.00	0.00	1.00

Table 6. Model-5D modal characteristics.

Mode No.	Period (s)	Angle	Translational Coefficient	Torsion Coefficient
1	0.7169	90.00	1.00	0.00
2	0.5751	0.00	1.00	0.00
3	0.4678	0.00	0.00	1.00

Table 7. Model-5V modal characteristics.

Mode No.	Period (s)	Angle	Translational Coefficient	Torsion Coefficient
1	0.6967	90.00	1.00	0.00
2	0.5546	0.00	1.00	0.00
3	0.4510	0.00	0.00	1.00

Table 8. Model-8K modal characteristics.

Mode No.	Period (s)	Angle	Translational Coefficient	Torsion Coefficient
1	1.0137	90.00	1.00	0.00
2	0.8086	0.00	1.00	0.00
3	0.6564	0.00	0.00	1.00

The ratio of the 1st torsional mode period to the 1st translational mode period for each structure is 0.63, 0.63, 0.65, 0.64, and 0.65, respectively. These values are all below the requirement specified in the technical specifications for the steel structures of tall buildings [29], which state that the ratio should not exceed 0.9. This indicates that the layout of each structure is reasonable and capable of effectively resisting lateral forces. From the structural modal period, it is known that the structural period varies with the change in structural form, but when the design parameters of the structure are the same, such as the length of the energy dissipation beam, beam–column bracing section, floor height, and number of floors, the periods of different forms of eccentrically braced structures are basically the same, indicating that the lateral stiffness is basically the same.

3. Pushover Analyses

A pushover analysis is a kind of static elastoplastic analysis combined with a response spectrum. In this method, a certain horizontal lateral load loading mode is adopted, and step-by-step increases in the horizontal lateral load are applied to the structure to push the structure to a target state or until the structure collapses. The deformation and internal forces of the structure are obtained, the elastic–plastic performance and lateral resistance of the structure are analyzed, and then the seismic performance is evaluated.

A pushover analysis is conducted on the designed structure. Horizontal loads are applied with an inverted triangle distribution during the analysis. Bi-directional analysis is used in this paper. The horizontal force is assumed to act in two orthogonal directions, the X-direction and the Y-direction. Because the stiffness of each eccentrically braced structure in the YZ plane is small and the longitudinal seismic capacity is weak, this paper only analyzes the unfavorable Y-direction. In the pushover analysis, the plastic hinge is rigid plastic and there is no elastic behavior. This is mainly because the pushover analysis aims to evaluate the structure's performance under ultimate loads, rather than considering its elastic behavior. In this paper, the end of the straight phase on the pushover capacity curve is considered the yield point of the structure. Before this, the whole structure is in the elastic state; afterwards, the energy dissipation beam segment begins to enter the elastoplastic phase. When the deformation of the plastic hinge reaches the maximum, unloading begins immediately, the structural stiffness decreases, and a steep drop occurs in the pushover capacity curve. In China's seismic code, the inter-story drift angle of the structure shall not be more than 1/50. Therefore, in this paper, the maximum inter-story drift angle of the structure of 0.02 is taken as the limit state of the pushover analysis.

3.1. Pushover Capacity Curve

For the structural example, the horizontal load with an inverted triangle distribution is applied, and only the first vibration mode and the seismic action dominated by shear deformation are analyzed by pushover. The pushover capacity curve is shown in Figures 3–5.

As can be seen from the pushover capacity curve, under the conditions of the same number of stories and component sections, the K-shaped eccentrically braced structure has the highest bearing capacity and stiffness. Followed by the V-shaped eccentrically braced structure, and with the increase in the number of floors, the difference becomes greater and greater. For the eccentrically braced structures of the same form, the bearing capacity and stiffness of the structure decrease with the increase in the number of floors. The trend of elastic–plastic development of each structure is basically the same. In the initial elastic phase, the bottom shear force and the top drift have a linear relationship. Subsequently, each structure goes into the elastoplastic stage, and the shear growth at the bottom slows down. Meanwhile, the top drift develops rapidly and eventually the structure reaches failure.

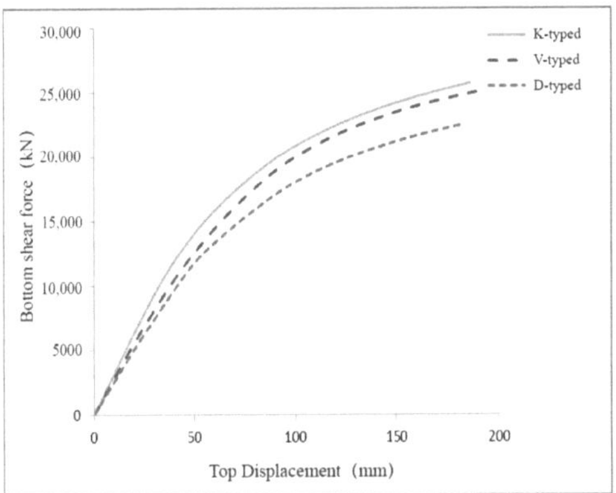

Figure 3. 3-story example pushover curve.

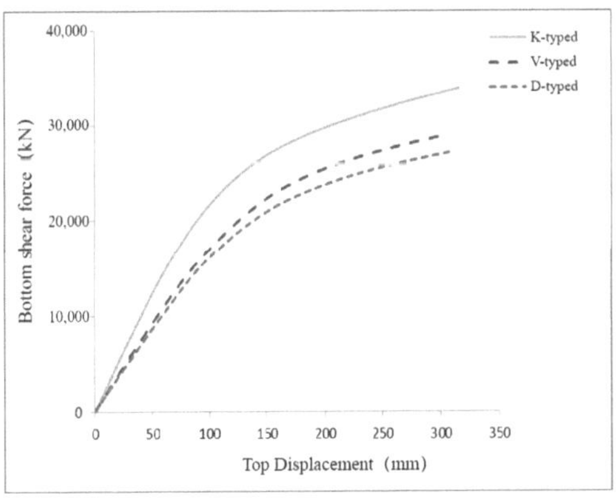

Figure 4. 5-story example pushover curve.

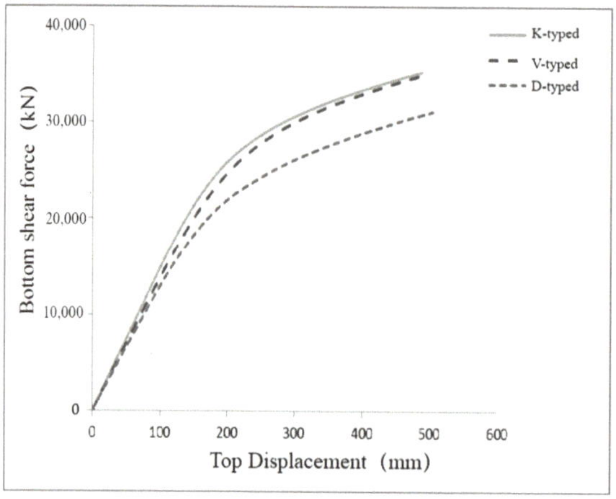

Figure 5. 8-story example pushover curve.

3.2. Structural Deformation Results

On the pushover capacity curve, we can obtain the corresponding performance points under small earthquakes and large earthquakes. Through the performance points and the deformation of different structures under different seismic strengths, we can judge whether the deformation of a structure under a particular seismic strength conforms to the provisions of the specifications. The inter-story drift angles of different structures under minor and major earthquakes are depicted in Figures 6–8.

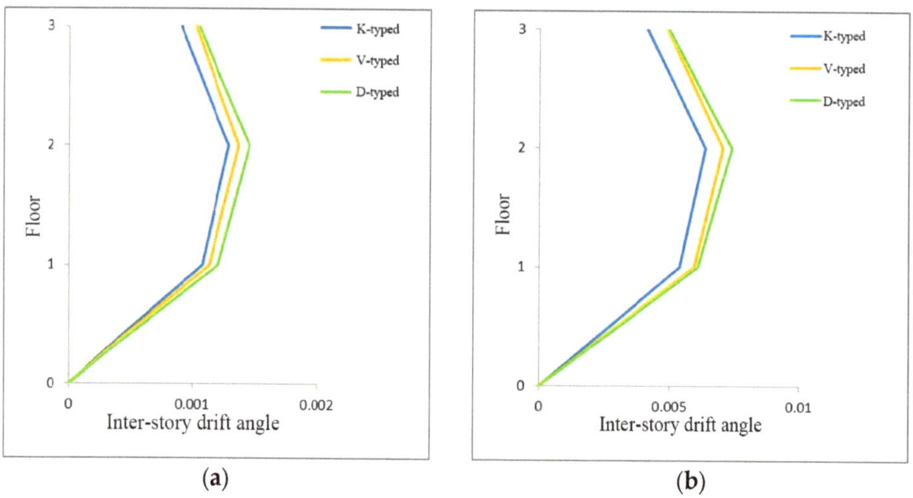

Figure 6. Inter-story drift angle analysis of 3-story examples. (**a**) Minor earthquake; (**b**) Major earthquake.

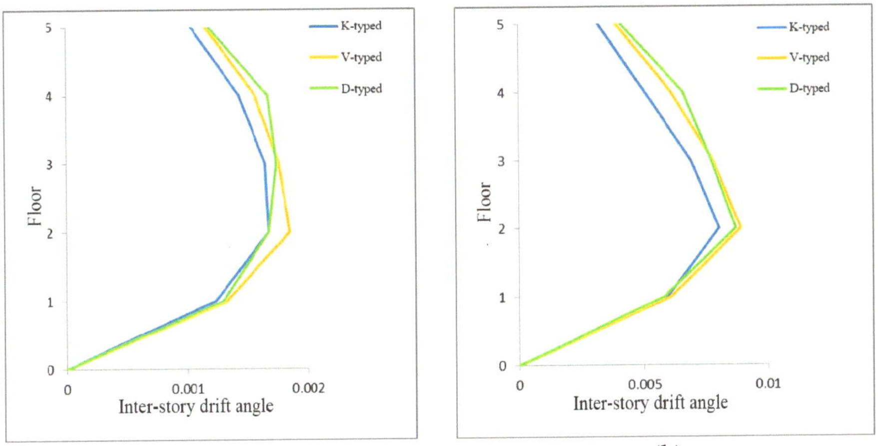

(a) (b)

Figure 7. Inter-story drift angle analysis of 5-story examples. (**a**) Minor earthquake; (**b**) Major earthquake.

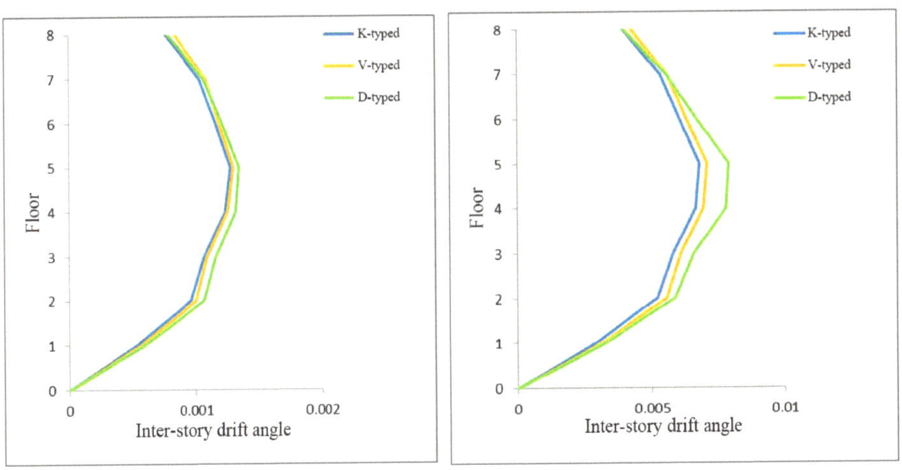

(a) (b)

Figure 8. Inter-story drift angle analysis of 8-story examples. (**a**) Minor earthquake; (**b**) Major earthquake.

In China, the limit of the inter-story drift angles of a steel structure under minor earthquakes is 1/250, and under major earthquakes is 1/50. As can be seen from the figure, the maximum inter-story drift angle of each structure under minor and major earthquakes meets the provisions of the Chinese resistance regulations and is far less than the specified limit requirements. Therefore, it can be proved that different forms of eccentrically braced structures have good seismic performance. Secondly, it can be seen that the largest inter-story drift angles of the K-shaped eccentrically braced structure are relatively small. This is also the reason why the pushover capacity curve of the K-shaped eccentric support structure is always located in the outermost story of the capacity curve of the three structural forms. At the same time, through the comparison of the results of the inter-story drift angle analysis, it can be clearly seen that the minimum inter-story drift angles of each structure appear in the bottom story of the structure. This shows that the bottom frame column of the structure has sufficient lateral stiffness, which can effectively prevent the appearance of a weak story at the bottom of the structure. The eccentric support structure can meet the expected goal of structural seismic design, has good seismic performance, and can be applied to engineering practice.

3.3. Development of Plastic Hinge under Pushover Analysis

Under the action of minor earthquakes, the structures are still in the elastic state, and no plastic hinges appear. When pushing to the major earthquake and limit state, taking the eight-story structure model as an example, the plastic hinge development of different structures is shown in Figures 9–11. B (pink) indicates the yield of the plastic hinge, C (yellow) indicates that the plastic hinge begins to lose its bearing capacity, and between B and C, IO (blue), LS (light blue), and CP (green) indicate the performance states of the plastic hinge for immediate occupancy, life safety, and collapse prevention, respectively.

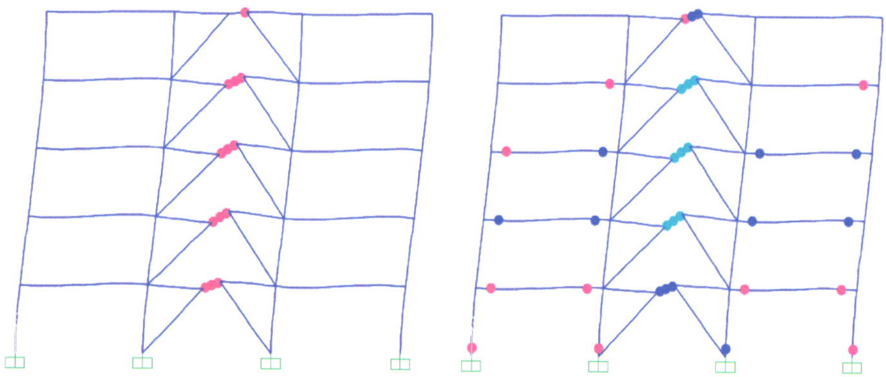
(a) (b)

Figure 9. Distribution of plastic hinges in 5-story K-shaped eccentrically braced structures. (**a**) Major earthquake; (**b**) Ultimate limit state.

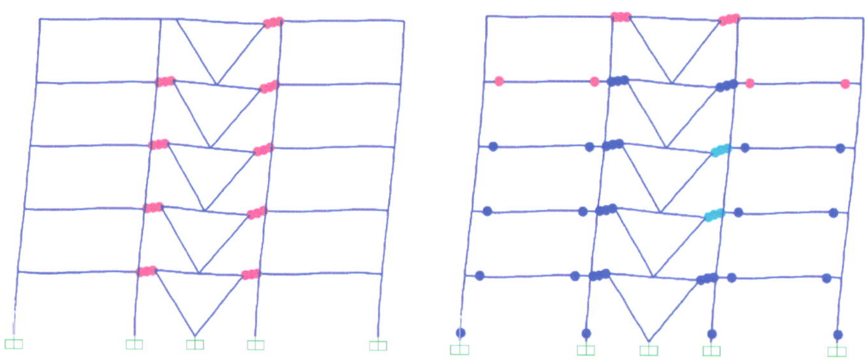
(a) (b)

Figure 10. Distribution of plastic hinges in 5-story V-shaped eccentrically braced structures. (**a**) Major earthquake; (**b**) Ultimate limit state.

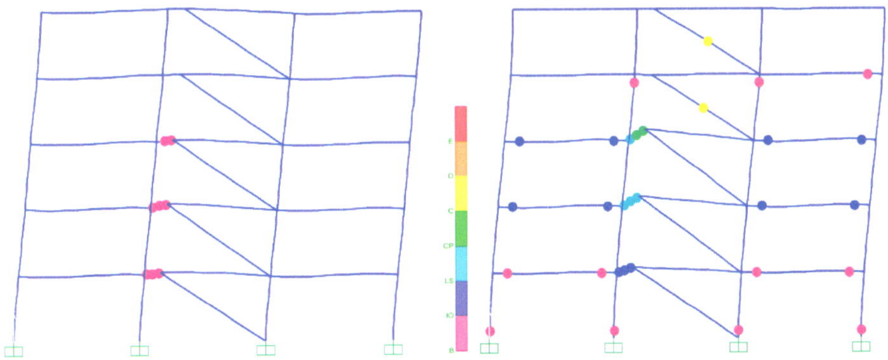

(a) (b)

Figure 11. Distribution of plastic hinges in 5-story D-shaped eccentrically braced structures. (**a**) Major earthquake; (**b**) Ultimate limit state.

From the pushover analysis, the plastic hinge development process of each structure is pushed to the rare earthquake and limit state, it can be seen that the plastic hinge development of different forms of eccentrically braced structures is basically the same. The energy dissipation beam section of the structure is the first line of defense against earthquakes. It first yields and enters the elastoplastic phase. In the process of structural yield, the energy dissipation beam section of each floor basically yields. The failure mode of the energy dissipation beam section is the shear yield type. In the shear yield of the web, the full section of the energy-consuming beam reaches the plastic state. Therefore, the plastic hinge development states of different positions of the energy dissipation beam section are the same. The frame beam of the structure is the second line of defense against earthquakes. The plastic hinge also begins to appear later, into the elastoplastic stage. When the structure is pushed to the limit state, the plastic hinge appears in the position of the structural column foot, which indicates that the structure has completed its yield. The whole yield process satisfies the traditional design concept of "strong column and weak beam". At the same time, the failure mechanism of the structure is transformed into the energy dissipation beam segment to the frame beam, and then to the frame column. This is precisely due to the eccentric support structure. In this way, the overall yield mechanism is satisfied, and the desired failure mode is achieved. This shows that the eccentric support structure has reasonable multiple seismic defense lines, so it is appropriate to use the eccentric support frame system in strong earthquake areas.

4. Response Analysis of Structural Ground Motion

4.1. Quantification of Structural Performance Index

To evaluate the exceedance probability of the structure's vulnerability in a damaged state, structural performance indicators must be established and quantified. In order to establish the performance index, it is essential to define a set of reference seismic fortification levels. Table 9 shows the fortification level of resistance in our country. In FEMA P-58 [33–35], the inter-story drift angle and inter-story drift acceleration are used to reflect the demand parameters of different components. Through experiment and theoretical analysis [36], it is found that the inter-story drift angle can reflect the deformation of inter-story members and the height of the floor well, and can reflect the damage state of the structure more intuitively. It is consistent with the checking calculation of the inter-story drift in the Code for Seismic Design of Buildings [17]. Therefore, the inter-story drift angle and floor acceleration are selected as the evaluation indexes of structural performance in this paper. The control target of the maximum inter-story drift angle of multi-story steel frame structures in China is shown in Table 10.

Table 9. Seismic design ground motion level in Code for Seismic Design of Buildings.

Earthquake Fortification Level	Frequent Earthquake (Minor Earthquake)	Basic Earthquake (Moderate Earthquake)	Rare Earthquake (Major Earthquake)	Extremely Rare Earthquake (Extreme Earthquake)
50-year exceedance probability	63%	10%	2%	0.1%
return period	50	475	2475	10,000

Table 10. Maximum inter-story drift angle limit in Code for Seismic Design of Buildings.

Performance Level	Intact	Slight Damage	Moderate Damage	Serious Damage
Limit regulation	1/300	1/200	1/100	1/55

At present, there is no unified standard for quantifying the index of eccentrically braced steel structures. Therefore, the performance of the eccentric support structure can be quantified by referring to the relevant example in Appendix M in the Code for Seismic Design of Buildings [17]: "when it is necessary to determine the service performance according to the seismic residual deformation, the inter-story drift reference index with different performance requirements". In this paper, the performance of eccentrically braced structures is divided into four levels: normal use (NO), immediate use (IO), life safety (LS), and collapse prevention (CP), as shown in Table 11. Taking the damage limit value of the performance level as the limit, the damage degree of the structure can be divided into five types. The five levels are intact, slightly damaged, moderately damaged, severely damaged, and collapsed.

Table 11. Performance level and quantitative index of the structure.

Performance Level	Normal Use	Immediate Use	Life Safety	Collapse Prevention
Demand	The structure and function of the building are perfect, and the deformation is far less than the elastic drift limit, so it can be used normally.	The structure and function of the building are basically intact, and the members may be slightly damaged, which can be used normally after repair, and the deformation is slightly larger than the limit of elastic drift.	There is slight plastic deformation, and the damage to non-structural components is in the range of ensuring personal safety.	If the building structure does not collapse, then it will be destroyed in an acceptable range.
Limit value of quantitative index	1/300	1/200	1/100	1/55

4.2. Selection and Amplitude Modulation of Seismic Waves

The non-linear response of building structures is closely related to seismic waves, and different seismic records can cause significant variations in structural responses. Therefore, selecting the appropriate seismic waves is crucial. The Code for Seismic Design of Buildings [17] proposes that during the time history analysis, acceleration time history curves should be selected based on site type and design earthquake grouping. The number of natural waves should not be less than two-thirds of the total amount. $S_a(T_1, \zeta\%)$ refers to the damped spectral acceleration corresponding to the basic period of elasticity of the structure. Because it greatly reduces the discrete type of analysis, this paper uses $S_a(T_1, \zeta\%)$ as the strength index. According to the time history curve and its response spectrum in the Code for Seismic Design of Buildings in China, among the seismic waves given in the report of ATC-63 [36] in the USA, 11 seismic waves satisfying the criteria were selected (Table 12) and their acceleration response spectrum curves are shown in Figure 12.

Table 12. Ground motion information selected.

Serial Number	Earthquake Magnitude	Name	Year	PGA/g	dt/s
EQ1	6.6	San_Fernando	1971	0.17	0.01
EQ2	6.5	Friuli-Italy-01	1976	0.35	0.005
EQ3	6.5	Imperial_Valley-06	1979	0.36	0.005
EQ4	6.5	Superstition_Hills-02	1987	0.45	0.01
EQ5	6.5	Superstition_Hills-02	1987	0.30	0.01
EQ6	6.9	Loma_Prieta	1989	0.44	0.005
EQ7	6.9	Loma_Prieta	1989	0.37	0.005
EQ8	7.3	Landers	1992	0.24	0.02
EQ9	6.9	Kobe-Japan	1995	0.24	0.01
EQ10	7.1	Hector_Mine	1999	0.27	0.01
EQ11	7.1	Hector_Mine	1999	0.15	0.01

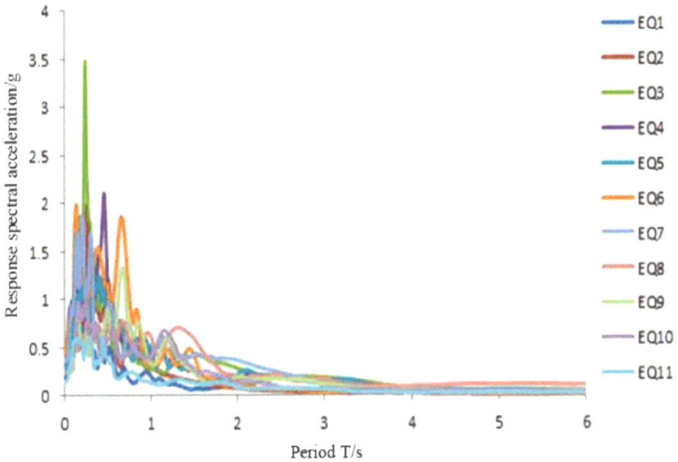

Figure 12. Seismic wave acceleration response spectrum.

In order to test whether the selected seismic wave is reasonable, the average spectrum of the selected seismic wave is compared with the code response spectrum (Figure 13). Figure 14 shows that the two response spectra are closer at the main period point of the structure (0.65 s~0.72 s). The average spectrum of the selected seismic wave is closest to the canonical response spectrum. The selected seismic wave and the canonical response spectrum are within 35% and 20% of each other, which is in line with the code of resistance. This shows that the selected seismic wave is more reasonable.

The scaling of ground motion and the selection of seismic records have significant impacts on inter-story drift angles and damage probabilities [37,38]. The scaling of seismic motion significantly impacts the dynamic response of structures. The scaling may cause bias for the response of buildings if the spectral shape is not compatible with the target spectrum. Depending on the site conditions, four seismic intensities are defined: multiple-occurrence earthquake (minor earthquake), basic earthquake (moderate earthquake), rare-occurrence earthquake (major earthquake), and extremely rare-occurrence earthquake (extreme earthquake). The acceleration values are 0.17 g, 0.5 g, 0.95 g, and 1.45 g, respectively. Each seismic wave is modulated to these four intensity levels by using the "single point amplitude modulation method", and the structural response is calculated by inputting the structure (Lu Dagang et al. [39]).

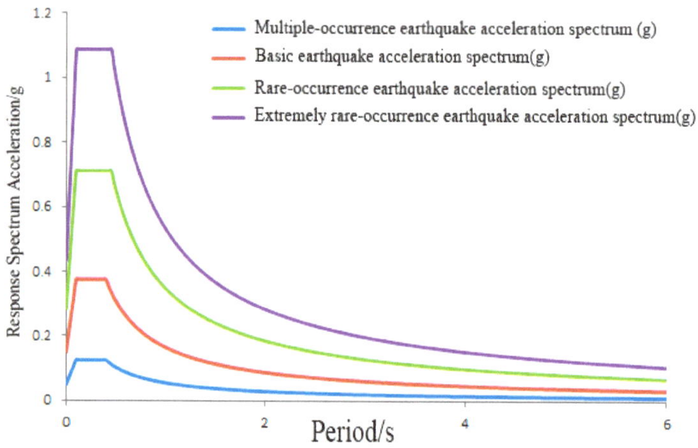

Figure 13. Response spectrum of four intensity levels.

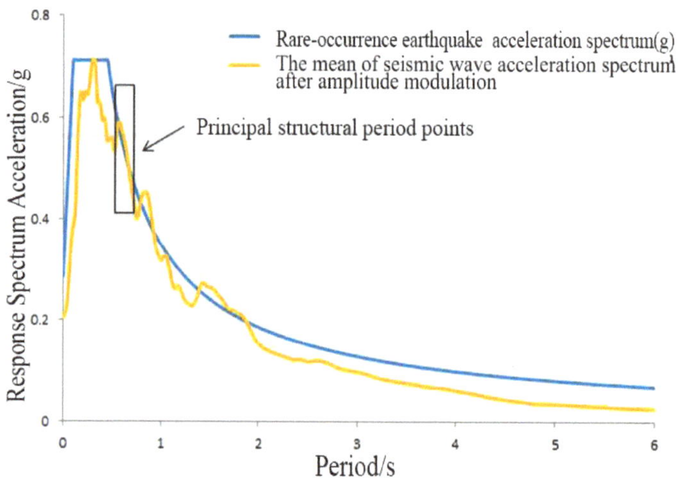

Figure 14. Comparison between average spectrum and code spectrum.

Taking the amplitude modulation of the five-story K-shaped eccentrically braced structure as an example, the amplitude modulation coefficients corresponding to the seismic waves in various places are shown in Table 13.

Table 13. Ground motion amplitude modulation coefficients.

Serial Number	Sa (g)	Minor Earthquake	Moderate Earthquake	Moderate Earthquake	Extreme Earthquake
EQ1	0.172	0.63	1.88	3.97	6.05
EQ2	0.346	0.31	0.93	1.97	3.01
EQ3	0.335	0.32	0.96	2.04	3.11
EQ4	0.420	0.26	0.77	1.62	2.48
EQ5	0.398	0.27	0.81	1.71	2.62
EQ6	0.075	1.44	4.30	9.09	13.89
EQ7	0.467	0.23	0.69	1.46	2.23
EQ8	0.525	0.21	0.62	1.29	1.98

Table 13. *Cont.*

Serial Number	Sa (g)	Minor Earthquake	Moderate Earthquake	Moderate Earthquake	Extreme Earthquake
EQ9	0.626	0.17	0.52	1.09	1.66
EQ10	0.303	0.36	1.07	2.25	3.43
EQ11	0.192	0.56	1.68	3.55	5.42

4.3. Results of Structural Analysis

4.3.1. Structural Failure Form

The failure forms of the plastic hinges of the three different types of structures under a minor earthquake, moderate earthquake, major earthquake, and maximum earthquake are shown in Figures 15–17. In this paper, we use the elastic–plastic state of the structural model under the EQ1 seismic wave as a specific example for explanation. Under the action of minor earthquakes, no plastic hinges appeared in any model member. The structure was still in an elastic state, so it was not analyzed. Under the moderate earthquake, a small number of plastic hinges appeared in each structure, among which the number of plastic hinges in the K-shaped eccentric braces was the least, concentrated in the middle of the structure. The highest number of plastic hinges occurred in the D-shaped eccentric support, and the plastic hinges occurring throughout the structure were evenly distributed. For V-shaped eccentric braces, the number of plastic hinges was in the middle, and the position was concentrated in the upper position of the structure. Under the action of major earthquakes, the structure entered an elastic–plastic state, and the plastic hinges of each eccentric support structure appeared on the energy-consuming beams, and the plastic deformation of the energy-consuming beams was uniformly distributed along the height, which basically reached the ideal damage mode. For beams, columns, and braces, there were no plastic hinges and they were still in the elastic stage, so there was no need to require too much plastic deformation capacity. Steel with higher strength can be used to reduce the cross-sectional area. The number and degree of plastic hinges of all structures under major earthquakes were further developed compared with those under major earthquakes.

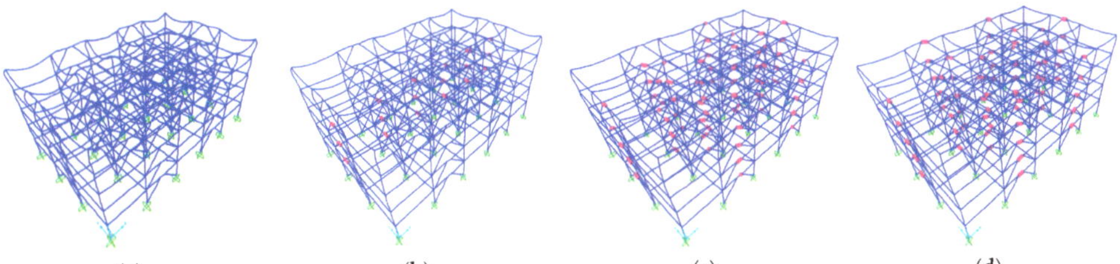

(a) (b) (c) (d)

Figure 15. Failure mode of K-shaped eccentrically braced structure. (**a**) Minor earthquake, (**b**) Moderate earthquake, (**c**) Major earthquake, and (**d**) Extreme earthquake.

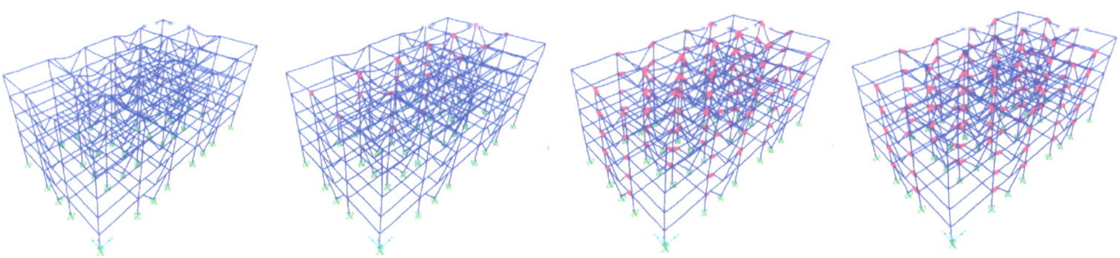

(a) (b) (c) (d)

Figure 16. Failure mode of V-shaped eccentrically braced structures. (**a**) Minor earthquake, (**b**) Moderate earthquake, (**c**) Major earthquake, and (**d**) Extreme earthquake.

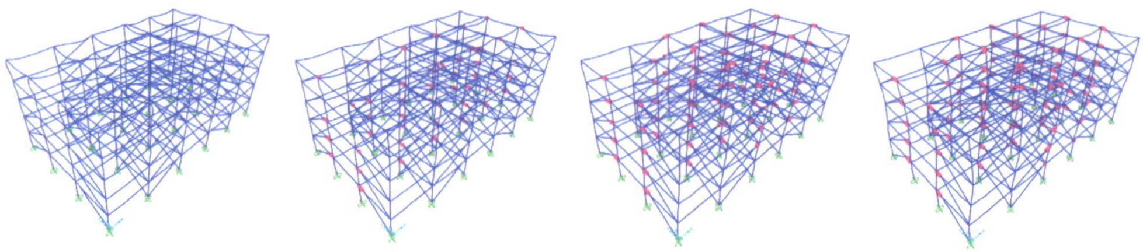

(a) (b) (c) (d)

Figure 17. Failure mode of D-shaped eccentrically braced structures. (**a**) Minor earthquake, (**b**) Moderate earthquake, (**c**) Major earthquake, and (**d**) Extreme earthquake.

4.3.2. Structural IDA Curve

IDA (incremental dynamic analysis) is a performance-based seismic analysis method with wide application value. The IDA curve records the whole process of the structure from elasticity to plasticity to collapse under the action of gradually increasing seismic strength.

IDA analysis involves inputting one or more seismic records into a structural model, where each seismic wave is "amplified" to different seismic intensity levels. The "amplified" seismic motion is then used for the elastoplastic analysis of the structure, resulting in a series of structural elastoplastic seismic responses and generating IDA curves that relate the seismic intensity to the damage indicators. Finally, the seismic performance of the structure can be evaluated according to the character points on the IDA curve.

Eleven seismic waves in accordance with the site conditions of the structure are selected (Table 12), the peak value of inter-story drift θ_{max} is selected as the damage index, and the spectral acceleration S_a is the intensity index. A series of ground shocks of different intensities are obtained after amplitude modulation and input into SAP2000 for a time range analysis to obtain the IDA curves. In this paper, three different forms of eccentrically braced structures are analyzed by non-linear time history, as shown in Figure 18. From the IDA curves of each frame structure, it can be seen that for small ranges of S_a, the IDA curve is in a state of linear increase, indicating that the structure is in the elastic stage; when S_a gradually increases, the slope of the IDA curve begins to decrease, indicating that the deformation of the structure is developing into the elastic–plastic stage; the slope at the end of the IDA curve is nearly 0, indicating that the structure finally collapses.

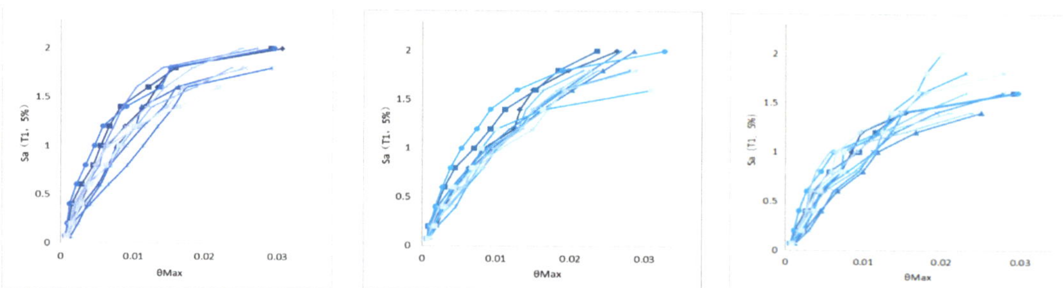

(a) (b) (c)

Figure 18. IDA curves for various structures. (**a**) K-shaped, (**b**) V-shaped, and (**c**) D-shaped.

At the same time, it can be seen that the IDA curves of the three types of structures shift to the right in turn, indicating that the stiffness of the structure decreases, the damage occurs when the ground motion is smaller, and the seismic capacity of the structure gradually becomes worse.

4.3.3. Structural Vulnerability Curve

A lognormal fragility function is fitted to the results of the incremental dynamic analyses using the maximum likelihood procedure proposed by Baker [40]. Next, the corresponding vulnerability functions are fitted to the four performance states of the structure, namely normal use (NO), immediate use (IO), life safety (LS), and collapse prevention (CP). The control target of the maximum inter-story drift angle of multi-story and high-rise steel frame structures in China is shown in Table 10. Through the analysis and integration of the results of the IDA analysis, the vulnerability curves of three different forms of eccentrically braced structures are obtained as shown in Figure 19.

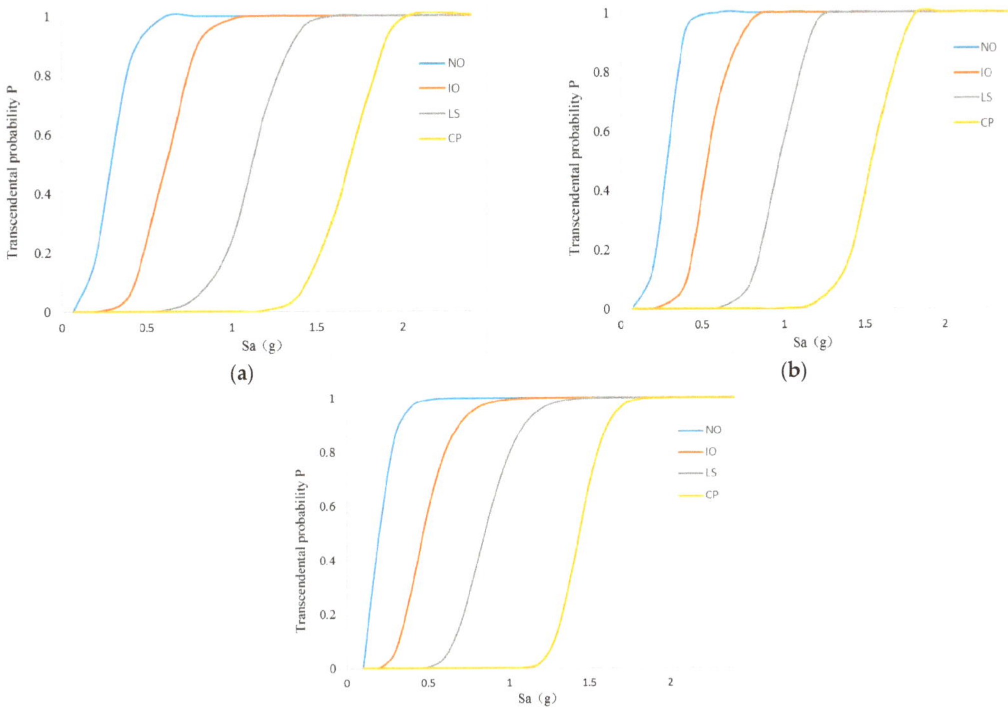

Figure 19. Fragility curve of each structure. (**a**) K-shaped, (**b**) V-shaped, and (**c**) D-shaped.

From Figure 19, it can be seen that the vulnerability curve of the structure under the four performance levels changes from steep to smooth, which shows that, in general, the structure will have at least minor damage, that is, it is easy to exceed the limit of elastic inter-story drift angles. However, with the gradual increase in the degree of damage, the structure gradually enters plasticity. In order to achieve the complete destruction of the structure, it is necessary to undergo a large variation in earthquake intensity amplitude. For K-shaped eccentrically braced structures, when the probability of reaching the four performance levels of normal use (NO), immediate use (IO), life safety (LS), and collapse prevention (CP) is 50%, the corresponding S_a is 0.30 g, 0.61 g, 1.12 g, and 1.68 g, respectively. For V-shaped eccentrically braced structures, when the probability of reaching the four performance levels is 50%, the corresponding S_a is 0.28 g, 0.55 g, 0.97 g, and 1.54 g, respectively. Figure 20 shows the collapse vulnerability curves of the three structures. The seismic strength of the three structures when they reach the median probability of preventing collapse is counted, as shown in Table 14. The results of the overall collapse vulnerability analysis of the structure show that the collapse probability of the three structures increases sequentially under the same response spectrum acceleration, indicating that the anti-collapse performance of the K-shaped eccentrically braced structure is the best, and that of the D-shaped eccentrically braced structure is the worst. The median collapse score of the three structures is 1.69 g, 1.54 g, and 1.44 g.

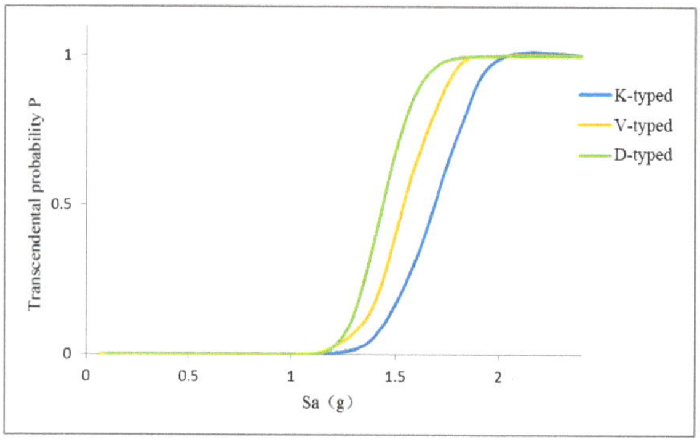

Figure 20. Collapse fragility curve of each structure.

Table 14. Fitting parameters of normal distribution of collapse fragility curve.

Structure Type	K-Shaped	V-Shaped	D-Shaped
Median collapse (g)	1.69	1.54	1.44
Standard deviation	0.15	0.13	0.14

5. Seismic Loss Assessment of Structures

5.1. FEMA P-58 Performance-Based Seismic Evaluation Theory of Buildings

FEMA P-58's structural seismic loss assessment utilizes the Monte Carlo method to randomly sample variables and compute structural loss outcomes, constituting an "implementation" process. Using this approach requires determining whether a structure collapses based on completing an IDA analysis. If collapse occurs, then repair costs and duration equal reconstruction costs and time. If no collapse happens, then the possibility of repair needs assessment. If irreparable, then the evaluation results match those described above; if repairable, then the damage extent is assessed based on fragility curves and response demand parameters, leading to loss assessment conclusions. FEMA P-58's ultimate goal is to establish a function relating structural performance metrics to exceedance probabilities.

The performance evaluation software PACT (Performance Assessment Calculation Tool) based on FEMA P-58 theory is an important tool to calculate and analyze the seismic performance of building structures. The program uses the building performance model to convert the structural analysis results into seismic performance, and the seismic performance is expressed by the maintenance cost. The FEMA P-58 building performance model is a collection of data representing building assets at risk during an earthquake. Building assets include structural systems and non-structural systems. The absolute floor acceleration and inter-story drift ratio are utilized to characterize the requirements of both structural and non-structural systems. The peak structural response parameters in the time history analysis are combined with the vulnerability function to determine the damage state of the building components, and the maintenance cost function is used to calculate the corresponding maintenance cost. In FEMA P-58 theory, the Monte Carlo method is used to simulate the influence of different structural response parameters (EDPs) on the results of the structural performance calculation.

5.2. Analysis Results of Collapse Vulnerability and Structural Response

5.2.1. Analysis Results of Inter-Story Drift Angles

The average value of the inter-story drift angle is comparable in building height, while the calculation results of the peak value of the inter-story drift angle are omitted. Therefore, this paper focuses on the analysis of the average drift angle between the stories of each structure. The results of the three different structural forms are shown below.

According to the analysis results of the drift angle between each story of each structure, it can be concluded that for the eccentric steel frame structure with five floors, the maximum drift angle between floors generally appears at the position of the second floor. The minimum inter-story drift angle of the structure generally occurs at the position of the first story. The first story of the structure has the smallest inter-story drift angle, which may be due to the fact that the column feet are rigidly connected and have a high stiffness. The inter-story drift angle of each structure increases at first and then decreases from the bottom to the top, indicating that the layout of each structure is more reasonable. According to the code, the inter-story drift limits of steel structures under frequent earthquakes and rare earthquakes are 1/250 and 1/50, respectively. According to Figure 21, the inter-story drift limit of the three structures under different earthquakes does not exceed the prescribed limit. The design of these three eccentric support structures is reasonable. It is in line with the concept of "no damage in minor earthquakes, repairable in moderate earthquakes, and no collapse in major earthquakes".

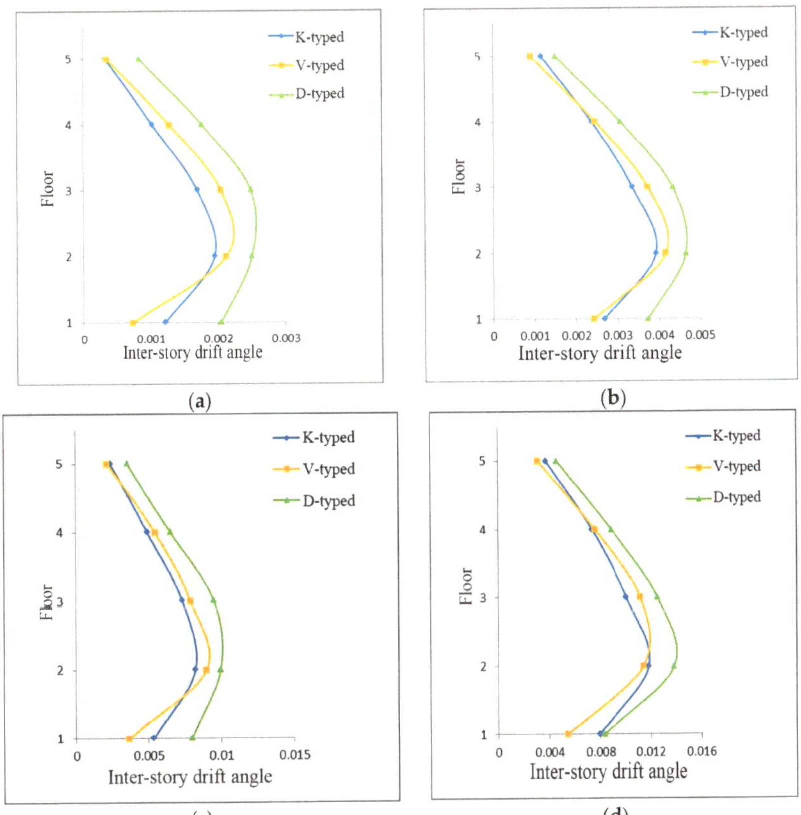

Figure 21. Mean inter-story drift analysis results of each structure. (**a**) Minor earthquake, (**b**) moderate earthquake, (**c**) major earthquake, and (**d**) extreme earthquake.

From Figure 21, it can be observed that under various seismic intensities, the mean inter-story drift angles of K-shaped, V-shaped, and D-shaped eccentrically braced frames progressively shift to the right. This indicates that the stiffness of K-shaped eccentrically braced frames is the highest and that of D-shaped eccentrically braced frames is the lowest. However, there is little difference between the V-shaped eccentrically braced frames and the K-shaped braces, which proves that the arrangement of braces also has a certain influence on the stiffness of eccentrically braced steel structures.

5.2.2. Analysis Results of Floor Peak Acceleration

Figure 22 shows the results of the acceleration analysis of each floor level of the three structures. All structures exhibit a progressive increase in floor acceleration from low to high, with the highest floor acceleration occurring on the uppermost floor, as determined by analyzing the floor acceleration data of various structures under varying earthquake intensities. We note that all structures exhibit varying rates of increase in floor accelerations from lower to upper floors. The acceleration of the K-shaped, V-shaped, and D-shaped eccentrically braced frames decreases with increasing strength, as can be seen from the peak acceleration analysis results of each structural floor. The average top acceleration response under frequent earthquakes is 0.16 g, 0.13 g, and 0.09 g, while the average top acceleration response under rare earthquakes is 0.61 g, 0.50 g, and 0.31 g. This is because the modal periods of the three structures increase in turn, so under the action of earthquakes, the acceleration response decreases, which is in line with the trend of the response spectrum curve.

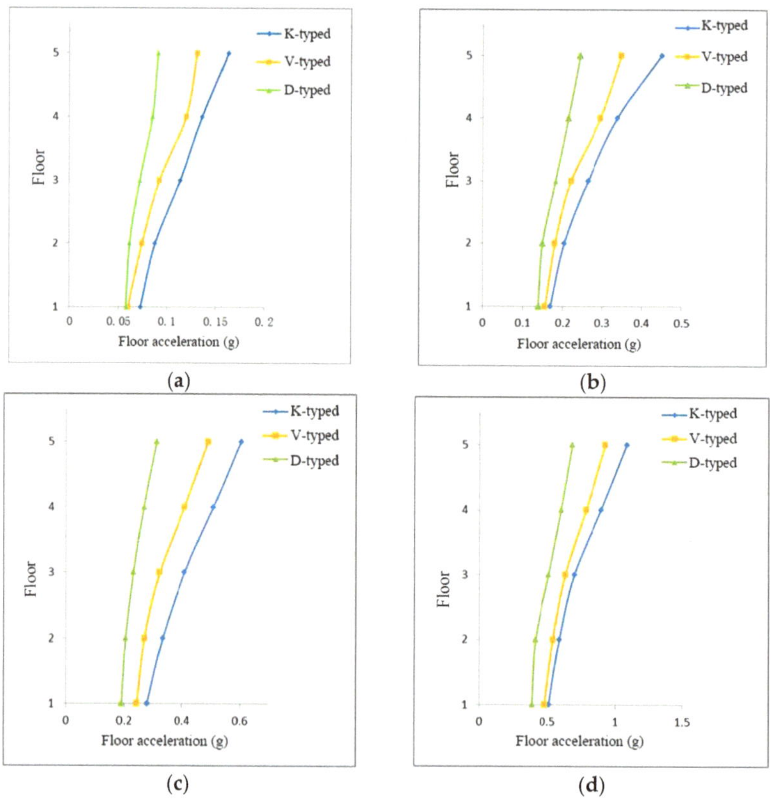

Figure 22. Analysis results of mean acceleration of each structural floor. (**a**) Minor earthquake, (**b**) moderate earthquake, (**c**) major earthquake, and (**d**) extreme earthquake.

5.3. Results of Earthquake Loss Assessment

The FEMA P-58 program is used to carry out 500 Monte Carlo analyses of each seismic state. After consultation, the replacement cost of the five-story structural building is set to 4.5 million US dollars, the replacement time is 350 days, and the maximum number of workers per unit area is 0.02 per square meter. The overall loss threshold is 0.5. The occupancy of the building reflects the additional cost of ongoing building operations, equipment, and some of the building features. The building model designed in this paper is an office building. For office buildings, the adjustment coefficient can be 1.0 when unoccupied and 1.2 when occupied. The three structures designed in this paper are all five-story office buildings, and the default population flow model provided in PACT is selected. The default value is the peak population density of 4 people/1000 sf, and the difference value of the model distribution is 0.2.

In this paper, a single collapse mode was selected. If the building collapses, then the probability of collapse is 1, and the mortality and injury rates of the population take the default values of 0.9 and 0.1.

After entering the various parameters of the structure into PACT, you can click the Evaluate Performance of the PACT panel for calculation, and finally, view the results of seismic loss in Examine Results.

The repair cost distribution curve from the PACT analysis is checked (see the median cost of structural maintenance and statistics in Figures 23–31). From Figures 23–25, the median repair costs of K-shaped eccentrically braced structures under small, moderate, large, and maximum earthquakes are 3.98, 24.39, 58.01, and 136.46 ten thousand dollars, respectively. The expenses of repairing structural members and non-structural components during significant earthquakes are 16.82 and 43.51 ten thousand dollars, respectively. These amounts represent 28% and 75% of the overall maintenance expenditures.

From Figures 26–28, the median repair costs of V-shaped eccentrically braced structures under small, moderate, large, and maximum earthquakes are 3.81, 19.03, 46.49, and 112.29 ten thousand dollars, respectively. Under major earthquakes, the repair costs of structural and non-structural components are 16.27 and 30.22 ten thousand dollars, accounting for 35% and 65% of the total maintenance costs, respectively.

From Figures 29–31, the median repair costs of V-shaped eccentrically braced structures under small, moderate, large, and maximum earthquakes are 4.90, 24.63, 75.18, and 141.95 ten thousand dollars, respectively. Structural and non-structural component repair costs during major earthquakes are 30.07 and 45.11 ten thousand dollars, representing 40% and 60% of the overall maintenance expenses, respectively.

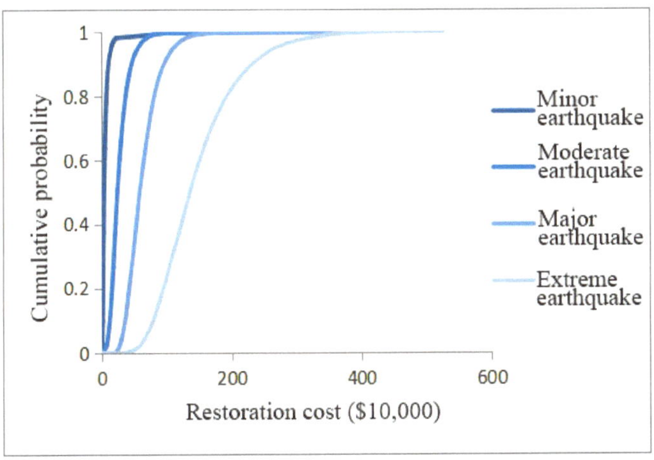

Figure 23. Probability distribution of repair costs of K-shaped eccentrically braced structures.

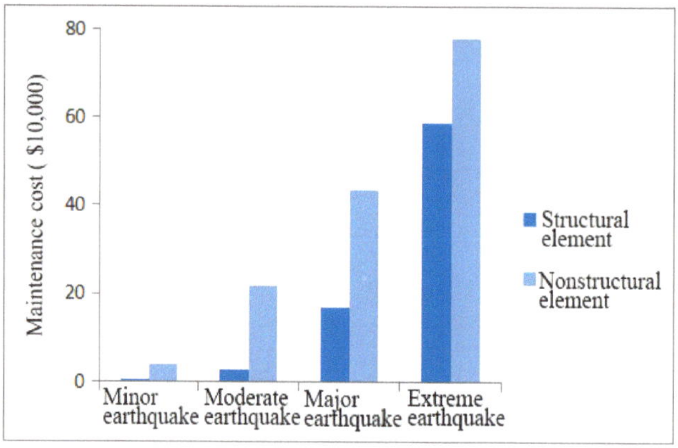

Figure 24. Distribution of repair costs of components of K-shaped eccentrically braced structures.

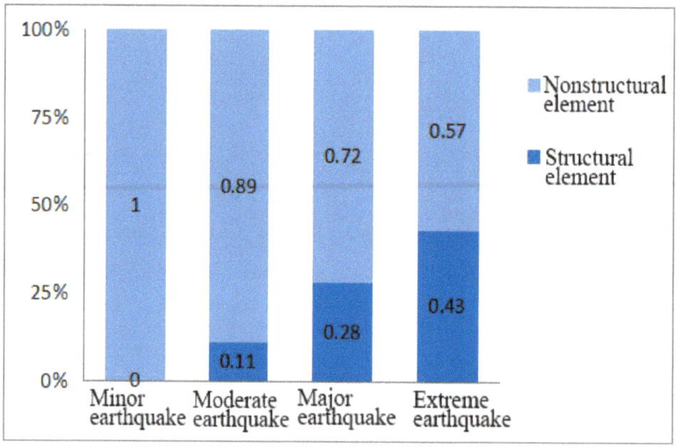

Figure 25. Proportion of repair costs of various components of K-shaped eccentrically braced structure.

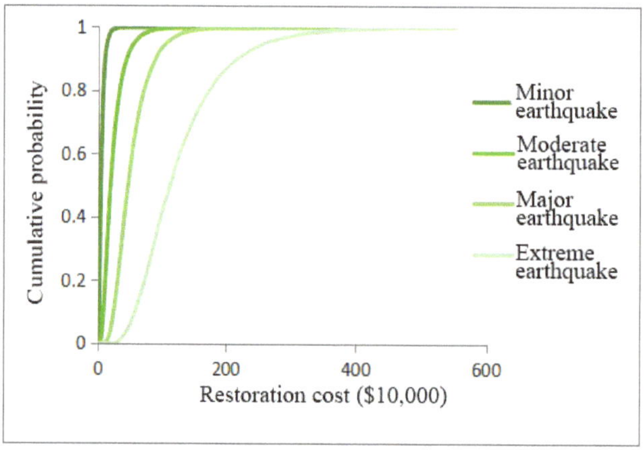

Figure 26. Probability distribution of repair costs of V-shaped eccentrically braced structures.

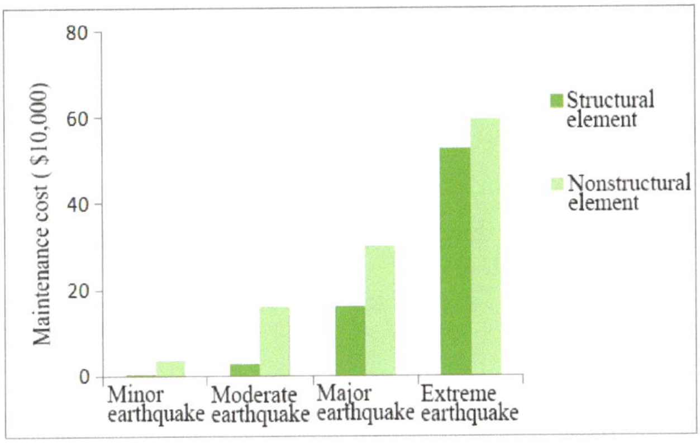

Figure 27. Distribution of repair costs of components of V-shaped eccentrically braced structures.

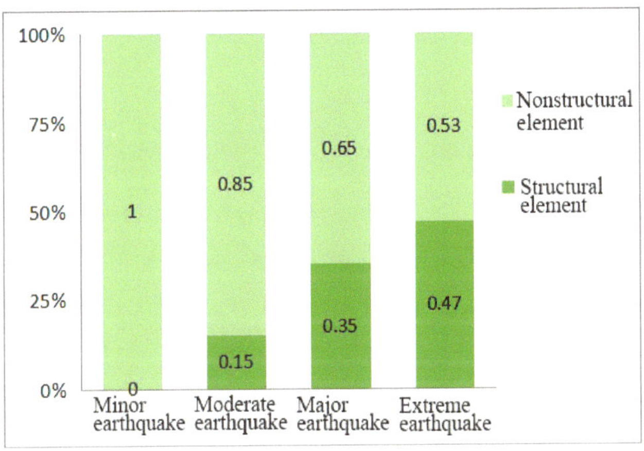

Figure 28. Proportion of repair costs of various components of V-shaped eccentrically braced structures.

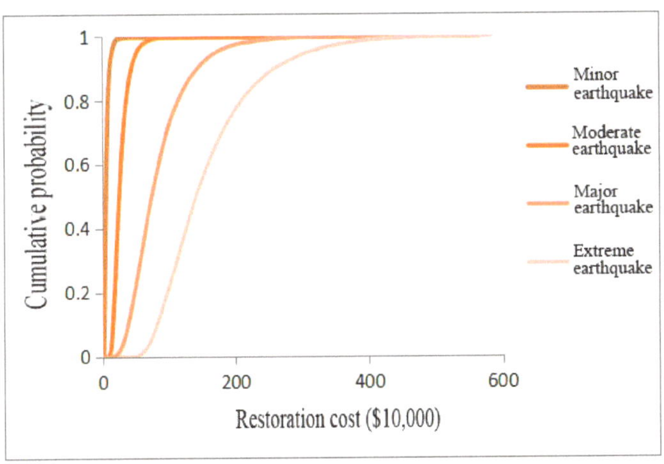

Figure 29. Probability distribution of repair costs of D-shaped eccentrically braced structures.

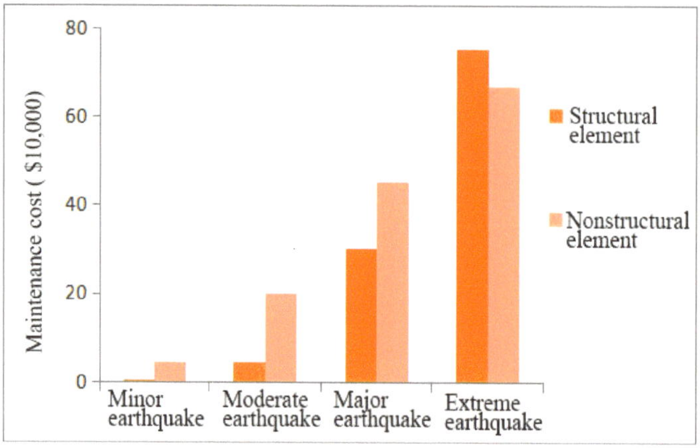

Figure 30. Distribution of repair costs of components of D-shaped eccentrically braced structures.

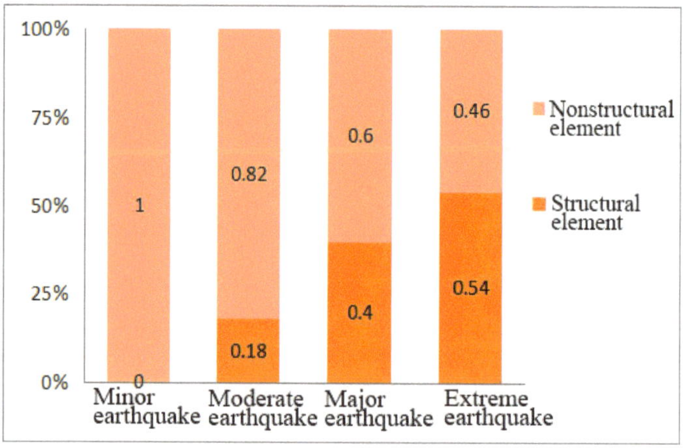

Figure 31. Proportion of repair costs of various components of D-shaped eccentrically braced structures.

According to the above earthquake loss results of maintenance costs, it can be found that the loss of V-shaped eccentrically braced structures is the smallest under the four earthquake intensities. Although, according to the results of the vulnerability analysis, the anti-collapse performance of the K-shaped eccentric brace is the best, but the vulnerability only takes the inter-story drift angles as the index. The loss is not only related to the inter-story displacement angle, but also to the floor acceleration, because non-structural components such as ceilings, elevators, and various pipelines take acceleration as the demand parameter and are acceleration-sensitive components. The central parts of the V-shaped eccentric brace are the angles of acceleration and inter-story drift. Generally speaking, the seismic loss of the V-shaped eccentric brace is the smallest. At the same time, it has been discovered that only non-structural members are lost in minor earthquakes. The structural members gradually lose strength as a result. For this reason, future engineering practices should also give careful consideration to the loss of non-structural members.

6. Conclusions

According to the concept of performance-based seismic engineering, the seismic loss analysis of eccentrically braced steel frame structures is of great significance for the selection of the structural layout. In this paper, different forms of eccentrically braced steel frame structures are designed, which are K-shaped, V-shaped, and D-shaped, respectively, and the vulnerability of the structure and earthquake loss are studied. The main conclusions are as follows:

Different forms of eccentrically braced structures show good seismic performance under the action of major earthquakes, in line with the design concept of "strong column, weak beam", and show a reasonable multi-seismic defense line.

The maximum inter-story drift angle of each structure under small earthquakes and large earthquakes is far less than the limit requirement stipulated in our country, which proves that different forms of eccentrically braced structures have good seismic performance. The whole yield process meets the design concept of "strong column and weak beam" in the traditional design, which reflects that the eccentrically braced structure has reasonable multi-seismic defense lines.

Different eccentrically braced structures show different plastic hinge failure modes under earthquake action, and the K-type structure has the best collapse resistance, the V-type structure is the second, and the D-type structure has the largest response. Using the energy-consuming capacity of energy-consuming beams can improve the overall seismic performance during structural yield.

Under different earthquake intensities, the failure modes of plastic hinges in each eccentrically braced model are also different. Under the action of minor earthquakes, plastic hinges do not appear in any member of the model, and the structure is still in an elastic state; under the action of major earthquakes, the plastic hinges of each model are mainly concentrated in the energy dissipation beam section of the structure, thus realizing the ideal failure mode of eccentrically braced structures. In the yield process of the structure, the energy dissipation capacity of the energy dissipation beam can be fully utilized, so that the seismic performance of the whole structure can be improved. From the collapse vulnerability curve, it can be concluded that the anti-collapse performance of the K-shaped eccentrically braced structure is the best, followed by the V-shaped. Among the three kinds of eccentric support structures, the D-type eccentric support structure has the most severe seismic response, and it has the worst collapse resistance. This is due to the poor symmetry of the D-type eccentric support structure.

Future designs should pay more attention to the impact of non-structural components and balance the engineering practice of different forms of eccentrically-braced structures.

From the vulnerability evaluation results, it is concluded that the anti-collapse performance of the K-shaped eccentrically braced steel frame is better, but from the point of view of earthquake loss, the loss of the V-shaped eccentrically braced structure is the smallest. This is because the earthquake loss is not only related to the inter-story drift angle, but also to the floor acceleration. In the process of earthquake loss calculation, non-structural components such as acceleration-sensitive components are also taken into account. This shows us that the loss of non-structural components should also be paid full attention to in the future design process. At the same time, we also need to realize that these three forms of eccentrically braced structures have their own advantages and disadvantages. How to choose designers in engineering practice needs to be considered with respect to the actual situation.

This paper evaluates the seismic performance of eccentrically braced steel frames from the perspectives of vulnerability and earthquake loss. However, there are areas where the considerations in this study are not comprehensive enough, and there are also difficulties in calculation and analysis. Some issues require further exploration:

This article only conducts earthquake loss analysis on eccentrically braced structures with five stories and three specific forms. It does not consider the effects of more structural forms, variations in material strength, or the length of energy dissipation beams on the structural response. These influencing factors require further exploration.

The vulnerability group and personnel mobility database in the PACT software are based on local conditions in California, USA. Using them to assess earthquake losses for structures designed according to Chinese standards may lead to significant limitations in the results. Therefore, substantial efforts are needed in collecting vulnerability component and population mobility data across China's provinces and municipalities. This is crucial for the development of earthquake loss assessment in China.

Author Contributions: Conceptualization, B.L.; Methodology, B.L.; Software, Y.L. and W.L.; Validation, J.L.; Formal analysis, J.Z.; Investigation, S.W.; Resources, G.N.; Data curation, Q.M.; Writing—original draft, B.L.; Writing—review & editing, Y.L. and J.Z. All authors have read and agreed to the published version of the manuscript.

Funding: This research received no external funding.

Data Availability Statement: The original contributions presented in the study are included in the article, further inquiries can be directed to the corresponding authors.

Conflicts of Interest: The authors declare that they have no known competing financial interests or personal relationships that could have appeared to influence the work reported in this paper.

References

1. Fujimoto, M.; Aoyagi, T.; Ukai, K.; Wada, A.; Saito, K. Structural characteristics of eccentric k-braced frames. *Trans. Archit. Inst. Jpn.* **1972**, *195*, 39–49. [CrossRef] [PubMed]
2. Roeder, C.; Popov, E.P. Eccentrically Braced Steel Frames for Earthquakes. *J. Struct. Div.* **1978**, *104*, 391–412. [CrossRef]
3. Hjelmstad, K.; Popov, E.P. Characteristics of Eccentrically Braced Frames. *J. Struct. Eng.* **1984**, *110*, 340–353. [CrossRef]
4. Tavakoli, H.R.; Afrapoli, M.M. Robustness analysis of steel structures with various lateral load resisting systems under the seismic progressive collapse. *Eng. Fail. Anal.* **2018**, *83*, 88–101. [CrossRef]
5. Yu, A. Experimental study on seismic behavior of EK and Y-shaped braces. *J. Xi'an Univ. Archit. Sci. Technol. (Nat. Sci. Ed.)* **1990**, *22*, 253–260.
6. Qian, J.; Chen, M.; Zhang, T. Experimental study and limit analysis of eccentrically braced steel frame under horizontal force. *Build. Struct.* **1993**, *4*, 3–9.
7. Bosco, M.; Rossi, P.P. Seismic behaviour of eccentrically braced frames. *Eng. Struct.* **2009**, *31*, 664–674. [CrossRef]
8. Wang, F.; Su, M.; Li, S.; Lian, M.; Zheng, X.; Tian, X.; Hong, M. Experimental study on seismic behavior of multi-story high-strength steel composite Y-shaped eccentrically braced steel frames. *J. Civ. Eng.* **2016**, *49*, 64–71.
9. Tian, X.; Su, M.; Li, S.; Yang, S. Parameter analysis of seismic performance of high-strength steel composite K-shaped eccentrically braced frames (I). *J. Guangxi Univ. (Nat. Sci. Ed.)* **2019**, *44*, 1542–1551.
10. Tian, X.; Su, M.; Li, S.; Yang, S. Parameter analysis of seismic performance of high-strength steel composite K-shaped eccentrically braced frames (II). *J. Guangxi Univ. (Nat. Sci. Ed.)* **2020**, *45*, 129–137.
11. Li, S.; Wang, Z.; Tian, J.; Li, X. Study on structural influence coefficient and displacement magnification factor of high-strength steel composite K-shaped eccentrically braced structure. *Prog. Build. Steel Struct.* **2022**, *24*, 31–40.
12. Özkılıç, Y.O.; Ün, E.M.; Topkaya, C. Frictional mid-spliced shear links for eccentrically braced frames. *Earthq. Eng. Struct. Dyn.* **2023**, *52*, 15. [CrossRef]
13. Özkılıç, Y.O. Optimized stiffener detailing for shear links in eccentrically braced frames. *Steel Compos. Struct.* **2021**, *39*, 35–50.
14. Özkılıç, Y.O.; Topkaya, C. Extended end-plate connections for replaceable shear links. *Eng. Struct.* **2021**, *240*, 112385. [CrossRef]
15. Özkılıç, Y.O.; Bozkurt, M.B.; Topkaya, C. Mid-spliced end-plated replaceable links for eccentrically braced frames. *Eng. Struct.* **2021**, *237*, 112225. [CrossRef]
16. Özkılıç, Y.O.; Zeybek, Ö.; Topkaya, C. Stability of laterally unsupported shear links in eccentrically braced frames. *Earthq. Eng. Struct. Dyn.* **2021**, *51*, 832–852. [CrossRef]
17. *GB 50011-2010*; Code for Seismic Design of Buildings. China Construction Industry Press: Beijing, China, 2016.
18. *ICC-IBC-2006*; International Building Code 2006. International Code Council INC: Country Club Hills, IL, USA, 2006.
19. Aslani, H.; Miranda, E. *Probabilistic Earthquake Loss Estimation and Loss Disaggregation in Buildings*; Report No., 157; John A. Blume Earthquake Engineering Center, Stanford University: Stanford, CA, USA, 2005.
20. Mitrani-Reiser, J. An Ounce of Prevention: Probabilistic Loss Estimation for Performance-Based Earthquake Engineering. Ph.D. Thesis, California Institute of Technology, Pasadena, CA, USA, 2007.
21. Ye, S.; Zhai, G. A summary of research on earthquake economic loss assessment. *Adv. Geogr.* **2010**, *29*, 684–692.
22. Zareian, F. *Simplified Performance-Based Earthquake Engineering*; Stanford University: Stanford, CA, USA, 2006.
23. Ramirez, C.M.; Miranda, E. *Building-Specific Loss Estimation Methods & Tools for Simplified Performance-Based Earthquake Engineering*; Report No. 157; John A. Blume Earthquake Engineering Center, Stanford University: Stanford, CA, USA, 2009.
24. Gobbo, G.D.; Williams, M.S.; Blakeborough, A. Seismic performance assessment of Eurocode 8-compliant concentric braced frame buildings using FEMA P-58. *Eng. Struct.* **2018**, *155*, 192–208. [CrossRef]
25. Zeng, X.; Liu, S.; Xu, Z.; Lu, X. Case study of earthquake economic loss prediction of campus buildings based on FEMA-P58 method. *Eng. Mech.* **2016**, *33* (Suppl. 1), 113–118.

26. Zhu, H.; Liang, X.; Dang, Y. Study on a new generation of seismic performance evaluation method of frame-shear wall structure based on seismic strength. *Vib. Shock* **2017**, *36*, 140148.
27. Yan, D. Seismic and Isolation Performance Evaluation of Reinforced Concrete Frame Structures Based on FEMA P58. Bachelor's Thesis, Institute of Engineering Mechanics, China Seismological Bureau, Beijing, China, 2019.
28. *GB 50017-2017*; Steel Structure Design Standard. China Construction Industry Press: Beijing, China, 2017.
29. *JGJ 99-2015*; Technical Specification for Steel Structure of Tall Buildings. China Construction Industry Press: Beijing, China, 2015.
30. *GB 50009-2012*; Code for Load of Building Structures. China Construction Industry Press: Beijing, China, 2012.
31. Beijing Zhuxinda Engineering Consulting Co., Ltd. *Chinese Version of SAP2000 Technical Guide and Engineering Application*; Renjiaotong Publishing House Co., Ltd.: Beijing, China, 2018.
32. *American Society of Civil Engineers: Prestandard and Commentary for Seismic Rehabilitation of Buildings*; Report No. FEMA 356; Federal Emergency Management Agency: Washington, DC, USA, 2002.
33. *FEMA P-58-1*; Seismic Performance Assessment of Buildings: Volume 1—Methodology. Federal Emergency Management Agency: Washington, DC, USA, 2012.
34. *FEMA P-58-2*; Seismic Performance Assessment of Buildings: Volume 2—Implementation Guide. Federal Emergency Management Agency: Washington, DC, USA, 2012.
35. *FEMA P-58-3*; Seismic Performance Assessment of Buildings: Volume 3—Provided Fragility Data. Federal Emergency Management Agency: Washington, DC, USA, 2012.
36. *ATC-63*; Quantification of Building Seismic Performance Factors, ATC-63 Project Report (90% Draft). FEMA P695/April 2008. Federal Emergency Management Agency: Washington, DC, USA, 2008.
37. Demir, A.; Kayhan, A.H.; Palanci, M. Response- and probability-based evaluation of spectrally matched ground motion selection strategies for bi-directional dynamic analysis of low- to mid-rise RC buildings. *Structures* **2023**, *58*, 105533. [CrossRef]
38. Demir, A.; Palanci, M.; Kayhan, A.H. Evaluation the effect of amplitude scaling of real ground motions on seismic demands accounting different structural characteristics and soil classes. *Bull. Earthq. Eng.* **2024**, *22*, 365–393. [CrossRef]
39. Lu, D.; Liu, T.; Li, S.; Yu, X. Analysis of the influence of target spectrum and amplitude modulation method on ground motion selection. *Earthq. Eng. Eng. Vib.* **2018**, *38*, 21–28.
40. Baker, J.W. Efficient analytical fragility function fitting using dynamic structural analysis. *Earthq. Spectra* **2015**, *31*, 579–599. [CrossRef]

buildings

Article

Study on Mechanical Properties of Steel Fiber-Reinforced Geopolymer Concrete under Multi-Axial Loads

Pengtao Wu [1,2,3], Xuan Wan [1], Qun Lu [1] and Yan Zhang [1,*]

1 Tianjin Key Laboratory of Civil Structure Protection and Reinforcement, Tianjin Chengjian University, Tianjin 300384, China; wupengtao0228@tcu.edu.cn (P.W.); wxdyx19980108@163.com (X.W.); zdlq585@126.com (Q.L.)
2 School of Civil Engineering, Tianjin University, Tianjin 300372, China
3 Tianjin Building Materials Science Research Academy Co., Ltd., Tianjin 300381, China
* Correspondence: zy_801010@163.com

Abstract: Steel fiber-reinforced geopolymer concrete (SFRGPC) is an inorganic cementitious material with environmentally friendly features. As compared to conventional concrete, SFRGPC has greater strength and durability, but it is brittle, making it similar to ordinary concrete. To date, the triaxial mechanical properties that regulate SFRGPC's structural performance at serviceable and ultimate-limit conditions remain poorly understood. In this study, we conducted experimental and theoretical analyses of these properties. Conventional triaxial testing is used to investigate the effects of varying steel fiber contents and ratio of length to diameter under different confinement pressures on SFRGPC's mechanical properties. The failure mode, maximal strength, stress–strain curve, maximum strain, and compressive toughness were analyzed and discussed. Under uniaxial compression, the failure mode of the SFRGPC specimens was a longitudinal split failure. The brittleness of the SFRGPC can be eliminated, and its resistance to breaking can be greatly improved by increasing the volume of steel fibers and the confining pressure in the mixture. The steel fiber content and ratio of length to diameter have obvious influence on the compressive strength of SFRGPC. As the steel fiber content increased, the compressive strength increased by 1.15–1.44 times; as the ratio of length to diameter increased, the compressive strength increased by 1.21–1.70 times. The increase in confining pressure can improve the compressive strength of concrete. With the increase in confining pressure, the increase trend of compressive strength becomes smooth. The confining pressure, steel fiber content, and steel fiber length have substantial influences on the compressive toughness index η_{c3}. Under increasing confining pressure, η_{c3} increases linearly; however, after confining pressure is higher than 5 MPa, η_{c3} tends toward a steady state when the confining pressure increases. Using numerical simulation, we also investigated the size effect of SFRGPC under triaxial load. The concrete cylinder's strength does not significantly decrease as its size increases.

Keywords: steel fiber-reinforced geopolymer concrete; triaxial; mechanical properties; numerical simulation

1. Introduction

In recent decades, concrete materials have been more and more widely used in building structures; with the global climate change and the increasingly serious environmental pollution problems, resource reuse, to achieve the "double carbon" goal has become a common concept of global development. The development of renewable energy can not only reduce the consumption of limited energy resources but also effectively reduce the emission of air pollutants, improve environmental quality, and enhance people's quality of life. The mechanical properties of geopolymer concrete (GPC) have been studied by many scholars. For instance, in kaolin-rich regions, the price of geopolymer concrete is higher than that of traditional Portland cement, while the amount of greenhouse gas produced by the formation of geopolymers from kaolin is 40% less than that of conventional cement [1–3]. In addition, some studies suggest that using a mixture of sodium hydroxide and sodium silicate as an alkali activator can significantly enhance GPC's properties as compared to using only NaOH [4,5]. It was investigated the durability and static properties of self-compacting geopolymer cementitious concrete made from fly ash, mineral particles, wollastonite, and graphene oxide [6]. Ghafoor et al. [7] studied the effects of two different Na_2SiO_3/NaOH ratios and the ratio of alkaline activator to fly ash (AA/FA) on the mechanical properties of solidified GPC using two locally produced fly ashes with different NaOH concentrations. Lincy et al. [8] added a small quantity of silica nanoparticles to an optimized GPC mixture to determine its additive impact on the performance of mixed GPC paver blocks.

At the early stage of the research, GPC was mixed without coarse aggregate. Although it had the advantages of high early strength and low carbon dioxide emission, its brittleness was particularly obvious. In addition, its tensile strength was low, so the application of GPC was limited [9]. Therefore, the method of fiber-reinforced concrete is used for reference, and various types of fibers are added to GPC to improve its bending strength and energy absorption capacity. The selection of fibers to use as reinforcement must take into account the following requirements [10]: (1) the compatibility between the material properties and the application; (2) a sufficient fiber–matrix interaction to transfer stress; and (3) an optimal length–diameter ratio to ensure effective post-cracking behavior.

With the addition of fibers to increase the strength and energy absorption capacity of GPC, many researchers began to focus on the use of various fibers to improve the mechanical properties of GPC. Ganesh [11] discovered that as the amount of glass fiber in GPC increased, the material's resistance and energy absorption capacity increased while its brittleness decreased substantially. Similarly, by measuring the physical and mechanical energies of steel fiber-reinforced geopolymer concrete (SFRGPC) [12], it was determined that the addition of fibers substantially enhanced the material's tensile strength. The structural energy of steel fiber and ceramic pellets as additives to GPC was investigated, indicating that the impact strength of the polymer can be considerably enhanced with these reinforcements [13]. Noushini [14] measured the mechanical and physical properties of polymer gel materials with various types of fibers, finding that polyolefin fiber fracturing was the most significant for the same volume of fiber. In other research, Liu et al. [15] discovered that an increase in fiber content can reduce the quantity of concrete and ease and that the fiber's ease decreases further with longer fibers. The smaller the fiber diameter and the longer the fiber, the stronger the concrete. Sharma et al. [16] concludes that the use of fiber-reinforced geopolymer concrete should be commercialized after the establishment of proper standards for manufacturing. The mechanical properties of fiber-reinforced geopolymer concretes were reviewed, and the development and application prospects of fiber-reinforced geopolymer concrete were introduced. Meskhi et al. [17] studied the application potential of geopolymer concrete in construction practice and evaluated it in detail. In order to improve the strength and durability of GPC and its sustainability, an optimal ratio of GPC based on glass fiber and waste basalt powder was proposed. Celik et al. [18] presented a comprehensive exploration of multiple parameters aimed at improving the strength, workability, setting time, and environmentally friendly properties of GPC. Özkılıç et al. [19] studied the influence of waste glass aggregate with fly ash in certain proportions by different amounts of molarity and waste glass aggregate proportion on GPC.

In practical engineering applications, engineering structures are often in a state of multi-axial complex load. Under multi-axial stress, the compressive strength, elastic modulus, and failure mode of concrete materials will change significantly. Therefore, it is neither reasonable nor reliable to guide engineering design only on the basis of the mechanical properties measured by uniaxial experiments.

Since the 1970s, a number of studies have concentrated on the triaxial properties of normal concrete (NC) [20], high-performance concrete (HPC), or the uniaxial properties of high-strength concrete or ultra-high-performance concrete (UHPC). Zhou et al. [21] observed the tensile brittle failure mode of high-performance concrete (HPC) specimens under tensile–compressive–compressive (T-C-C) loading. They found that UHPC's triaxial compressive strength and ductility increase with confinement pressure [22]. In addition, their tests showed that the shear and expansion failure modes of UHPC are realized effectively, and the maximal axial strain increases linearly with the confining pressure. In relevant research, the failure of cylindrical specimens of UHPC was considerably delayed compared to ultra-high-strength concrete (UHSC) [23]. In contrast to fiber-reinforced geopolymer composite samples, Khan et al. [24] found that the confining pressure significantly affects the compressive strength of HSG materials. In another study, the constitutive relationships and failure criteria of entirely recycled concrete (TRC) under triaxial compression at high temperature were investigated [25]. Zhang et al. [26] experimentally and numerically investigated the triaxial mechanical behavior of a reactive powder cement slurry prepared with an alcohol-based shrinkage reducer.

In order to further study the strengthening properties of steel fiber on concrete materials, numerous researchers have explored the experimental triaxial compression performance of steel fiber-reinforced concrete (SFRC) [27–29] and found that with an increase in the confining pressure and fiber content, the compressive strength, tensile strength, Poisson's ratio, failure mode, and deformation of concrete are evidently altered. Wang et al. [30] systematically analyzed the effects of varying contents and confining pressures on the triaxial compressive strength of SFRC. Wang et al. [31] analyzed the triaxial strength and deformation characteristics of SFRC with different steel fiber volume ratios under three distinct strain powers and established a set of spatial failure criteria for SFRC. However, the triaxial mechanical properties of SFRGPC have been rarely studied.

Therefore, it is particularly important to study the triaxial mechanical properties and static constitutive relationships of ultra-high-performance concrete materials. Examining the mechanical properties of SFRGPC under uniaxial and multi-axial stress is necessary to derive accurate constitutive models. This study presents the results of uniaxial and triaxial compression tests conducted on SFRGPC and analyzes the mechanical behavior of SFRGPC under various stress conditions. The test results demonstrate the effects of confinement conditions on the compressive strength and ductility, stress–strain curves, and failure modes of SFRGPC. The specific application of SFRGPC in other practical scenarios is supported by test data. This research provides crucial mechanical parameters for the structural design of geopolymer concrete under complex stress conditions.

2. Experiments Program

2.1. Materials

To enhance the uniformity of the generated SFRGPC samples, this study employed the following material components: cementitious materials (slag powder, silica fume, fly ash, silica powder, the mixture ratio is 0.72:0.07:0.12:0.09), an alkaline activator (sodium silicate solution, sodium hydroxide), quartz sand, and steel fibers (Table 1, Figure 1), and superplasticizer. Table 2 shows the resulting mixture ratio that satisfied the requirements after experimenting with numerous mixtures. In addition, the table displays the composition of the SFRGPC used in the present study. To decrease the binder and internal porosities, improve the gradation of the geopolymer-based concrete aggregates, and increase compactness, we used three distinct steel filaments. Quartz sand can be used in geopolymer concrete to adjust the water–binder ratio, enhance the concrete's density and strength, and provide strong resistance against acid corrosion. These experiments tested fine (70–140 mesh), medium (50–70 mesh), and coarse (>70 mesh) ISO-standard quartz sands. The superplasticizer is a polycarboxylic acid superplasticizer with a solid content of 40%.

Unlike conventional HPC, quartz sand conforming to ISO standards was readily available. Additionally, ultrafine industrial waste powder, such as fly ash and mineral powder, was utilized to supplant a portion of the silica particles. As shown in Table 2, ultrafine industrial waste powder (silica fume, fly ash, silica powder, and mineral powder) comprised approximately 44% of the binder, while the proportion of expensive silica fume was only 4%, and the water–binder ratio was 0.1. Since the production of cement and fine quartz sand requires more energy and resources and the output of silica fume is limited and more expensive than that of fly ash, silica powder, and mineral powder, the UHPC used in this test demonstrates energy and cost savings.

Steel fiber is a form of ultra-light, copper-based steel wire that is available in flat, hooked, wavy, and spiral configurations. It has a tensile strength exceeding 4000 MPa. Steel fiber can improve the tensile strength and deformation capacity of concrete, providing an optimal balance between workability and strong mechanical properties. The diameter of the steel fibers used in this experiment was 0.12 mm, and their lengths were 6, 10, and 15 mm.

Table 1. Mechanical properties of steel fibers.

Steel Fiber	Elastic Modulus (MPa)	Tensile Strength (MPa)	Diameter (mm)	Length (mm)	Aspect Ratio
MF06	2.1×10^5	4295	0.12	6	50
MF10	2.1×10^5	4295	0.12	10	83
MF15	2.1×10^5	4295	0.12	15	125

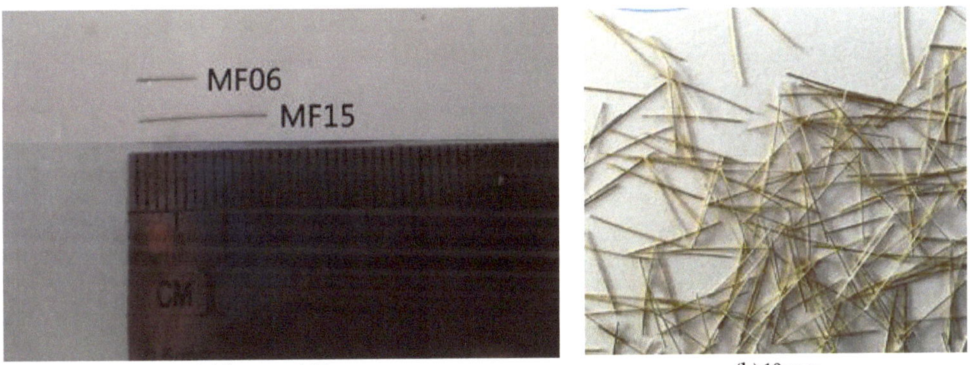

(**a**) 6 mm and 15 mm (**b**) 10 mm

Figure 1. Steel fiber.

Table 2. Mixture proportions of SFRGPC samples.

Group	Steel Fiber	Steel Fiber Volume Fraction V_f (%)	Cementitious (kg/m^3)	Quartz Sand (kg/m^3)	Basic Activator (kg/m^3)	Superplasticizer (kg/m^3)
S0	--	0	1292	950	699	9.8
S1	MF06	2.5	1292	950	699	9.8
S2	MF10	2.5	1292	950	699	9.8
S3	MF15	1.0	1292	950	699	9.8
S4	MF15	2.0	1292	950	699	9.8

2.2. Specimens

Silica fume, fly ash, mineral powder, quartz sand, and additional raw materials were added to a mixer and mixed for five minutes. After thoroughly combining the granular ingredients, we added a pre-blended solution of the alkaline stimulant, water, and water-reducing agent, followed by the addition of the steel fiber. After completely incorporating the steel fiber into the concrete, we continued mixing for three minutes. The specimens were cured at 20 °C and a relative humidity of greater than 95%. After 24 to 48 h, the sample was demolded and stored for 28 days in an indoor curing chamber. After curing, SFRGPC specimens were extracted using an automatic coring machine, and their two planes were polished to meet the test requirements. To test with a uniform distribution of steel fibers, we took sections from the center of the rectangular specimens so that they accurately reflect the mechanical properties after curing. The final specimens are depicted in Figure 2. Each group consists of three specimens, the failure mode and stress–strain curve selected are the most representative.

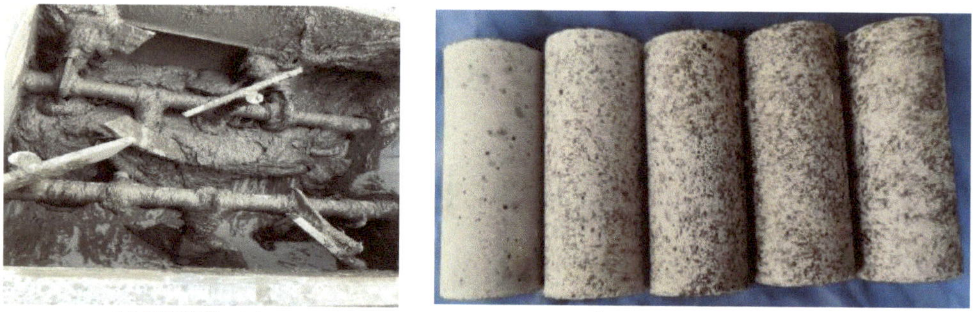

(**a**) SFRGPC mixing (**b**) Compressive specimens

Figure 2. Specimens of SFRGPC for uniaxial and triaxial tests.

2.3. Experimental Setup

This experiment used an RMT-150C (The equipment was developed and produced by Wuhan Institute of Rock and Soil Mechanics, Chinese Academy of Sciences), a computer-controlled, three-axis, electro-hydraulic servo pressure testing device (Figure 3). The test is carried out according to the test standard recommended by the International Association of Rock Mechanics [32]. The RMT-150C's loading mechanism consists of two separate loading devices: (1) a hydraulic actuator with servo control that exerts an axial force of up to 1000 kN and (2) a high-pressure container that uses hydraulic oil to uniformly apply confining pressure to the whole sample surface. A constricting pressure of up to 50 MPa was applied to the specimen's surface. The specimen's axial deformation was measured using a linear variable differential transformer (LVDT). The average recorded deformation was used to represent the axial distortion.

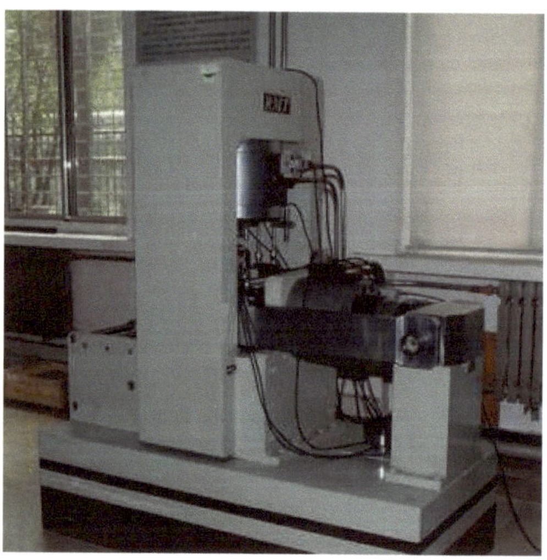

Figure 3. RMT 150C system.

Figure 4 depicts the stress state of the sample under conventional triaxial compression. To measure uniaxial compression, we employed the displacement control method with a uniaxial loading rate of 0.02 mm/min.

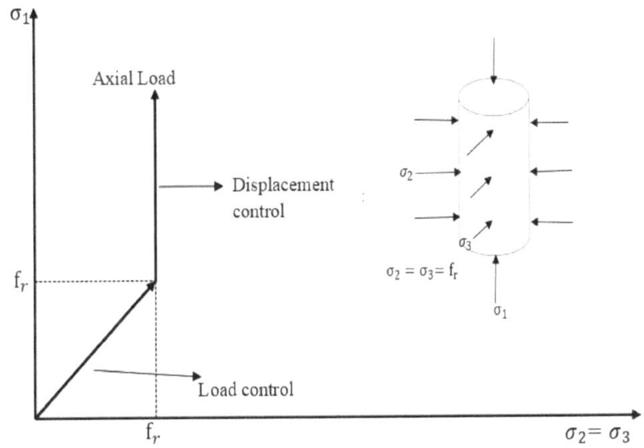

Figure 4. Development of stress in the triaxial compression test.

The confining pressure and axial load were simultaneously applied to the surface of the geopolymer concrete specimen ($\sigma_1 = \sigma_2 = \sigma_3$, σ_1, σ_2 and σ_3 correspond to the principal stresses of the X, Y, and Z axes, respectively) using the force control method to test the conventional triaxial compression. Figure 4 shows the stress state of the sample under conventional triaxial compression. After maintaining the confining pressure below the set value for 10 s to achieve a constant confining pressure, the axial loading rate was altered to 1 kN/s on the top surface of the SFRGPC specimen to apply axial stress up to 80% of the ultimate strength. The load was then administered using the displacement control method at a loading rate of 0.02 mm/min until failure. The tested confinement pressures ranged were 5, 10, 15, 20, 30, and 40 MPa.

3. Experimental Results

3.1. Failure Modes

Figure 5 describes the failure patterns of GPC under various confining pressure conditions. All fracture surfaces were relatively planar, with no bonding effects. At the outset of the uniaxial compression test, a vertical crack parallel to the loading direction appeared in the middle of the specimen. As the load increased, one or more fractures developed. The specimen's failure mode was a longitudinal split failure. Under axial load, the specimen was axially compressed, while the radial direction was subject to tension. With the increase in axial stress, the radial dimension expanded. When the tensile stress exceeded the ultimate tensile strength, tiny fractures began to develop in the specimens. As the stress increased, the cracks progressively expanded and lengthened, and a small amount of concrete spalling occurred. Eventually, the developed test specimen split obliquely through cracking, resulting in the specimen's destruction, which occurred when the confining pressure was between 5 and 20 MPa and the development direction of the oblique fracture was 60 to 70 degrees relative to the horizontal. As the confining pressure rose, the damage patterns became oblique rupture failures, and the angle of crack development tended to decrease marginally.

Figures 6–9 depict the failure patterns of the SFRGPC specimens under varying confining pressures. The addition of steel fibers substantially altered the failure modes of the specimens. After the addition of steel fiber, the integrity of the specimen improved, and the fractures occurring in the specimen were smaller. During the uniaxial compression test, the SFRGPC specimens were compressed axially and tensioned tangentially. As axial stress increased, the radial expansion of the SFRGPC specimen commenced. When the tensile stress exceeded the ultimate tensile strength, micro-fractures appeared. In response to the increasing tension, the cracks grew and penetrated the specimen, which was ultimately destroyed. Because of the lateral restraint of the confining pressure and the bridging effect of the steel fiber, the test specimens expanded radially during the triaxial test. The specimens displayed oblique shear failure, and their fractures were relatively fine. The original integrity was largely preserved, and they did not fracture into two or more fragments like the specimens lacking steel fiber. Thus, the steel fiber increased the ductility of the GPC, allowing the specimen to absorb more energy during the failure process.

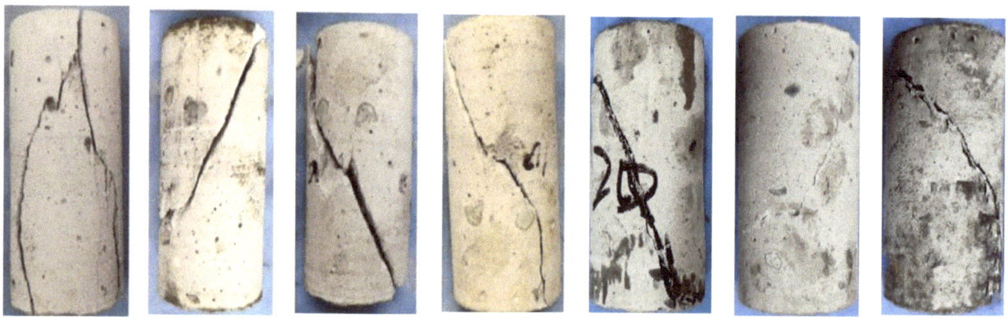

0 MPa 5 MPa 10 MPa 15 MPa 20 MPa 30 MPa 40 MPa

Figure 5. Failure patterns of GPC specimens under different confining pressure conditions.

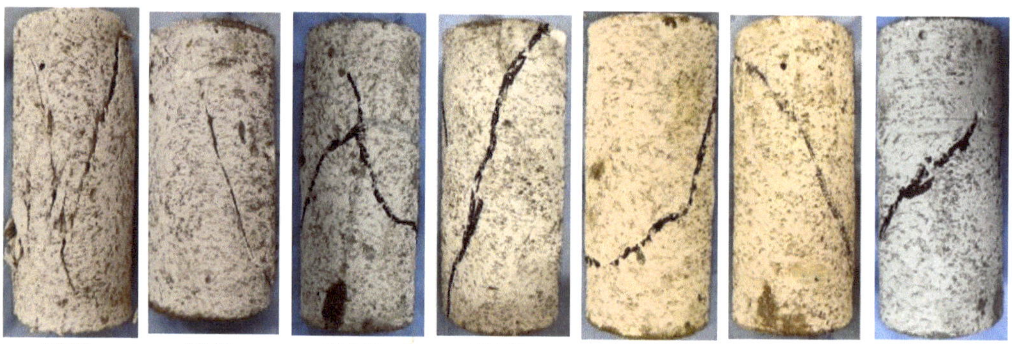

0 MPa 5 MPa 10 MPa 15 MPa 20 MPa 30 MPa 40 MPa

Figure 6. Failure patterns of the SFRGPC specimens with 1.0% MF15.

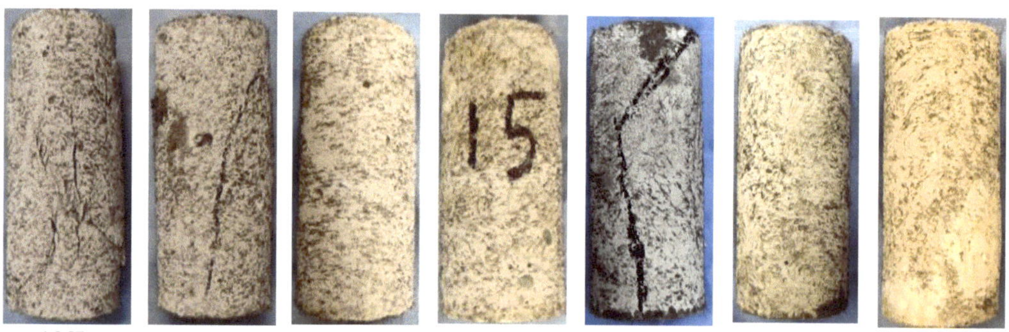

0 MPa 5 MPa 10 MPa 15 MPa 20 MPa 30 MPa 40 MPa

Figure 7. Failure patterns of the SFRGPC specimens with 2.0% MF15.

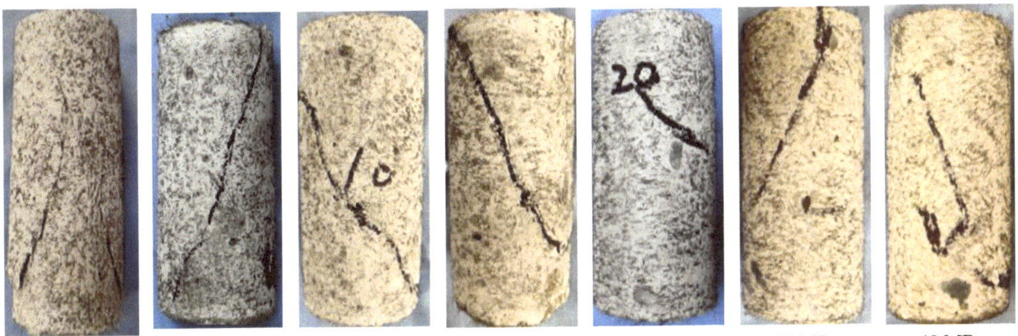

0 MPa 5 MPa 10 MPa 15 MPa 20 MPa 30 MPa 40 MPa

Figure 8. Failure patterns of the SFRGPC specimens with 2.5% MF06.

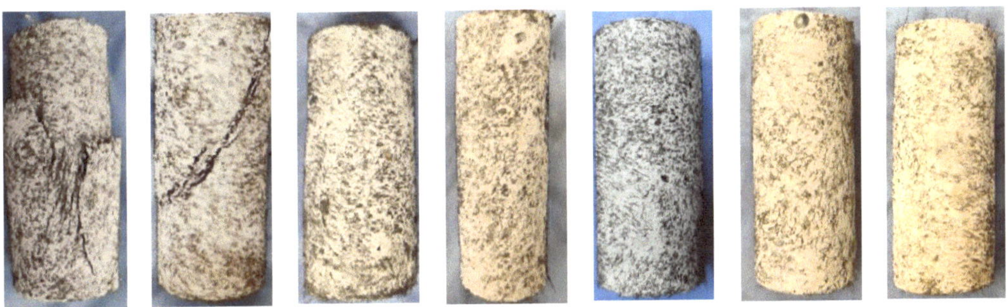

0 MPa 5 MPa 10 MPa 15 MPa 20 MPa 30 MPa 40 MPa

Figure 9. Failure patterns of the SFRGPC specimens with 2.5% MF10.

3.2. Stress–Strain Curves

Figure 10 depicts the complete axial stress–strain contours of the SFRGPC specimens subjected to various confining pressures. Figure 10a shows that the GPC exhibited a characteristic brittle failure curve when subjected to multi-axial compression. As the confining pressure increased, the strength and deformation of the GPC specimens increased by varying degrees, and the confining pressure limited the lateral deformation of specimens to some degree. Figure 10b–e illustrate that the peak stress and peak strain of the SFRGPC specimens increased substantially with the confining pressure. These outcomes indicate that the peak tension and peak strain increase with the increased addition of steel fiber content. Therefore, steel fiber can considerably improve the SFRGPC's strength and ductility. However, when the steel fiber exceeds a particular control content, the influence of the peak stress and peak strain decreases and stabilizes.

Analysis of the results reveals that the confining pressure had a greater effect on the tensile strength of the SFRGPC specimens. For specimens containing varying amounts of steel fiber, the triaxial compressive strength increased with the confining pressure. As the confining pressure increased, the specimens' lateral deformation was further constrained. The specimen was compressed further as the axial load increased, and the stress–strain curve exhibits an increasing trend. Consequently, the triaxial compression strength is represented by its first yield point, and the corresponding strain cannot be considered the maximum strain. The respective strain is not considered as the peak strain and is not enumerated in Table 3.

Without the addition of steel fiber, the respective increases in strength under various confining pressures of 5, 10, 15, 20, 30, and 40 MPa were 83%, 115%, 170%, 225%, 297%, and 374%. At an MF15 fiber volume ratio of 1.0%, the respective increments under various confining pressures were 95%, 144%, 233%, 308%, 349%, and 407%. The increments in various confining pressures were 111%, 171%, 221%, 276%, 341%, and 421% when the MF15 fiber volume ratio increased to 2.0%. At an MF06 fiber volume ratio of 2.5%, the respective increases in confining pressure were 101%, 173%, 218%, 254%, 298%, and 371%. Further increasing the MF10 fiber volume ratio to 2.5% resulted in increases of 110.4%, 178%, 258%, 290%, 386%, and 507%, respectively.

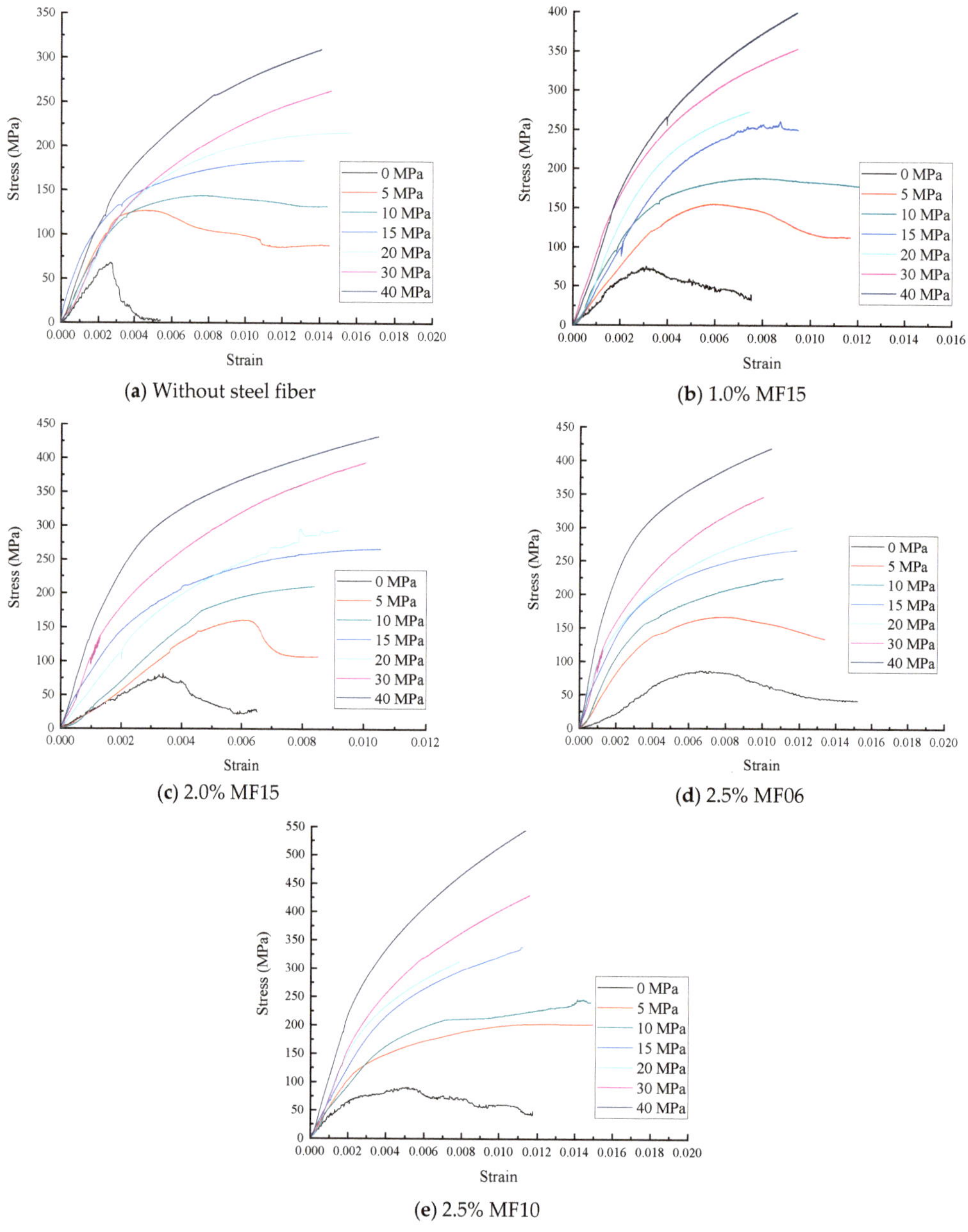

Figure 10. Stress–strain curves of SFRGPC specimens under different confining pressures.

Table 3. Triaxial compression test results.

Steel Fiber	V_f (%)	Confining Pressure (MPa)	Strength (MPa)	Peak Strain	Steel Fiber	V_f (%)	Confining Pressure (MPa)	Strength (MPa)	Peak Strain
Without steel fiber	0	0	68.33	0.0025	MF06	2.5	0	82.96	0.0040
		5	125.0	0.0055			5	166.32	0.0085
		10	146.87	0.0081			10	226.17	0.0101
		15	184.77	0.0145			15	264.20	0.0116
		20	222.39	---			20	293.28	---
		30	271.46	---			30	330.17	---
		40	323.75	---			40	390.33	---
MF15	1.0	0	78.63	0.0035	MF10	2.5	0	87.32	0.0052
		5	153.45	0.0058			5	197.72	0.0145
		10	192.11	0.0082			10	243.08	0.0147
		15	261.73	---			15	312.96	---
		20	320.46	---			20	340.79	---
		30	353.44	---			30	423.97	---
		40	398.99	---			40	530.34	---
MF15	2.0	0	83.95	0.0039					
		5	158.47	0.0063					
		10	207.63	0.0084					
		15	256.59	0.0100					
		20	301.03	---					
		30	327.59	---					
		40	403.34	---					

3.3. Failure Criterion

The peak stress increases linearly with the confining pressure, according to the Mohr–Coulomb failure criterion, expressed as

$$\frac{\sigma_1}{f_c} = a + k\frac{\sigma_3}{f_c} \tag{1}$$

where σ_1 is the peak stress, f_c is the uniaxial compression strength, a and k are the empirical coefficients fitted according to the experimental data related to the concrete material, and σ_3 is the confining pressure. The data from the above table are input into the formula, and the results are depicted in Figure 11a. The linear variation does not adequately explain the increase in peak SFRGPC stress with confining pressure, as shown in the graph. Therefore, the Mohr–Coulomb failure criterion (Formula (1)) is rewritten as an exponential function:

$$\frac{\sigma_1}{f_c} = 1 + k\left(\frac{\sigma_3}{f_c}\right)^a \tag{2}$$

where k and a are empirical coefficients.

As shown in Figure 11b and Formulas (3)–(7), as compared to the linear relationship previously proposed, this exponential function can more accurately predict the peak stress of SFRGPC under various confining pressures, steel fiber types, and steel fiber contents. The empirical coefficients k and a are affected by confining pressure and uniaxial compressive strength. This function can be used to predict the triaxial strength through confining pressure and uniaxial compressive strength in subsequent studies, which provides a certain basis for structural design.

$$\text{No Fiber} \quad \frac{\sigma_1}{f_c} = 1 + 5.686\left(\frac{\sigma_3}{f_c}\right)^{0.782} \quad R^2 = 0.99 \tag{3}$$

$$\text{1.0\% MF15} \quad \frac{\sigma_1}{f_c} = 1 + 6.570\left(\frac{\sigma_3}{f_c}\right)^{0.653} \quad R^2 = 0.95 \tag{4}$$

$$2.0\%\ \text{MF15} \quad \frac{\sigma_1}{f_c} = 1 + 6.072\left(\frac{\sigma_3}{f_c}\right)^{0.650} \quad R^2 = 0.98 \tag{5}$$

$$2.5\%\ \text{MF06} \quad \frac{\sigma_1}{f_c} = 1 + 5.548\left(\frac{\sigma_3}{f_c}\right)^{0.569} \quad R^2 = 0.99 \tag{6}$$

$$2.5\%\ \text{MF10} \quad \frac{\sigma_1}{f_c} = 1 + 8.571\left(\frac{\sigma_3}{f_c}\right)^{0.708} \quad R^2 = 0.99 \tag{7}$$

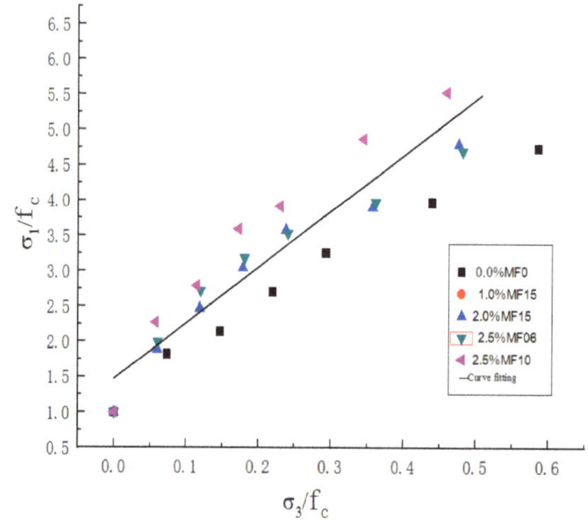

(**a**) Mohr–Coulomb failure criterion

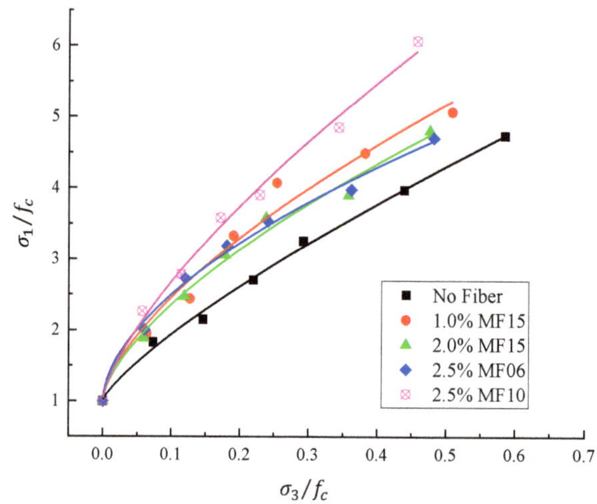

(**b**) Improved Mohr–Coulomb failure criterion

Figure 11. Comparison of peak stress fit and experimental values.

4. Discussion

4.1. Failure Pattern

The SFRGPC specimens' mode of failure can be determined by comparing steel fibers of the same 15 mm length and respective contents of 1% and 2% (Figures 6 and 7). The failure mode of the specimen was affected by the length of the steel fiber and steel fiber content. In this instance, all specimens were longitudinally fractured and damaged, and the failure behaviors did not vary significantly. The direction of the oblique fracture was 60 to 70 degrees relative to the horizontal. As the confining pressure rose, the damage patterns became oblique rupture failures, and the angle of crack development tended to decrease marginally. Although the specimens' failure mode changed to oblique shear failure as the confining pressure increased, the shear angle (i.e., the angle between the oblique crack and the horizontal plane) of the specimen with a 2.0% steel fiber content was smaller than that with a 1.0% steel fiber content. When the confining pressure exceeded 20 MPa, no surface cracks were evident on the specimen containing 2.0% steel fibers, whereas the specimen containing 1.0% steel fibers displayed obvious oblique shear cracks. Within a given volume, the more added steel fiber, the more energy the specimens can assimilate and the greater their ductility. The test results indicate that a 2% steel fiber content is optimal.

Comparing the failure patterns of specimens S1 and S2 under uniaxial compression (Figures 8 and 9) reveals that both specimens failed in a similar manner, with multiple irregular diagonal fractures. As the confining pressure increased, the specimen's failure pattern changed to oblique shear failure, but specimen S2 had a smaller shear angle than specimen S1. When the confining pressure exceeded 10 MPa, specimen S2 was not damaged, its length shortened, its diameter expanded, and its resistance to damage was greater than that of specimen S1, which continued to develop diagonal cracks.

4.2. Peak Stress

Under varied confining pressures, the trend of the stress–strain curve is evidently distinct, as shown in Figure 10. As the stress increased under uniaxial load, the strain changed swiftly, and the resulting stress–strain curve is steep with distinct peaks. When confining pressure was applied, as the tension gradually increased, the strain was more gradual with no prominent peak point. The section of the curve that consists of a straight line is shorter, whereas the ascending section is longer. The descending portion of the curve decreases more slowly, indicating greater ductility, and the specimen's failure is relatively prolonged. This demonstrates that, under confining pressure, internal fracture and radial deformation of the specimen are constrained, resulting in a gradual increase in concrete strain. The contours still have a descending section when the confining pressure is less than 15 MPa. At confining pressures greater than 15 MPa, the tension and strain continued to increase, with no descending section. In addition, the confining pressure increased the elastic modulus, peak stress, peak strain, and area covered by the stress–strain curve. The results indicate that confinement pressure can drastically alter the brittle failure of SFRGPC.

At a confining pressure, the principal compressive stress and axial strain both increase proportionally with the increase in fiber content, and the curve trend is roughly the same. However, the stress–strain curves of S4 are more extensive than those of S3, demonstrating that steel fiber has a constraining effect on the specimen, inhibiting lateral deformation. With a constant confining pressure and steel fiber content, as the length of the steel fiber increases, the peak strain and peak tension of the specimen also increase.

The steel fiber content and ratio of length to diameter have obvious influence on the compressive strength of SFRGPC. As the steel fiber content increased, the compressive strength increased by 1.15–1.44 times, as the ratio of length to diameter increased, the compressive strength increased by 1.21–1.70 times. The increase in confining pressure can improve the compressive strength of concrete. With the increase in confining pressure, the increase trend of compressive strength becomes smooth.

4.3. Compression Toughness

The area under the stress–strain curve is an index commonly used to determine the compressive toughness of concrete materials [33]. Figure 12 illustrates the definition of the compressive toughness index. In the ascending portion of the stress–strain curve, the critical stress is defined as 85% of the maximal stress at point A. Point B represents the critical strain corresponding to the critical stress. On the strain coordinate axis, points D and F correspond to strains C and E, respectively, on the stress–strain curve. The indices of compressive toughness, η_{c2} and η_{c3}, can then be defined as follows:

$$\eta_{c2} = \frac{S_{OACD}}{S_{OAB}} \tag{8}$$

$$\eta_{c3} = \frac{S_{OAEF}}{S_{OAB}} \tag{9}$$

where S_{OAB}, S_{OACD}, and S_{OAEF} represent the respective areas enclosed by curves OAB, OACD, and OAEF.

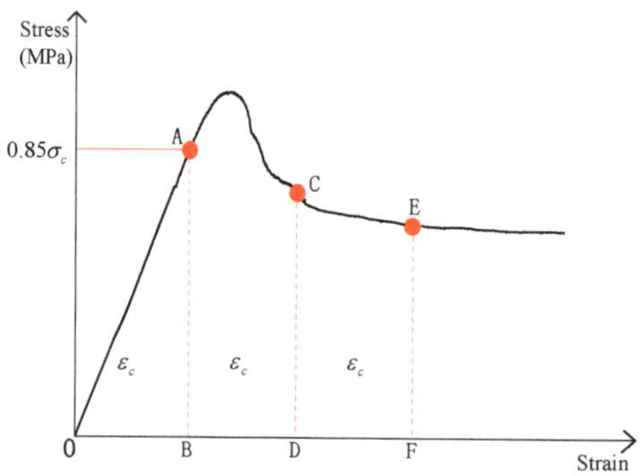

Figure 12. Schematic diagram defining the compressive toughness index.

As shown in Figure 10, when the confining pressure exceeds 10 MPa, the stress increases slowly and does not appear to decrease as the strain increases. Therefore, Table 4 contains compressive toughness index data for only three confining pressures: 0, 5, and 10 MPa.

Table 4. Specimens' compression toughness indices.

V_f (%)	Fiber Length (mm)	Confining Pressure (MPa)	σ_c (MPa)	Critical Stress (MPa)	Critical Strain	S_{OAB}	η_{c2}	η_{c3}
0	0	0	68.47	58.20	0.0020	0.0539	2.56	2.78
		5	117.10	99.45	0.0031	0.152	3.30	5.34
		10	143.85	122.27	0.0036	0.249	2.96	4.98
1.0	15	0	83.31	70.81	0.00278	0.0904	2.52	3.35
		5	149.94	127.45	0.00371	0.187	2.91	4.51
		10	188.16	159.93	0.00372	0.339	2.95	5.22
2.0	15	0	81.57	69.33	0.00283	0.108	2.81	3.15
		5	158.95	135.11	0.0035	0.257	3.63	6.04
		10	202.95	172.50	0.0059	0.481	3.39	5.79
2.5	6	0	86.71	73.70	0.0026	0.084	---	---
		5	164.69	139.98	0.0043	0.374	2.81	4.63
		10	226.30	192.35	0.0054	0.597	2.96	4.99
2.5	10	0	83.86	71.28	0.0037	0.157	2.51	3.36
		5	202.58	172.19	0.0060	0.689	2.712	4.43
		10	255.20	216.92	0.0086	1.117	2.88	4.84

With various steel fiber contents, ratio of length to diameter, and confining pressure conditions, the critical compressive toughness of SFRGPC varies significantly, as shown in Figure 13. The relationship between the confining pressure and the essential compressive toughness exhibits a linear growth pattern. As shown in Table 4, the distinction between compression and compressive toughness index is more intuitive. Consequently, the compressive toughness index can better capture the influence of confining pressure, steel fiber length, and steel fiber content on the compressive toughness of SFRGPC specimens.

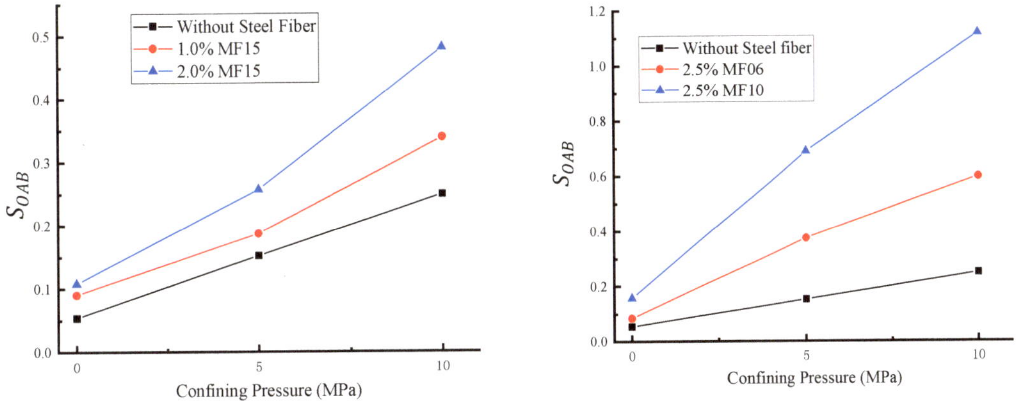

(**a**) Different steel fiber volumes (**b**) Different steel fiber types

Figure 13. S_{OAB}—confining pressure relationship curve.

As depicted in Figure 14a, η_{c3} increases linearly with confining pressure; however, once the confining pressure reaches a certain strength, η_{c3} does not increase significantly and tends to be stable.

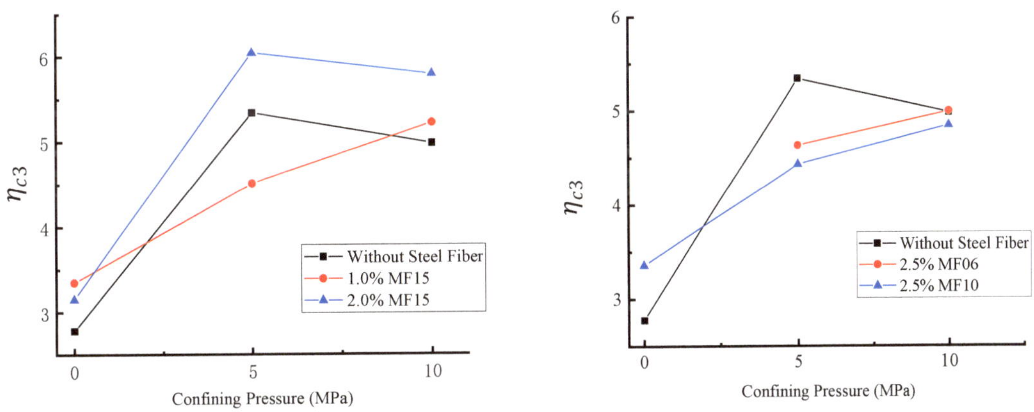

(**a**) Different steel fiber volumes (**b**) Different steel fiber types

Figure 14. η_{c3}—confining pressure relationship curve.

As depicted in Figure 14b, under the same confining pressure condition, a decrease in η_{c3} is not apparent as the steel fiber content increases, indicating a nonlinear decrease. In the process of concrete pouring, due to the agglomeration effect of steel fiber added, the compactness of SFRGPC will be reduced and small bubbles will be produced compared with GPC. In the course of the test, due to the reason of compactness, the stress–strain curve will change to a certain extent, resulting in obvious and unclear compressive toughness changes.

5. Numerical Simulation

5.1. Modeling Method and Verification

The finite element modeling approach utilized in this investigation was validated and verified through the development of numerical models of SFRGPC specimens subjected to triaxial stress. The results of the tests are compared to determine if the specified material properties, contact method, element size, and method of applying load were accurate.

In this study, the SFRGPC is modeled using the CONCRETE_DAMAGE_Rel3 (MAT_072R3) solid element and material model in LS-DYNA. The MAT_072R3 model is a plastic damage model that depicts the strength development and damage evolution of concrete through three independent strength surfaces: yield strength surface F_y, maximum strength surface F_m, and residual strength surface F_r. In addition, users can also define their own strain rate–dynamic increase coefficient curves and equations of state [34,35].

This investigation used a hexahedral solid element with eight nodes to model concrete, and mesh refinement experiments were conducted. The initial mesh size of concrete was estimated to be 5 × 5 × 5 mm. Once the load–deformation behavior simulated with this mesh size was deemed acceptable, the mesh was refined to 2.5 × 2.5 × 2.5 mm and 1 × 1 × 1 mm. The numerical convergence study indicates that the data of mesh sizes of 2.5 and 1 mm are closer to the experimental curve, and the average difference between the simulation results of two different mesh sizes is less than 2%, as shown in Figure 15. However, the calculation time for the 1 mm mesh was significantly longer. Consequently, the 2.5 mm mesh size was utilized for further analysis and parameterization.

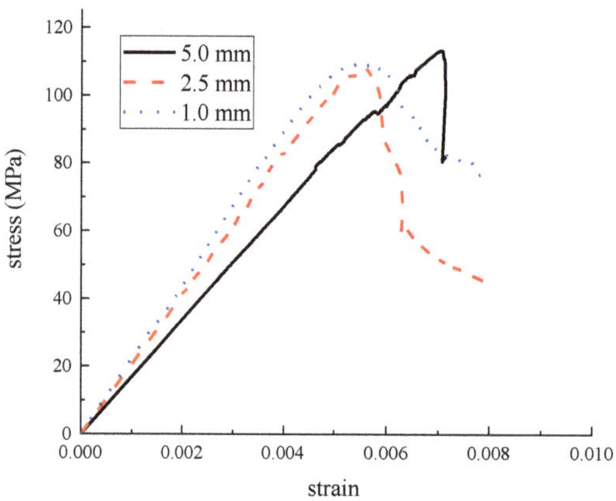

Figure 15. Results of mesh size convergence study.

The user can also automatically generate model parameters that can be checked and modified. Table 5 outlines the parameter values used in this study.

Table 5. Key parameters of CONCRETE_DAMAGE_Rel3 (MAT_072R3) model for SFRGPC.

Density (kg/m^3)	Poisson's Ratio	f_c' (MPa)	f_t (MPa)	b_1	b_2	b_3	Omega
2400	0.19	87	5.45	0.85	2.89	1.88	0.75

The findings of the experiments and simulations of SFRGPC specimens subjected to triaxial strain are shown in Figures 16 and 17, respectively. The transverse fractures created in the numerical model accurately represent the failure mechanism when subjected to triaxial force. The connections between the stress and strain occurring in SFRGPC specimens are shown graphically in Figure 17. The patterns of growth and the location of the curve's inflection point when subjected to triaxial pressures are virtually the same in both the computational results and the experimental data.

Therefore, the numerical model can accurately represent the failure mode and stress–strain curves of SFRGPC specimens subjected to triaxial stresses, confirming the model's dependability.

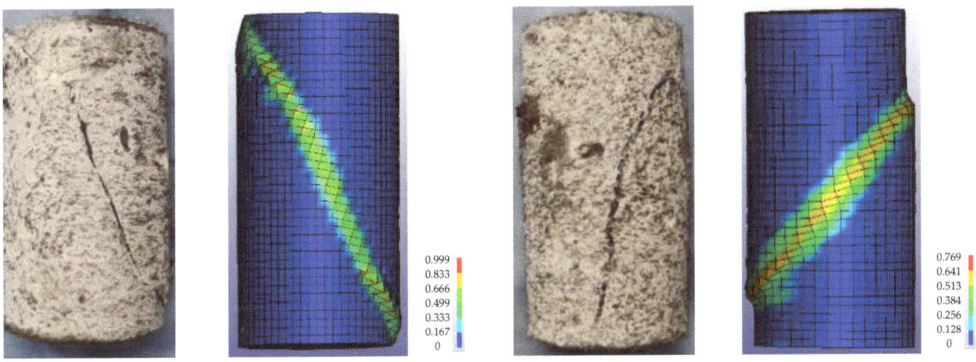

(**a**) 1.0% MF15 (**b**) 2.0% MF15

Figure 16. Effective Plastic Strain of test and simulation results.

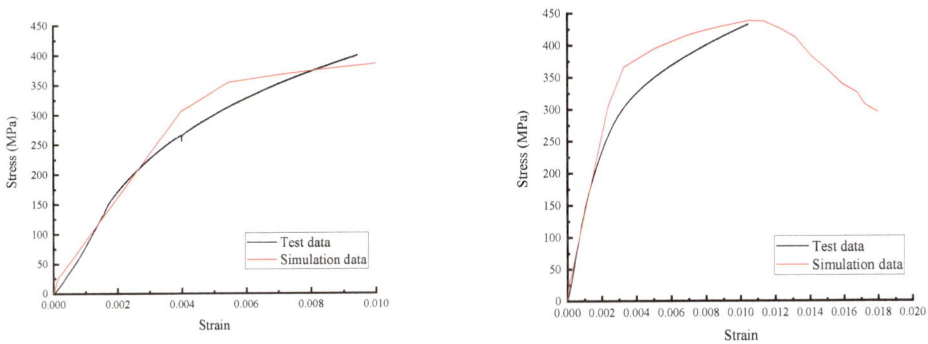

(**a**) 1.0% MF15 (**b**) 2.0% MF15

Figure 17. Comparison of stress–strain curves for experimental tests and simulations.

5.2. Size Effect

5.2.1. Failure Patterns

Figures 18 and 19 illustrate the failure patterns of SFRGPC specimens with varied diameters (50 and 100 mm) and a uniform aspect ratio of 0.5 when subjected to various confining pressures (40, 70, and 110 MPa).

Figure 18 depicts the failure modes of ∅50 × 100 mm SFRGPC specimens with varying steel fiber contents and confining pressures (From blue to red, the damage degree of the specimen is more obvious). As the confining pressure increases, the area of stress clouds expands, and a vertical fracture parallel to the loading direction appears in the middle of the specimen during the early stage of loading, followed by the formation of one or more main cracks that penetrate the specimen. All numerical specimen models subjected to uniaxial compression exhibited excellent ductility. The lower two-thirds of the specimen model incurs substantial damage when the confining pressure exceeds 110 MPa. When the confining pressure is increased, the cylinder gradually expands and extends longitudinally, causing oblique cracking through the existing cracks until failure.

Comparing the failure patterns under 40 and 70 MPa confining pressures, the cracks are progressively distributed throughout the cylinder, not just at the bottom. At a pressure of 110 MPa, the cylinder is damaged, and the longitudinal deformation increases as the circumferential pressure approaches the uniaxial compressive strength.

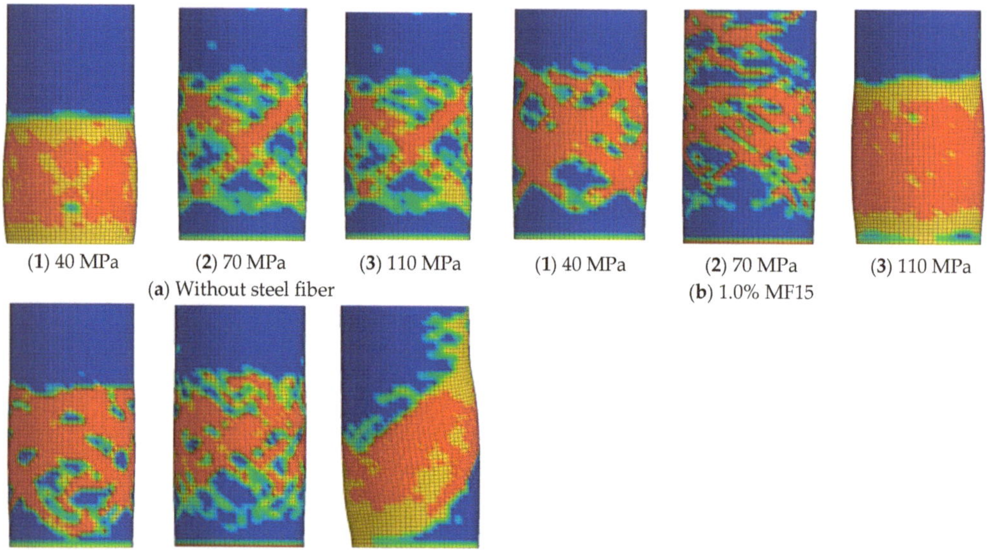

(1) 40 MPa (2) 70 MPa (3) 110 MPa
(a) Without steel fiber

(1) 40 MPa (2) 70 MPa (3) 110 MPa
(b) 1.0% MF15

(1) 40 MPa (2) 70 MPa (3) 110 MPa
(c) 2.0% MF15

Figure 18. Failure patterns of ∅50 × 100 mm concrete cylinders under different confining pressures.

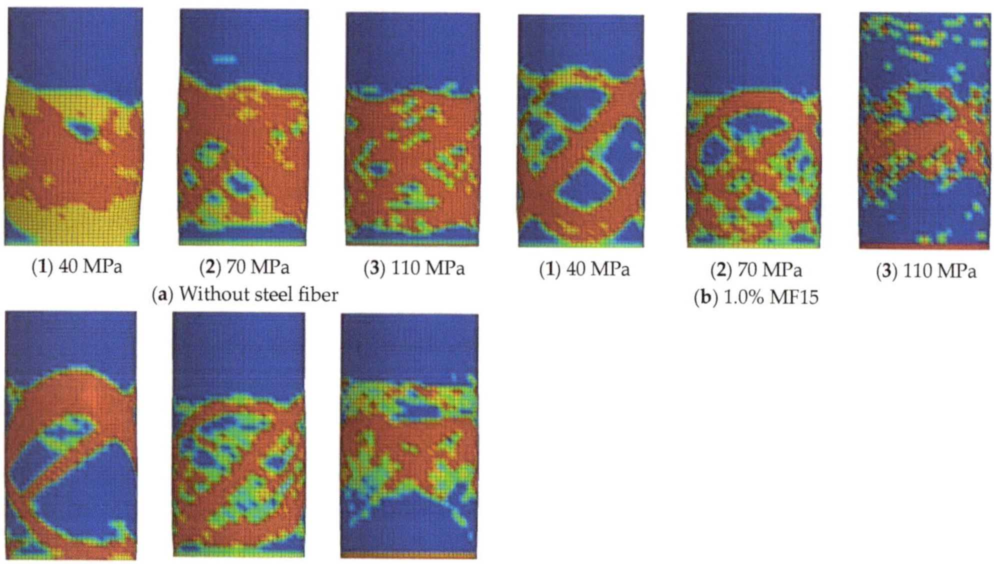

(1) 40 MPa (2) 70 MPa (3) 110 MPa
(a) Without steel fiber

(1) 40 MPa (2) 70 MPa (3) 110 MPa
(b) 1.0% MF15

(1) 40 MPa (2) 70 MPa (3) 110 MPa
(c) 2.0% MF15

Figure 19. Failure patterns of ∅100 × 200 mm concrete cylinders under different confining pressures.

Figure 19 presents the failure modes of ∅100 × 200 mm SFRGPC models with varying steel fiber contents and confining pressures. As the confining pressure increases, the failure modes become increasingly concentrated at the center for all models, as depicted in the figure. Low confining pressures result in the formation of fractures. With the steel fibers, the SFRGPC cylinders exhibit fewer cracks than GPC without steel fiber. Thus, the steel fibers improve the ductility of the GPC and allow it to absorb additional energy during the failure process.

In conclusion, when the size of the specimen increases at the same confining pressure, a gradual decrease occurs in the specimen's strength. The damage caused by the failure state of a specimen made of the same material progressively accumulates from deformation to stress and migrates to the specimen's center.

5.2.2. Stress–Strain Curve

As depicted in Figure 20, under the same confining pressure, the concrete cylinder's strength does not significantly decrease as its size increases. The confining pressure restricts its lateral deformation to some degree. With the decrease in stress and peak strain, the deformation reaches its maximum value, and as the volume ratio of steel fiber increases, the internal stress progressively decreases. Although the addition of steel fiber can improve the tensile strength and ductility of SFRGPC, after it exceeds a certain threshold, the effect of size on the specimen's peak tension and peak strain is diminished. Since the modeling is based on the test data, there may be some defects in the production process of the specimen, so the data change significantly in the numerical simulation. In the follow-up study, we will optimize the numerical model and further establish a microscopic model to highlight the strengthening effect of steel fiber.

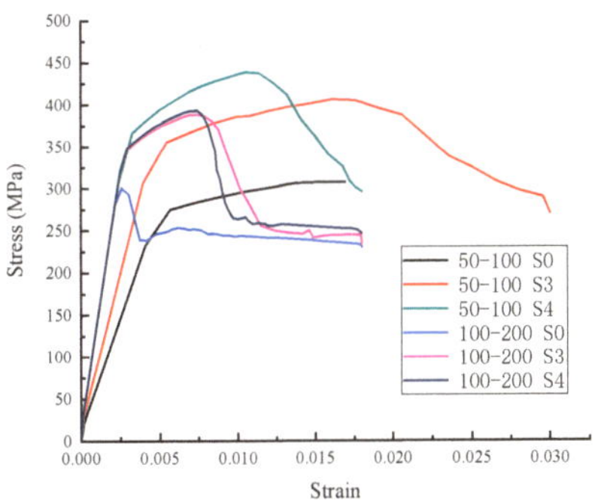

(**a**) 40 MPa

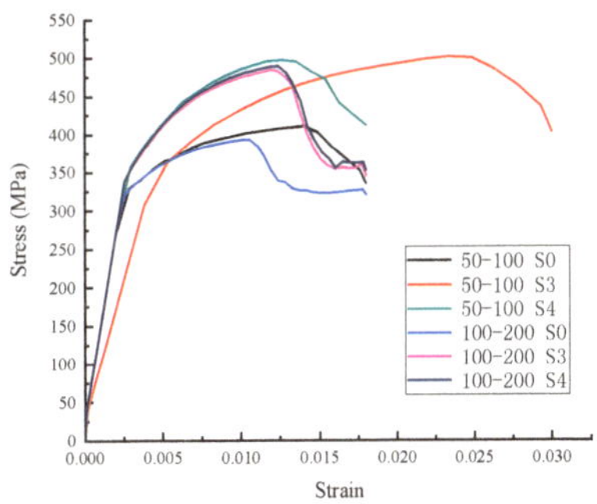

(**b**) 70 MPa

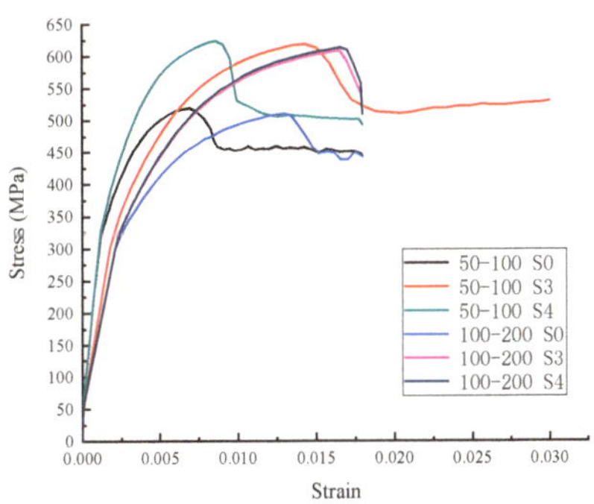

(**c**) 110 MPa

Figure 20. Stress-strain curves of specimens with different sizes and materials under the same confining pressures.

6. Conclusions

This study investigates the relationships of stress, strain, and compressive toughness with confining pressure, steel fiber volume fraction, and steel fiber length in SFRGPC. The material model, generated in LS-DYNA R11.2.2 software, was validated by the test data. The results will better guide the application of SFRGPC in the future application. The key findings are as follows:

1. Under uniaxial compression, with the increase in steel fiber content, the failure mode of the SFRGPC specimens gradually developed into ductile failure.
2. Under multi-axial compression, with the confining pressure increased, a corresponding increase in the angle between the failure crack and the longitudinal axis of the specimens occurred. As the confining pressure and steel fiber content increased, the brittleness of the SFRGPC can be completely eliminated, and its resistance to breaking can be greatly improved.
3. The steel fiber content and ratio of length to diameter have obvious influence on the compressive strength of SFRGPC. As the steel fiber content increased, the compressive strength increased by 1.15–1.44 times; as the ratio of length to diameter increased, the compressive strength increased by 1.21–1.70 times. The increase in confining pressure can improve the compressive strength of concrete. With the increase in confining pressure, the increase trend of compressive strength becomes smooth. The relationship between the peak stress and the confining pressure is linear and proportional.
4. The confining pressure, steel fiber content, and steel fiber length have substantial influences on the compressive toughness index η_{c3}. Under increasing confining pressure, η_{c3} increases linearly; however, after confining pressure is higher than 5 MPa, η_{c3} tends toward a steady state when the confining pressure increases.
5. By modifying the parameters of the material model, a uniform numerical model was established, and the simulation results matched the experimental data.

Author Contributions: Conceptualization, P.W.; methodology, P.W. and Y.Z.; software, X.W. and Y.Z.; validation, P.W.; investigation, Y.Z.; resources, P.W.; data curation, X.W.; writing—original draft preparation, X.W. and Y.Z.; writing—review and editing, P.W.; visualization, Q.L.; supervision, Q.L.; project administration, P.W. All authors have read and agreed to the published version of the manuscript.

Funding: The research presented herein is jointly supported by the National Natural Science Foundation of China (Grant Nos. 52308518 and 52208281) and the Natural Science Foundation of Tianjin, China (Grant No. 23YDTPJC00100).

Data Availability Statement: The data presented in this study are available on request from the corresponding author. The data are not publicly available due to authors need to apply for a patent.

Acknowledgments: The test result was finished in Tianjin Key Laboratory of civil structure protection and reinforcement, Tianjin Chengjian University.

Conflicts of Interest: Author Pengtao Wu was employed by the company Tianjin Building Materials Science Research Academy Co., Ltd. The remaining authors declare that the research was conducted in the absence of any commercial or financial relationships that could be construed as a potential conflict of interest.

References

1. Nguyen, H.T.; Pham, T.K.; Promentilla, M.A.B. Development of Geopolymer-Based Materials from Coal Bottom Ash and Rice Husk Ash with Sodium Silicate Solutions. In Proceedings of the 4th Congrès International de Géotechnique—Ouvrages—Structures, Ho Chi Minh City, Vietnam, 26–27 October 2017; Springer: Singapore, 2017.
2. Mcguire, E.M.; Provis, J.L.; Duxson, P.; Crawford, R.H. Geopolymer Concrete: Is There an Alternative and Viable Technology in the Concrete Sector which Reduces Carbon Emissions. In Proceedings of the Concrete: Building A Sustainable Future, Perth, Australia, 22 October 2011.
3. Davidovits, J. Geopolymer Cement a review. *Geopolymer Sci. Tech.* **2013**, *21*, 1–11.
4. Morsy, M.S.; Alsayed, S.H.; Al-Salloum, Y.; Almusallam, T. Effect of Sodium Silicate to Sodium Hydroxide Ratios on Strength and Microstructure of Fly Ash Geopolymer Binder. *Arab. J. Sci. Eng.* **2014**, *39*, 4333–4339. [CrossRef]

5. Nematollahi, B.; Sanjayan, J. Effect of different superplasticizers and activator combinations on workability and strength of fly ash based geopolymer. *Mater. Des.* **2014**, *57*, 667–672. [CrossRef]
6. Arora, S.; Jangra, P.; Lim, Y.Y.; Pham, T.M. Strength, durability, and microstructure of self-compacting geopolymer concrete produced with copper slag aggregates. *Environ. Sci. Pollut. Res.* **2022**, *30*, 666–684. [CrossRef]
7. Ghafoor, M.T.; Khan, Q.S.; Qazi, A.U.; Sheikh, M.N.; Hadi, M.N.S. Influence of alkaline activators on the mechanical properties of fly ash based geopolymer concrete cured at ambient temperature. *Constr. Build. Mater.* **2021**, *273*, 121752. [CrossRef]
8. Lincy, G.A.; Velkennedy, R. Experimental optimization of metakaolin and nanosilica composite for geopolymer concrete paver blocks. *Struct. Concr.* **2020**, *22*, E442–E451.
9. Yoo, D.Y.; Banthia, N. Mechanical properties of ultra-high-performance fiber-reinforced concrete: A review. *Cem. Concr. Compos.* **2016**, *73*, 267–280. [CrossRef]
10. Ranjbar, N.; Zhang, M. Fiber reinforced geopolymer composites: A review. *Cem. Concr. Compos.* **2019**, *107*, 103498. [CrossRef]
11. Ganesh, A.C.; Muthukannan, M. Development of high performance sustainable optimized fiber reinforced geopolymer concrete and prediction of compressive strength. *J. Clean. Prod.* **2020**, *282*, 124543. [CrossRef]
12. Moradikhou, A.B.; Esparham, A.; Avanaki, M.J. Physical & mechanical properties of fiber reinforced metakaolin-based geopolymer concrete. *Constr. Build. Mater.* **2020**, *251*, 118965.
13. Liu, J.; Wu, C.; Liu, Z.; Li, J.; Xu, S.; Liu, K.; Su, Y.; Chen, G. Investigations on the response of ceramic ball aggregated and steel fibre reinforced geopolymer-based ultra-high performance concrete (G-UHPC) to projectile penetration. *Compos. Struct.* **2021**, *255*, 112983. [CrossRef]
14. Noushini, A.; Hastings, M.; Castel, A.; Aslani, F. Mechanical and flexural performance of synthetic fibre reinforced geopolymer concrete. *Constr. Build. Mater.* **2018**, *186*, 454–475. [CrossRef]
15. Liu, Y.; Zhang, Z.; Shi, C.; Zhu, D.; Li, N.; Deng, Y. Development of ultra-high performance geopolymer concrete (UHPGC): Influence of steel fiber on mechanical properties. *Cem. Concr. Compos.* **2020**, *112*, 103670. [CrossRef]
16. Sharma, U.; Gupta, N.; Bahrami, A.; Özkılıç, Y.O.; Verma, M.; Berwal, P.; Althaqafi, E.; Khan, M.A.; Islam, S. Behavior of Fibers in Geopolymer Concrete: A Comprehensive Review. *Buildings* **2024**, *14*, 136. [CrossRef]
17. Meskhi, B.; Beskopylny, A.N.; Stel'makh, S.A.; Shcherban', E.M.; Mailyan, L.R.; Shilov, A.A.; El'shaeva, D.; Shilova, K.; Karalar, M.; Aksoylu, C.; et al. Analytical Review of Geopolymer Concrete: Retrospective and Current Issues. *Materials* **2023**, *16*, 3792. [CrossRef]
18. Çelik, A.İ.; Özkılıç, Y.O.; Bahrami, A.; Hakeem, I.Y. Effects of glass fiber on recycled fly ash and basalt powder based geopolymer concrete. *Case Stud. Constr. Mater.* **2023**, *19*, e02659. [CrossRef]
19. Özkılıç, Y.O.; Çelik, A.İ.; Tunç, U.; Karalar, M.; Deifalla, A.; Alomayri, T.; Althoey, F. The use of crushed recycled glass for alkali activated fly ash based geopolymer concrete and prediction of its capacity. *J. Mater. Res. Technol.* **2023**, *24*, 8267–8281. [CrossRef]
20. Kufper, H. Behavior of Concrete under Biaxial Stresses. *Aci J.* **1969**, *66*, 656–666.
21. Zhou, J.; Pan, J.; Ma, H.; Zhao, J.; Li, Z. Behavior of high-performance concrete under multiaxial tensile-compressive loading. *Constr. Build. Mater.* **2020**, *260*, 119887. [CrossRef]
22. Wang, Y.Z.; Wang, Y.B.; Zhao, Y.Z.; Li, G.Q.; Lyu, Y.F.; Li, H. Experimental study on ultra-high performance concrete under triaxial compression. *Constr. Build. Mater.* **2020**, *263*, 120225. [CrossRef]
23. Ren, G.M.; Wu, H.; Fang, Q.; Liu, J.Z.; Gong, Z.M. Triaxial compressive behavior of UHPCC and applications in the projectile impact analyses. *Constr. Build. Mater.* **2016**, *113*, 1–14. [CrossRef]
24. Khan, M.Z.N.; Hao, Y.; Hao, H.; Shaikh, F.U.A.; Liu, K. Mechanical properties of ambient cured high-strength plain and hybrid fiber reinforced geopolymer composites from triaxial compressive tests. *Constr. Build. Mater.* **2018**, *185*, 338–353. [CrossRef]
25. Meng, E.; Yu, Y.; Zhang, X.; Su, Y. Experimental and theoretical research on the mechanical performance of totally recycled concrete under triaxial compression after high temperatures. *Constr. Build. Mater.* **2020**, *261*, 120012. [CrossRef]
26. Zhang, K.; Zhao, L.Y.; Ni, T.; Zhu, Q.Z.; Shen, J.; Fan, Y.H. Experimental investigation and multiscale modeling of reactive powder cement pastes subject to triaxial compressive stresses. *Constr. Build. Mater.* **2019**, *224*, 242–254. [CrossRef]
27. Chern, J.C.; Yang, H.J.; Chen, H.W. Behavior of steel fiber reinforced concrete in multiaxial loading. *Aci Mater. J.* **1993**, *89*, 32–40.
28. Lu, X.; Hsu, C. Behavior of high strength concrete with and without steel fiber reinforcement in triaxial compression. *Cem. Concr. Res.* **2006**, *36*, 1679–1685. [CrossRef]
29. Farnam, Y.; Moosavi, M.; Shekarchi, M.; Babanajad, S.K.; Bagherzadeh, A. Behaviour of Slurry Infiltrated Fibre Concrete (SIFCON) under triaxial compression. *Cem. Concr. Res.* **2010**, *40*, 1571–1581. [CrossRef]
30. Wang, Z.; Zhu, B. Strength and Toughness Characteristic of Steel Fiber Reinforced Concrete in Triaxial Compression. *J. Build. Mater.* **2012**, *15*, 301–305+311.
31. Wang, Z.L.; Zhu, H.H.; Wang, J.G.; Zhu, B. Experimental Study on Macroscopic Mechanical Behavior of SFRC under Triaxial Compression. *Mech. Adv. Mater. Struct.* **2012**, *19*, 653–662. [CrossRef]
32. *The ISRM Suggested Methods for Rock Characterization, Testing and Monitoring: 2007–2014*; International Society for Rock, Echanics, Commission on Testing Methods: Lisbon, Portugal, 2015.
33. Wu, P.; Wu, C.; Liu, Z.; Xu, S.; Li, J.; Li, J. Triaxial strength and failure criterion of ultra-high performance concrete. *Adv. Struct. Eng.* **2022**, *25*, 1893–1906. [CrossRef]

34. Malvar, L.J.; Crawford, J.E.; Wesevich, J.W.; Simons, D. A plasticity concrete material model for DYNA3D. *Int. J. Impact Eng.* **1997**, *19*, 847–873. [CrossRef]
35. Crawford, J.E.; Wu, J.; Choi, H.J.; Magallanes, J.M.; Lan, S. *Use and validation of the release III K&C concrete model in LS-DYNA*; Karagozian & Case: Glendale, CA, USA, 2012.

buildings

MDPI

Article

Experimental Study on Axial Compression of Bamboo Scrimber Cold-Formed Thin-Walled Steel Composite Special-Shaped Columns

Chao Lei [1], Yuhao Wu [1], Bingyang Yang [1], Bingbing Wang [1], Jianqiang Han [1,2,*] and Xiuyan Fu [1]

1 College of Civil and Architectural Engineering, North China University of Science and Technology, Tangshan 063210, China; 15116323777@163.com (C.L.); wu2393461360@163.com (Y.W.); fuxiyan@ncst.edu.cn (X.F.)

2 Key Laboratory of Earthquake Engineering and Disaster Prevention of Hebei Province, Tangshan 063210, China

* Correspondence: hjq@ncst.edu.cn; Tel.: +86-15032587758

Abstract: As one of the four key sectors for energy saving and emissions reduction, the construction industry faces ongoing high energy consumption and emissions. To support China's sustainable development, urgent promotion of green construction and energy-saving measures is necessary. This led to the proposal of nine specimens of L-shaped, T-shaped, and cross-shaped engineered bamboo, cold-formed thin-walled steel, and their combinations for axial compression tests to study the effect of bamboo–steel structures on axial compression performance. The results showed that the load-bearing capacity of the three bamboo–steel composite columns increased by 19.5–21.4% compared to the sum of steel composite and L-shaped bamboo composite columns, significantly enhancing overall stability and deformation capacity. The synergy between steel and engineered bamboo effectively addressed the instability issues of steel structures with large width-to-thickness ratios. Using Abaqus finite element software for simulation, the stress distribution at failure and load-displacement curves were closely aligned with experimental outcomes. The study presents a formula for calculating the axial compression capacity of cold-formed thin-walled steel-engineered bamboo composite columns, with theoretical and experimental discrepancies within 13.28%, offering a theoretical basis for the design of engineered bamboo–steel composite columns.

Keywords: cold-formed thin-walled steel; reorganized bamboo; special-shaped column; axial compression

1. Introduction

In recent years, with the rapid development of China's economy, the scale of the construction industry has been expanded and the technical strength has been obviously improved. As one of the four key sectors for energy-saving and emissions reduction, the construction industry faces ongoing high energy consumption and emissions [1]. To support the objectives of China's sustainable development, urgent promotion of green construction and energy-saving measures is necessary. With vast resources and a large population, China has been engaged in housing construction since ancient times. In recent years, with the continuous updating of China's smelting process and the continuous increase of steel production, China has become a steel power. With the unique advantages of raw materials, steel structure has a wider range of applications. The cold-formed thin-walled steel structure system has been applied in many forms in China. With the advantages of light structural mass, good anti-seismic performance, flexible and diversified cross-section forms, easy processing, and environment-friendly and recyclable building materials, etc., it has wide applicability [2]. In recent years, logging has been strictly prohibited in China, and there is a large demand for timber. Meanwhile, bamboo, as an original product in China, has numerous types, strong adaptability, wide distribution, and many advantages. Raw bamboo is convenient to obtain, low in price, and short in maturity duration, and it is an excellent raw material for construction [3–7].

With the constant improvement of specifications for cold-formed thin-walled steel and bamboo scrimber, the study of cold-formed thin-walled steel has developed from the ground floor to high-rise buildings, and domestic and foreign scholars are devoted to studying the physical properties of bamboo scrimber and cold-formed thin-walled steel composite structures [8,9]. In the study of the built-in reinforced bamboo scrimber column, it is found that the ultimate bearing capacity, rigidity, and ductility of the specimen can be improved by increasing the reinforcement ratio of the specimen. When the stirrup ratio is not changed, the increase in slenderness ratio will lead to a decrease in rigidity, ductility, and ultimate bearing capacity of the specimen, further causing the failure state to change from adhesive layer failure to buckling failure [10]. The bearing capacity of the steel–bamboo composite structure is in proportion to the slenderness ratio of the specimen and the width–thickness ratio of the section. The two materials have an obvious combination effect, and the specimen shows good bearing capacity and ductility, which indicates that the two materials collaborate well [11–13]. The bamboo scrimber improves the problem of easy instability for the cold-formed thin-walled steel section due to the large width–thickness ratio, and the cold-formed thin-walled steel also inhibits the deformation and failure of the bamboo scrimber [14–18]. In the case of loading the same load, the weight of reconstituted bamboo is lighter than that of other woods, reducing the self-weight of the building and having unique advantages as a load-bearing component [19,20].

Combined with relevant research in China and abroad, this paper proposes bamboo scrimber cold-formed thin-walled steel composite special-shaped column specimens of L-shape, T-shape, and cross-shape. All the contact surfaces of L-shaped cold-formed thin-walled steel and bamboo scrimber are bonded with epoxy resin adhesive, and the bonded specimen is reinforced with bolts to ensure the integrity of the composite special-shaped column. The specific form of the composite column is shown in Figure 1. Through the axial compression test, the axial compression bearing capacity of each special-shaped column is obtained. In the paper, the failure mechanism of the bamboo–steel composite special-shaped column is obtained by exploring the experimental phenomena and the failure status as well as analyzing the experimental data, and a reasonable formula for calculating the axial compression bearing capacity is put forward by comparing the improvement in the overall stability and deformation capacity of the specimen from the bamboo–steel composite special-shaped column. The structure of the steel–bamboo composite special-shaped column combines the advantages of the integral aesthetic sense, the flexible function design, and the excellent bearing performance of the building so that the construction industry in China will enter a brand-new period of progress in the future, and the composite structure will inevitably have a wider application range and better development.

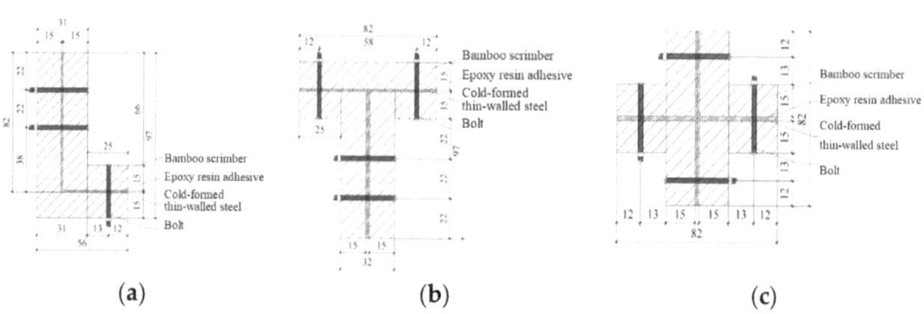

Figure 1. The specific size of the composite column. (**a**) Section of L-shaped bamboo–steel composite special-shaped column; (**b**) Section of T-shaped bamboo–steel composite special-shaped column; (**c**) Section of cross-shaped bamboo–steel composite special-shaped column.

2. Experiment Overview

2.1. Design of Experiment

In the experiment, nine composite special-shaped columns of L-shaped, T-shaped, and cross-shaped bamboo scrimber composite special-shaped columns, cold-formed thin-walled steel composite special-shaped columns, and bamboo scrimber cold-formed thin-walled steel composite special-shaped columns are designed, as shown in Table 1. The thickness of the steel is 1 mm, and the length of the specimen is 1200 mm. Place the polished steel profile and the reorganized bamboo board on a horizontal surface and place the side to be coated with glue on it. Mix the epoxy resin glue HB-826 according to the ratio of 1:1; within 10 min, the epoxy resin glue evenly coats in the reorganization of the bamboo board and the steel section, and the thickness of the glue coating is about 1 mm. Then, with the reorganization of the bamboo board and steel according to the design of the splicing, the use of fixtures will be fixed so that the steel and reorganization of bamboo between the epoxy resin adhesive is evenly distributed and will overflow, the excess epoxy resin adhesive wiped away, placed for 24 h. After the completion of the combination of the components, the electric drill will be used to drill the bolts into design position (bolt size of M5 mm × 50 mm, the vertical spacing is 200 mm). When the bolts are just, all in the member of the internal stop so that each bolt is into the member of the same depth, this will ensure the integrity of the combination of components during the test. For the specific dimensions, see Table 1.

Table 1. Design parameters of bamboo–steel composite special-shaped columns.

Specification	No.	Specimen Size/(mm)	Slenderness Ratio
L-shaped column	L-G-Z	82 × 41 × 1	71.8
	L-Z-Z	96 × 55 × 30 × 30	62.1
	L-G-Z-Z	97 × 56 × 31 × 31	38.4
T-shaped column	T-G-Z	82 × 82 × 2 × 1	61.3
	T-Z-Z	80 × 66 × 30 × 30	46.7
	T-G-Z-Z	82 × 66 × 31 × 32	45.4
Cross-shaped column	S-G-Z	82 × 82 × 2 × 2	50.0
	S-Z-Z	80 × 80 × 30 × 30	44.4
	S-G-Z-Z	82 × 82 × 32 × 32	43.1

2.2. Material Property Test

The bamboo scrimber plate in the composite column adopts phyllostachys pubescens as the raw material, and the cold-formed thin-walled steel adopts the model of Q235. The mechanical properties are measured again for the materials in the uniform batch used in the text.

2.2.1. Compressive Strength Test of Bamboo Scrimber Along the Grain

The compression specimens of bamboo scrimber along the grain in this test are designed according to the "Standard for Methods Testing of Timber Structures" (GB/T50329-2012) [21] and "Bamboo Scrimber" (GB/T40247-2021) [22]. The specimens have the dimensions of 15 mm × 25 mm × 105 mm, with the reference number KY1~KY6, and there are six specimens in total. The section size of the specimen is shown in Figure 2. The WAW-300 electro-hydraulic servo universal testing machine is used for carrying out the loading test, and displacement loading is adopted. The initial load is 5% of the failure load, and the specimen is uniformly loaded at the loading speed of 4.5 mm/min; the loading time is stipulated in 30–90 s. Before loading, the specimen was placed in a constant temperature environment and dried, the force sensor was placed vertically at the bottom of the testing machine, and the specimen was placed on the sensor. The axial line of the specimen coincided with the center of the reaction frame, and the displacement was loaded at a uniform speed until the specimen was damaged.

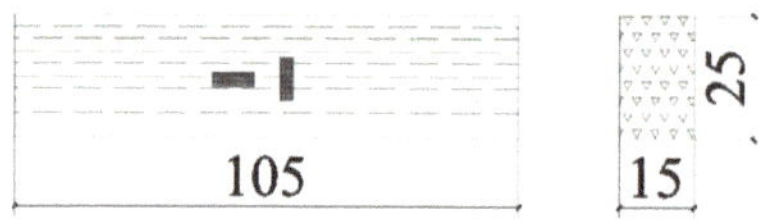

Figure 2. Compression specimens along the grain.

For the compression specimen of bamboo scrimber along the grain, there are mainly two failure modes of creasing failure and "Y"-shaped failure. The failures of the compression specimens are shown in Figure 3. In the elastic stage, the stress increases uniformly with the strain, and it presents a linear increase integrally; when entering the elastic-plastic stage, the stress increases slowly with the strain, with a gentler slope for the curve; and in the plastic stage, the slope remains basically unchanged, the strain changes quickly, and finally the specimen fails. The stress–strain curve of the compression specimen is as shown in Figure 4.

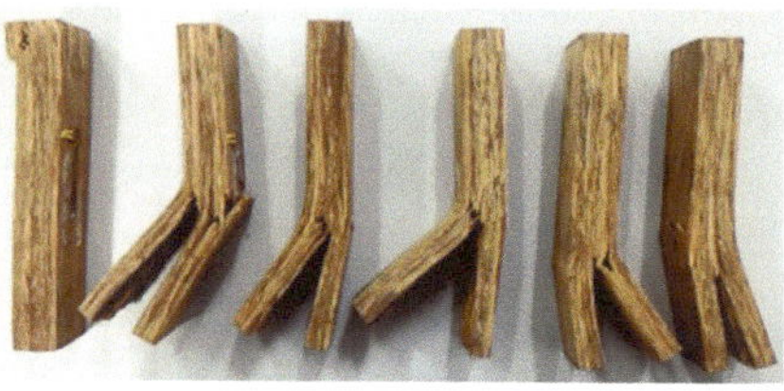

Figure 3. Failure state of bamboo scrimber compressive specimen.

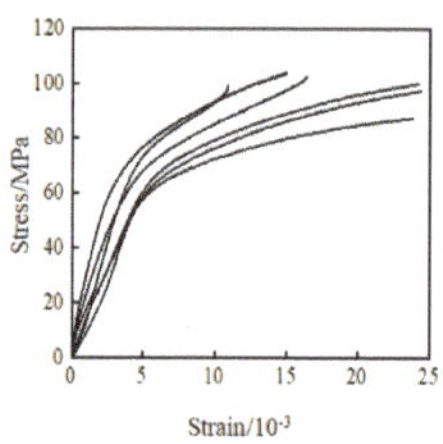

Figure 4. Stress–strain curve of bamboo scrimber compressive specimen.

Calculate the elastic modulus and compressive strength for the compression specimen of bamboo scrimber along the grain according to the specification of "Bamboo Scrimber", and calculate the compressive elastic modulus Ec according to Formula (1):

$$E_c = \frac{\Delta P}{bh\Delta\varepsilon} \tag{1}$$

wherein ΔP is the load difference at the linear stage, $\Delta\varepsilon$ is the strain difference corresponding to the load difference, b is the width of the specimen, and h is the thickness of the specimen.

The compressive strength is calculated according to Formula (2):

$$\sigma_c = \frac{P_{max}}{bh} \tag{2}$$

wherein P_{max} is the maximum value for compression failure of the specimen, b is the width of the specimen, and h is the thickness of the specimen.

The average value for compressive strength of the bamboo scrimber along the grain is 98.49 MPa, and the average value for elastic modulus is 15,006.01 MPa. According to the requirements in the specification of "Bamboo Scrimber", the bamboos in this batch are high-class products with a compressive strength of grade 120Ec. Table 2 shows the compression test results of the bamboo scrimber along the grain.

Table 2. Results of compression test of bamboo scrimber along the grain.

No.	Ultimate Load/kN	Compressive Strength/MPa	Compressive Elastic Modulus/MPa
KY1	36.61	97.63	14,620.33
KY2	32.75	87.33	11,149.61
KY3	39.01	104.03	21,667.00
KY4	37.52	100.05	8960.23
KY5	37.23	99.28	18,289.34
KY6	38.49	102.64	15,349.53
Average value	36.94	98.49	15,006.01
Standard deviation	2.23	5.94	4219.78
Coefficient of variation	6.04%	6.03%	28.12%

2.2.2. Tensile Strength Test of Bamboo Scrimber Along the Grain

The tensile specimens of bamboo scrimber along the grain in this test are designed according to "Bamboo Scrimber" (GB/T40247-2021) [22] and the "Method of Testing in Tensile Strength Parallel to Grain of Wood" (GB/T1938-2009) [23]. The specimens have the dimensions of 15 mm × 7 mm. Six tensile specimens of bamboo scrimber along the grain are processed in total, with the reference number KL1~KL6, and the size of the specimen is shown in Figure 5. The WAW-300 electro-hydraulic servo universal testing machine is used for carrying out the loading test, and displacement loading is adopted. The specimen is constantly loaded at the loading speed of 3 mm/min. The loading time is stipulated to be from 30 to 90 s. Before loading, Caffert glue is applied to the strain gauge on the specimen for protection. After the specimen is placed and dried in a constant temperature environment, it is vertically fixed in the middle of the chuck of the testing machine. The axial line of the specimen coincides with the center of the upper and lower chuck, and then the test is completed.

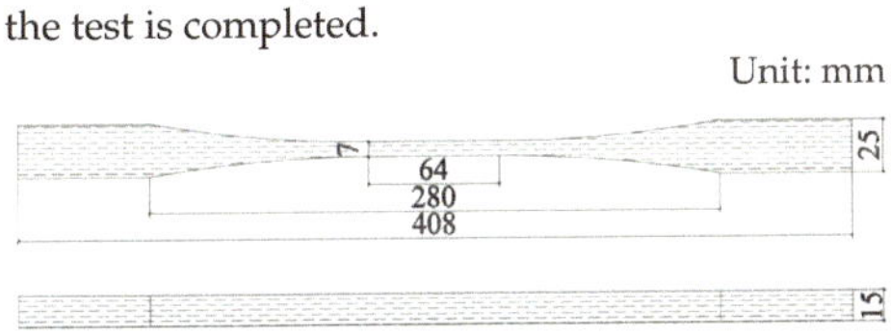

Figure 5. Tensile specimens along the grain.

For the tensile specimens of bamboo scrimber along the grain, there are mainly three failure modes of diagonal-crack failure, V-shaped failure, and Z-shaped failure. The failures of the tensile specimens are shown in Figure 6. The test of the tensile specimen is divided into two stages. In the linear stage, the curve slope is constant, and the strain increases uniformly with the increase of stress; when the specimen reaches the maximum load, the specimen rapidly fails, and the load drops rapidly. The stress–strain curve of the tensile specimen is shown in Figure 7.

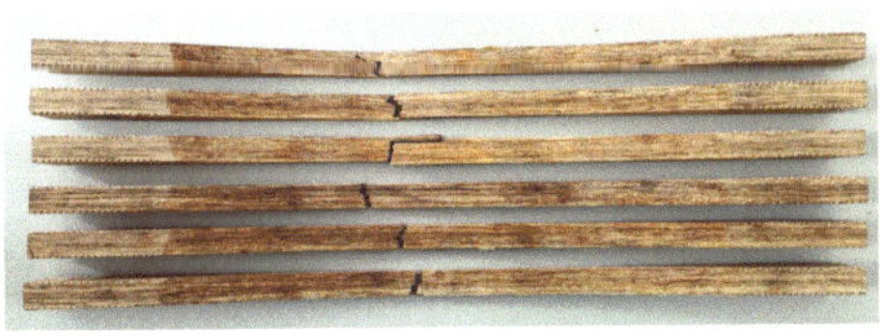

Figure 6. Failure state of bamboo scrimber tensile specimen.

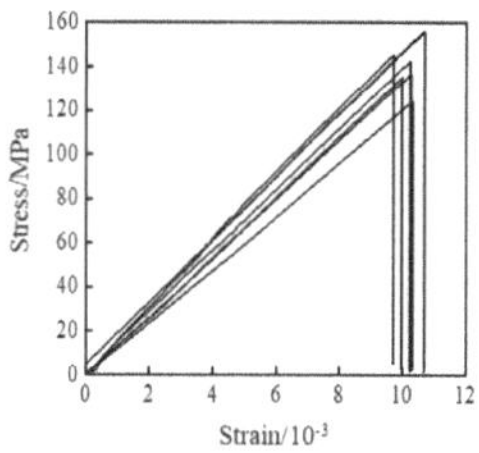

Figure 7. Stress-strain curve of recombinant bamboo tensile specimen.

The elastic modulus and the tensile strength for the tensile specimen of bamboo scrimber along the grain are calculated according to the specification of "Bamboo Scrimber", and the tensile elastic modulus is calculated according to the Formula (3):

$$E_t = \frac{\Delta P}{bh\Delta\varepsilon} \quad (3)$$

wherein ΔP is the load difference at the linear stage, $\Delta\varepsilon$ is the strain difference corresponding to the load difference, b is the width of the specimen, and h is the thickness of the specimen.

The tensile strength is calculated according to Formula (4):

$$\sigma_t = \frac{P_{max}}{bh} \quad (4)$$

wherein $Pmax$ is the maximum value for tensile failure of the specimen, b is the width of the specimen, and h is the thickness of the specimen.

The average value for tensile strength of the bamboo scrimber along the grain is 139.99 MPa, and the average value for elastic modulus is 13,877.80 MPa. According to the requirements in the specification of "Bamboo Scrimber", the bamboos in this batch are high-class products with a tensile strength of grade 120Et. Table 3 shows the tensile test results of the bamboo scrimber along the grain.

Table 3. The results of the tensile test of bamboo scrimber along the grain.

No.	Ultimate Load/kN	Tensile Strength/MPa	Tensile Elastic Modulus/MPa
KL1	14.33	136.48	13,353.97
KL2	16.37	155.90	14,343.47
KL3	14.19	135.14	13,170.17
KL4	15.28	145.53	16,958.27
KL5	14.98	142.67	13,430.44
KL6	13.04	124.19	12,010.69
Average value	14.70	139.99	13,877.80
Standard deviation	1.03	9.80	1536.64
Coefficient of variation	7.00%	7.00%	11.07%

2.2.3. Tensile Strength Test of Cold-Formed Thin-Walled Steel

The specimens used in the test are designed and processed according to the "Technical Code of Cold-formed Thin-Wall Steel Structures" (GB 50018-2002) [24], and three groups of tensile specimens are made, with a thickness of 1.0 mm. The tensile specimen is shown in Figure 8. The WDW-100 electro-hydraulic servo universal testing machine is used to complete the tensile test. The specimens, numbered G1, G2, and G3, are constantly loaded with force at the loading rate of 120 N/s until failed, and the loading time is ensured to be about 60 s. The failure state of the specimens is shown in Figure 9.

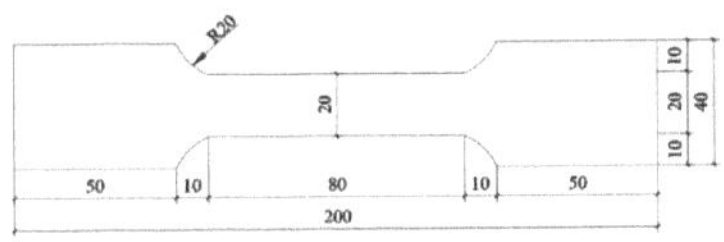

Figure 8. Steel tensile specimens.

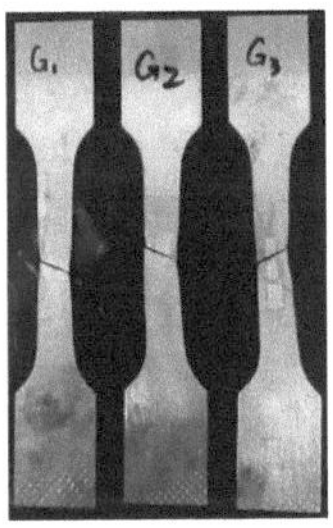

Figure 9. Failure state of steel tensile specimens.

Before loading the epoxy resin adhesive coated in the specimen on the strain gauge for protection, the specimen will be placed in a constant temperature environment after drying to maintain the vertical fixed in the middle of the test machine chuck; the specimen rolling direction axis and the upper and lower center of the chuck coincide with the distance between the chuck for the specimen of the original distance, the use of force loading until the destruction of the specimen, the record of the destruction of loads.

At the initial stage of loading, there is no obvious change in the specimen. With the increase of the load, the obvious necking phenomenon can be observed in the middle area of the specimen, and finally, a crisp sound is heard, and the specimen fails. For the cold-formed thin-walled steel tensile specimens, all failures are located in the middle of the specimens where the strain gauges are pasted. Table 4 shows the tensile test results of cold-formed thin-walled steel.

Table 4. Steel tensile test results.

No.	Ultimate Load/kN	Tensile Strength/MPa	Tensile Elastic Modulus/MPa
G1	6.49	324.59	169,747.23
G2	7.45	372.25	183,378.95
G3	7.31	365.33	137,287.24
Average value	7.08	354.06	163,471.14
Standard deviation	0.42	21.03	19,333.10
Coefficient of variation	5.98%	5.94%	11.83%

2.3. *Test Scheme and Arrangement of Measuring Points*

The specimen is subjected to the axial compression test on a 200 t electro-hydraulic servo pressure testing machine. The length of the specimen is 1200 mm. The upper bearing plate of the testing machine is a hinged support, and the lower bottom plate is provided with a self-made hinged support. The test adopts displacement control, and the loading rate is 0.005 mm/s. When loading to the ultimate load, continue to load, and stop when the load drops to 50% of the ultimate load. In order to better measure the stress–strain of the specimen, the test will be arranged in the strain gauge at the column height of 1/2 in the external reorganization of the bamboo, and the internal cold-formed thin-walled steel sections will be pasted on the same position of the strain gauge; at the same time, in the external reorganization of the bamboo strain gauge on the same height of the arrangement of the displacement meter, to prevent contact with the strain gauge resulting in inaccurate measurement data, will be placed in the displacement meter pointer on the side of the strain gauge. Displacement and strain are collected with the Gantner data acquisition instrument. The layout of the cross-shaped strain gauges and the displacement gauges are as shown in Figure 10.

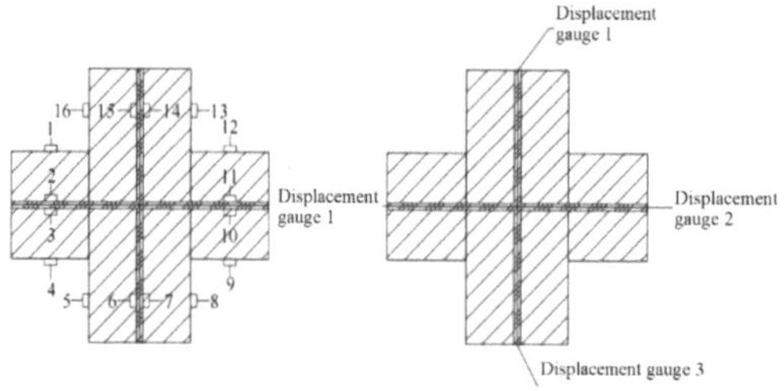

Figure 10. Layout of strain gauges and displacement meters for cross-shaped steel–bamboo composite columns.

In the preparation stage, the strain gauges and displacement gauges pasted on the specimen were connected to the collector one by one, and the strain gauges and displacement gauges were checked on the test computer to see if they were normal. In this test, the force transducer is placed in the center of the lower base plate of the testing machine, the homemade hinge support is placed in the center above the force transducer, and a layer of fine sand is laid on the upper surface of the hinge support to ensure that the specimen is subjected to a uniform force during the test.

During the test phase, the combined column is placed in the middle position of the hinge support, the distance between the top plate of the hydraulic press and the specimen is adjusted to about 10 mm, the combined column is physically aligned, and the top plate of the hydraulic press is adjusted to contact with the combined column at the end of the alignment.

Set the preload to about 10% of the estimated ultimate load, check whether the displacement gauge and strain gauges work well, and adjust the position of the combined column by observing the numerical size of all the strain gauges to ensure that the combined column is axially pressurized. The test adopts displacement control, with a loading rate of 0.005 mm/s, loading to the ultimate load in order to get the falling section of the load-displacement curve; continue to load until the load falls to 85% of the ultimate load. When loading stops, the test is over.

3. Test Results and Analysis

3.1. Test Phenomenon

The specimen L-G-Z is an L-shaped steel column. During the loading process, the specimen has obvious distortional buckling of the wave shape. When the specimen is loaded to about 5 kN, the middle part of the flange is bent. The ultimate bearing capacity of the final specimen is 5.7 kN, at which the bending and buckling failure occurs. The failure of the specimen is shown in Figure 11.

The specimen L-Z-Z is an L-shaped bamboo scrimber column. When it is loaded to about 79 kN, the specimen is observed to start bending, and a slight sound of adhesive cracking is heard. When the specimen is continuously loaded to 81 kN, it reaches the ultimate bearing capacity, obvious bending occurs, and the bending instability failure finally occurs. The failure of the specimen is shown in Figure 12.

The specimen L-G-Z-Z is an L-shaped steel–bamboo scrimber column. When the load reaches about 40 kN, the steel inside the specimen is subjected to wave buckling, with a slight sound of adhesive cracking occasionally. When the specimen is continuously loaded to 61 kN, the buckling amplitude of the steel inside the specimen increases, the frequency of the adhesive cracking sound increases, and the specimen is observed to start bending integrally. When the load reaches about 105 kN, the specimen reaches the ultimate bearing capacity, and bending instability and glue failure finally occur. The failure of the specimen is shown in Figure 13.

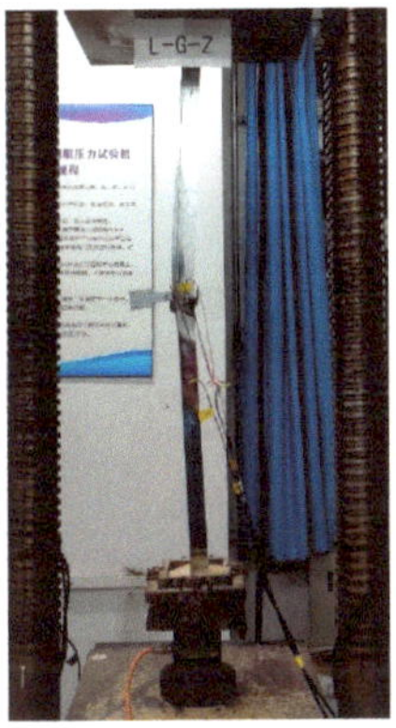

Figure 11. L-G-Z destroying figure.

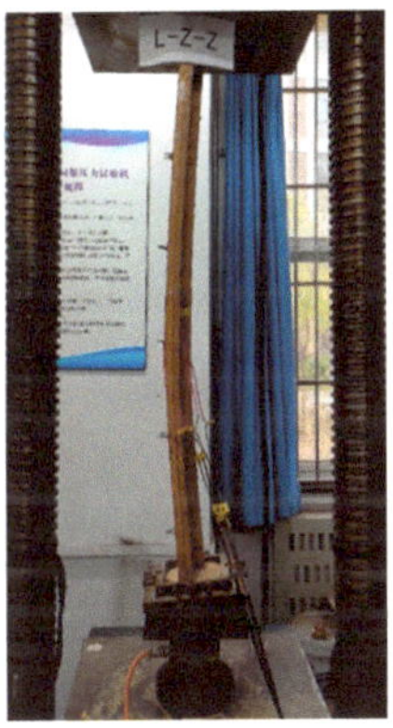

Figure 12. L-Z-Z destroying figure.

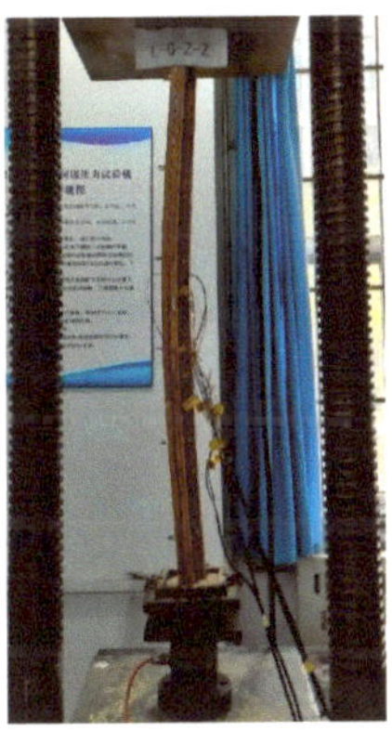

Figure 13. L-G-Z-Z destroying figure.

The specimen T-G-Z is a T-shaped steel column. When the specimen is loaded to about 4.6 kN, the flange on one side of the specimen begins to bend, and a gap appears at the middle-lower end of the two L-shaped steels. When the specimen is continuously loaded to about 8 kN, the flange on the other side of the specimen begins to bend, and the web bends towards the flange direction. When the load reaches about 14 kN, the specimen reaches the ultimate bearing capacity, and distortional buckling occurs in the middle part on one side of the flange. The final failure mode of the specimen involves distortional buckling and flexural-torsional buckling, and the failure of the specimen is shown in Figure 14.

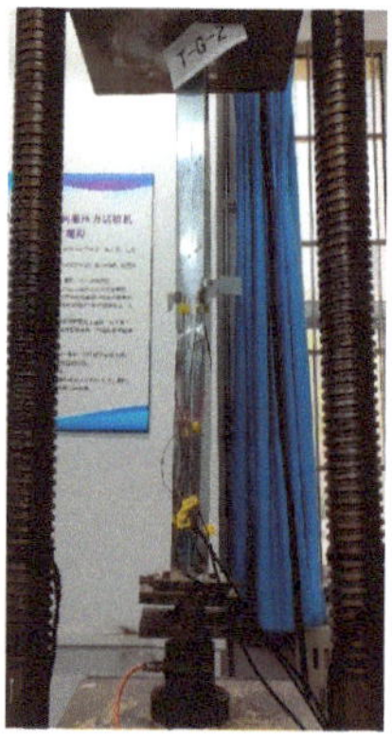

Figure 14. T-G-Z destroying figure.

The specimen T-Z-Z is a T-shaped bamboo scrimber column, and there is no phenomenon in the early loading stage. When the specimen is loaded to about 139 kN, the specimen makes a slight sound of glue failure and begins to bend integrally. When the specimen is continuously loaded to about 171 kN, the specimen reaches the ultimate bearing capacity, the overall bending effect is obvious, and the specimen is subjected to overall bending failure. The failure of the specimen is shown in Figure 15.

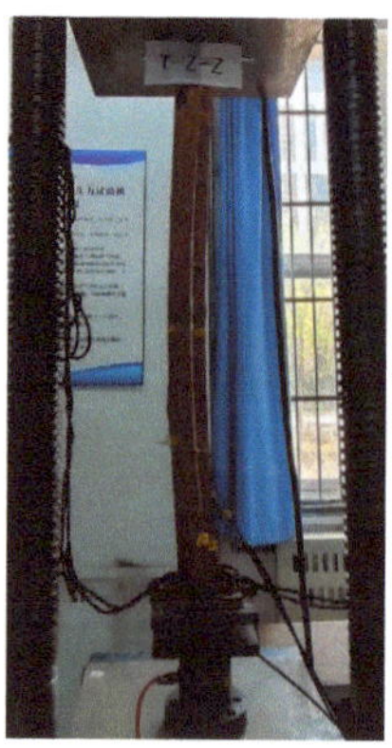

Figure 15. T-Z-Z destroying figure.

The specimen T-G-Z-Z is a T-shaped steel–bamboo scrimber column. When the specimen is loaded to about 73 kN, the steel in the middle of the web begins to buckle, and the specimen is slightly bent. When it is continuously loaded to about 105 kN, the steel in the middle of the flange on one side of the specimen begins to buckle, and the force basically increases linearly. When the specimen is loaded to about 190 kN, load fluctuation occurs, and consequently, the load-bearing capacity continues to increase. It is observed that the gap between the flange steels is relatively large, and the buckling is serious. The specimen has obvious buckling integrally. When the load reaches about 221 kN, the specimen reaches the ultimate bearing capacity, and the ultimate failure of the specimen is instability failure, glue failure, and plate-buckling failure. The failure of the specimen is shown in Figure 16.

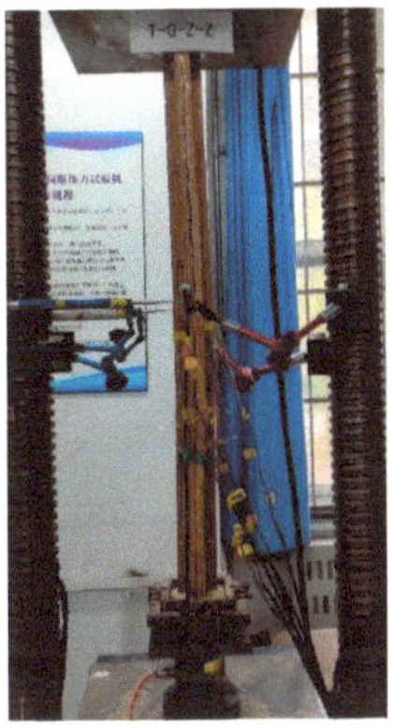

Figure 16. T-G-Z-Z destroying figure.

The specimen S-G-Z is a cross-shaped steel column. When the load reaches about 6 kN, a gap begins to appear between the rear flange and the upper part of the right flange, and weak buckling occurs in the local part. When the load reaches about 15 kN, the axial displacement increases, the gap between the two flanges continuously increases, and the distortional buckling is obvious. The wave-type buckling phenomenon occurs in the front flange, and the sound is given out continuously under continued loading. When the load reaches about 22 kN, the specimen is twisted integrally, the bearing capacity is continuously increased, and the twisting angle is also continuously increased. When the load reaches about 31 kN, the specimen reaches the ultimate bearing capacity, and finally, the specimen undergoes local buckling failure and flexural-torsional buckling failure. The failure of the specimen is shown in Figure 17.

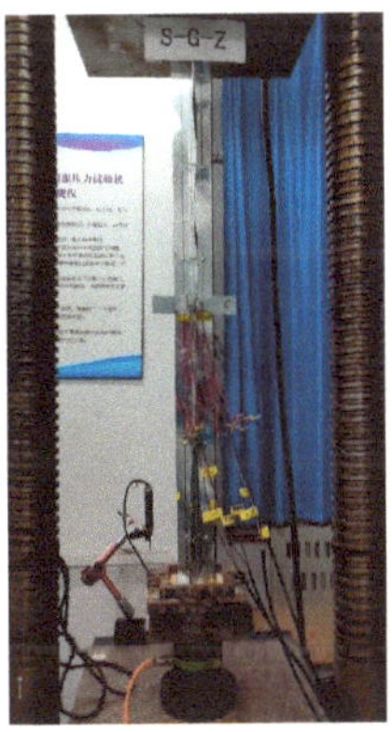

Figure 17. S-G-Z destroying figure.

The specimen S-Z-Z is a cross-shaped bamboo scrimber column, and there is no obvious change in the early and middle loading periods of the specimen. When the specimen is loaded to about 90 kN, a weak sound of adhesive cracking appears. With the continuous increase of the bearing capacity, the adhesive cracking sound continuously appears. When the loading reaches about 113 kN, the specimen begins to bend integrally, but the bending is not obvious. When the specimen is loaded to about 120 kN, the specimen reaches the ultimate bearing capacity, and finally, the specimen is subjected to instability failure integrally. After unloading, the specimen basically returns to normal without any damage to the appearance. The failure of the specimen is shown in Figure 18.

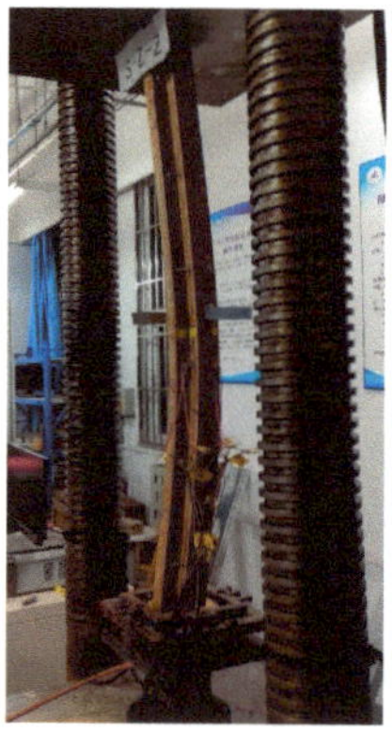

Figure 18. S-Z-Z destroying figure.

The specimen S-G-Z-Z is a cross-shaped steel–bamboo scrimber column. There is no obvious phenomenon in the early and middle loading periods of the specimen. When the specimen is loaded to about 93 kN, the sound of adhesive cracking appears. With the continuous increase of the load, the weak sound of adhesive cracking appears occasionally. When the load reaches about 135 kN, the steel plate inside the front flange is severely buckled, and the steel plate inside the rear flange begins to buckle. When the load reaches about 179 kN, the steel plate inside the specimen has wave-type buckling, the gap of the front flange is relatively large, and the other flanges have no obvious buckling effect. When the specimen is loaded to about 181 kN, it reaches the ultimate bearing capacity, and the overall bending phenomenon is obvious. Continue to loading, and the bearing capacity begins to slowly decrease and the test is completed once the bearing capacity drops within the set load range. After unloading, the specimen has a good recovery effect integrally as well as good elastic recovery capacity and toughness, and the ultimate failure of the specimen is instability failure, steel plate buckling, and glue failure. The failure of the specimen is shown in Figure 19.

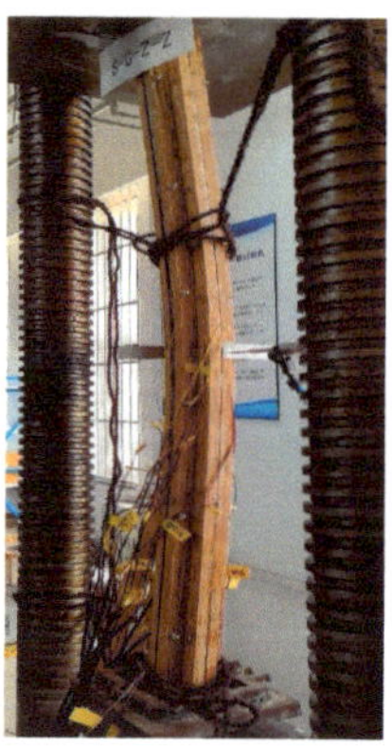

Figure 19. S-G-Z-Z destroying figure.

3.2. Load-Displacement Relationship Curve

It can be seen from Figure 20 and Table 5 that the bearing capacity of the L-shaped steel–bamboo composite special-shaped column is 1.21 times the sum for the L-shaped steel composite special-shaped column and the L-shaped bamboo composite special-shaped column, which indicates that the bearing capacity of the L-shaped steel–bamboo composite column is increased by 21.36%, and the steel and bamboo scrimber has a good composition effect, which can improve the bearing capacity of the composite specimen. In the early stage of the test, the lateral displacement of the specimen changes little, and the load-displacement curve is basically a linear curve. When the load is increased to about 70% of the ultimate load, the lateral displacement will obviously increase. After reaching the ultimate load, the lateral displacement continues to increase, and the load drops within the set range of the test. At this time, the L-shaped steel composite special-shaped column has obvious buckling, while the L-shaped bamboo and the L-shaped steel–bamboo composite special-shaped column have no obvious failure, and both specimens have instability failure.

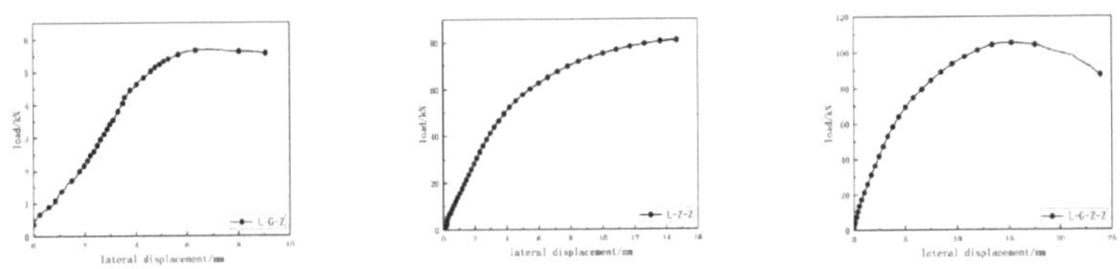

(a) (b) (c)

Figure 20. Load-lateral displacement relationship curve of L-shaped composite special-shaped column. (**a**) L-G-Z load-lateral displacement; (**b**) L-Z-Z load-lateral displacement; (**c**) L-G-Z-Z load-lateral displacement.

Table 5. Test results of L-shaped composite columns.

No.	λ	P_t/kN	Failure Phenomena
L-G-Z	71.8	5.68	Local buckling + flexural-torsional buckling
L-Z-Z	62.1	80.99	Instability failure + glue failure
L-G-Z-Z	38.4	105.18	Instability failure + glue failure + plate buckling

It can be seen from Figure 21 and Table 6 that the bearing capacity of the T-shaped steel–bamboo composite special-shaped column is 19.01% higher than that of the T-shaped steel composite special-shaped column and the T-shaped bamboo composite special-shaped column. In the early loading stage, the specimen is in the linear stage, and the lateral displacement changes little. When the load reaches about 85% of the ultimate load, the lateral displacement begins to increase rapidly, the specimen is bent and deformed integrally, and the lateral displacement in the column is the largest. After the ultimate load is reached, the load will decrease slowly, and the lateral displacement will continue to increase. From Figure 21c, it can be seen that the load-lateral displacement curve of the specimen occasionally fluctuates, which indicates that with the increasing of the load, there is continuous glue failure between the steel and the bamboo scrimber. Finally, the T-shaped steel composite special-shaped column is subjected to flexural-torsional buckling failure, while the T-shaped bamboo and the T-shaped steel–bamboo composite special-shaped columns have instability failure.

It can be seen from Table 7 the bearing capacity of the cross-shaped steel–bamboo composite special-shaped column is 19.52% higher than the sum of that for the cross-shaped steel composite special-shaped column and the cross-shaped bamboo composite special-shaped column. It can be seen from Figure 22a that, due to the flexural-torsional buckling failure of the cross-shaped steel special-shaped column during the test, the load increases irregularly, and the ultimate failure is flexural-torsional failure. It can be seen from Figure 22b that, before the cross-shaped bamboo special-shaped column is loaded to about 20 kN, there is basically no lateral displacement. When the specimen is loaded continuously, it reaches the linear stage, and the load-lateral displacement curve keeps a linear growth relationship. When the loading is continued to 70% of the ultimate load, the curve slope gradually decreases, the specimen has obvious overall bending, and the ultimate failure is bending instability failure. It can be seen from Figure 22c that the cross-shaped steel–bamboo composite special-shaped column has no obvious lateral displacement before it is loaded to about 30 kN. When the specimen is loaded continuously, the load-lateral displacement develops with a large slope. When the load reaches about 70% of the ultimate load, the lateral displacement gradually and rapidly increases, and finally, the overall bending instability failure occurs.

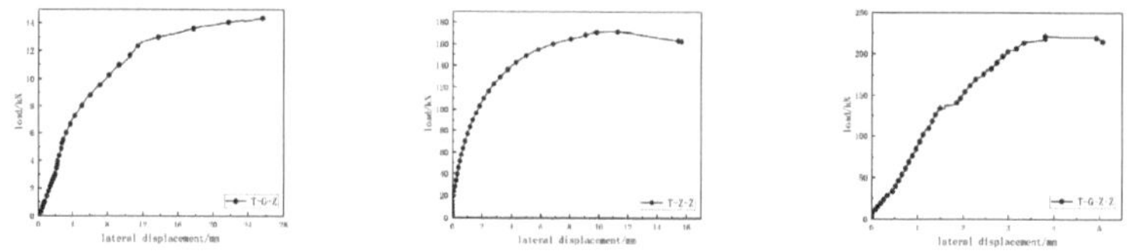

(a) (b) (c)

Figure 21. Load-lateral displacement relationship curve of T-shaped composite special-shaped column. (**a**) T-G-Z load-lateral displacement; (**b**) T-Z-Z load-lateral displacement; (**c**) T-G-Z-Z load-lateral displacement.

Table 6. Test results of T-shaped composite columns.

No.	λ	P_t/kN	Failure Phenomena
T-G-Z	61.3	14.82	Distortional buckling + flexural-torsional buckling
T-Z-Z	46.7	171.51	Instability failure + glue failure
T-G-Z-Z	45.4	221.76	Instability failure + glue failure + plate buckling

Table 7. Test results of cruciform composite special-shaped columns.

No.	λ	P_t/kN	Failure Phenomena
S-G-Z	50.0	31.62	Distortional buckling + flexural-torsional buckling
S-Z-Z	44.4	120.31	Instability failure + glue failure at the end
S-G-Z-Z	43.1	181.58	Instability failure + glue failure + fiber tear

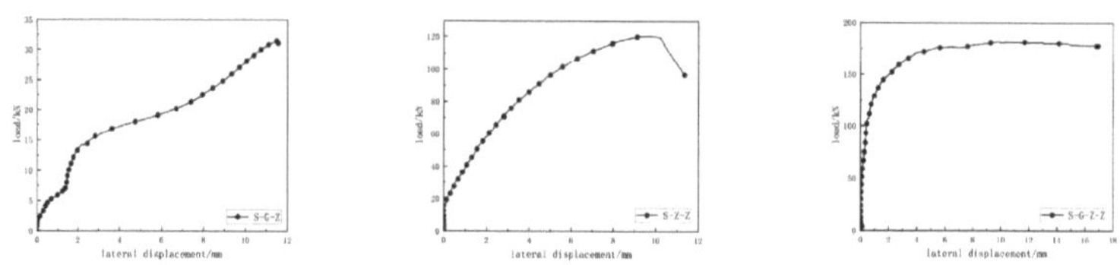

(a) (b) (c)

Figure 22. Load-lateral displacement curve of the cross-shaped composite special-shaped column.(**a**) S-G-Z load-lateral displacement; (**b**) S-Z-Z load-lateral displacement; (**c**) S-G-Z-Z load-lateral displacement.

3.3. Load–Strain Relationship Curve

From the load–strain relationship in Figure 23a, it can be seen that the L-shaped steel special-shaped column is in the elastic stage before being loaded to 50% of the ultimate load, and all strains increase linearly. When the load reaches about 4 kN, the specimen is transformed into the elastic-plastic stage; steel 1 and steel 2 of the strain gauge reach the yield load, the strain increases rapidly compared with the previous stage, and the strain of the specimen continues to increase for a period of time after the load reaches the ultimate load.

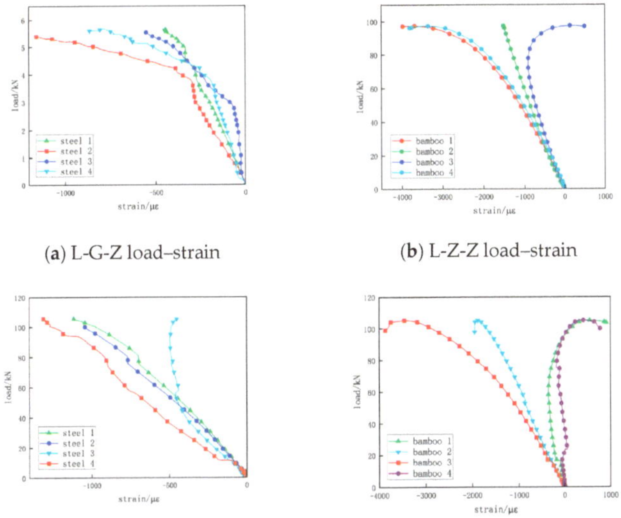

(**a**) L-G-Z load–strain (**b**) L-Z-Z load–strain

(**c**) L-G-Z-Z steel load–strain (**d**) L-G-Z-Z bamboo load–strain

Figure 23. Load–strain relationship curve of T-shaped composite special-shaped column.

From the load–strain relationship in Figure 23b, it can be seen that the strain of the bamboo scrimber is larger than that of the steel. At the initial stage of loading, the specimen is in the elastic stage, and the strain increases uniformly with the increase of the load; when the load reaches about 50% of the ultimate load, bamboo 1 and bamboo 2 of the strain gauge are compressed, bamboo 3 is in a linear growth trend, bamboo 4 is in tension, and the specimen begins to bend integrally. When the loading is continued, the slope of load–strain begins to decrease constantly, the strain rapidly increases, and the overall bending deformation occurs. When the specimen reaches the ultimate load, the bearing capacity of the specimen slowly decreases with the increase of the vertical displacement, which indicates that the bamboo scrimber is not subject to brittle failure, and the bamboo scrimber structure has good elastic recovery capability and toughness.

It can be seen from Figure 23c,d that, under the same load, the strain of the bamboo scrimber is greater than that of steel. At the initial stage of loading, the strain curves of steel and bamboo scrimber are in the linear stage; as the load increases to 60% of the ultimate load, they reach the elastic-plastic stage, and difference occurs in the four surfaces. Bamboo 1 and bamboo 4 of the strain gauges are in tension, while bamboo 2 and bamboo 3 of the strain gauges are in compression, and the specimen undergoes bending deformation. After loading to the ultimate load, the strain of the specimen continuously increases. After being loaded in the later stage, the stress of the specimen is borne by the bamboo scrimber. Through comparison, the load-bearing capacity of the steel–bamboo composite column is obviously higher than that of the steel column and the bamboo column, which shows that steel and bamboo collaborate well.

It can be seen from Figure 24a that the T-shaped steel special-shaped column is in the elastic stage before being loaded to about 40% of the ultimate load, the strain of the strain gauge increases linearly with the increase of the load, and the specimen begins to bend and twist. When it is loaded to about 12 kN, the bending and torsion phenomenon of the specimen is intensified; steel 1 of the strain gauge is in tension, and the rest of the steel is in compression.

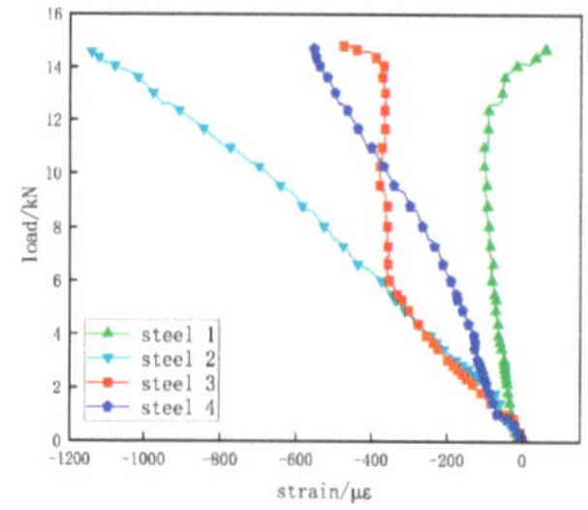

(**a**) T-G-Z load–strain

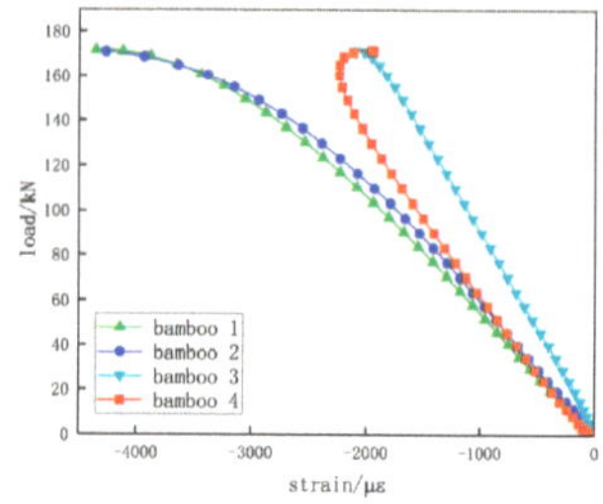

(**b**) T-Z-Z load–strain

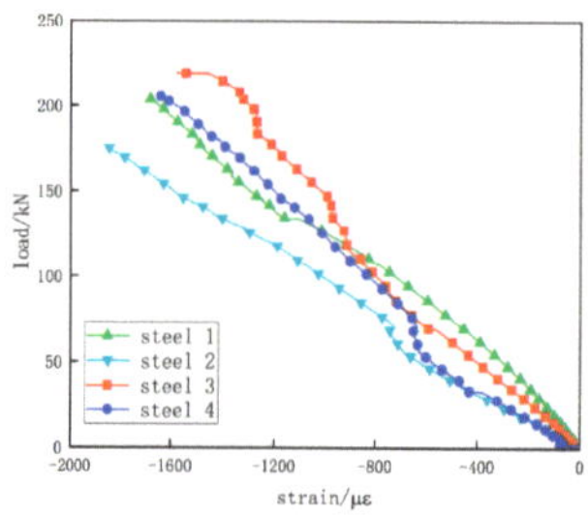

(**c**) T-G-Z-Z steel load–strain

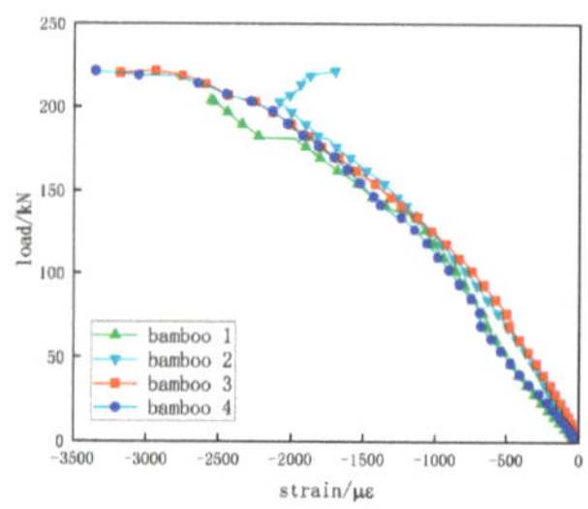

(**d**) T-G-Z-Z bamboo load–strain

Figure 24. Load–strain relationship curve of T-shaped composite special-shaped column.

It can be seen from Figure 24b that the T-shaped bamboo special-shaped column is in the elastic stage before being loaded to about 60% of the ultimate load; all strains increase linearly, and the overall bending effect is not obvious. When the loading is continued, the specimen is transformed into the elastic-plastic stage, the slope of the load–strain curve for bamboo 1 and bamboo 2 begins to decrease slowly, the strain begins to increase rapidly, and the specimen has an obvious bending phenomenon integrally. When the load reaches the ultimate value, all the strain gauges are compressed, and the specimen is subject to overall instability failure.

It can be seen from Figure 24c,d that in the loading process of a T-shaped steel–bamboo composite special-shaped column, steel and bamboo scrimber have the same strain development trend, which is basically maintained in the elastic stage, indicating that steel and bamboo scrimber work together under the action of epoxy resin adhesive and bolt. As the glue failure occurs constantly in the loading process of the test, the load–strain curve of steel shows an uneven growth and all the bamboo load–strain curves are regarded as overlap in the elastic stage, which indicates that the specimen is in the axial compression state.

It can be seen from Figure 25a that the strain value of the specimen is always negative and always under compression. During the loading process, the specimen is basically in the elastic stage, accompanied by flexural-torsional buckling and distortional buckling, and the curve shows an irregular change.

It can be seen from Figure 25b that the cross-shaped bamboo special-shaped column is in the elastic stage until it is loaded to about 70% of the ultimate load. When the loading is continued, the curve slope begins to decrease, presenting two different development trends. The two curves of the same development trend basically coincide, and the specimen has overall bending deformation.

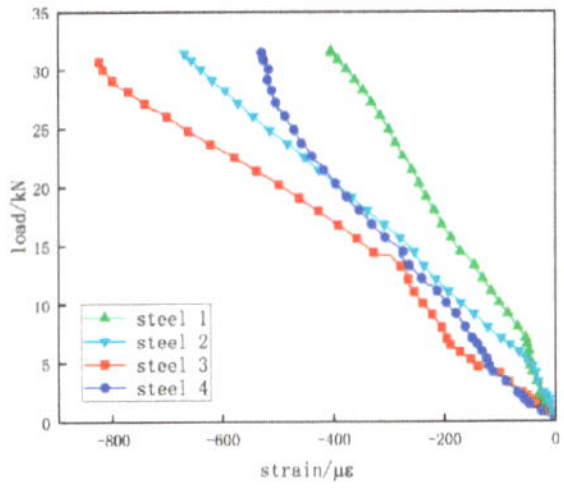

(**a**) S-G-Z load–strain

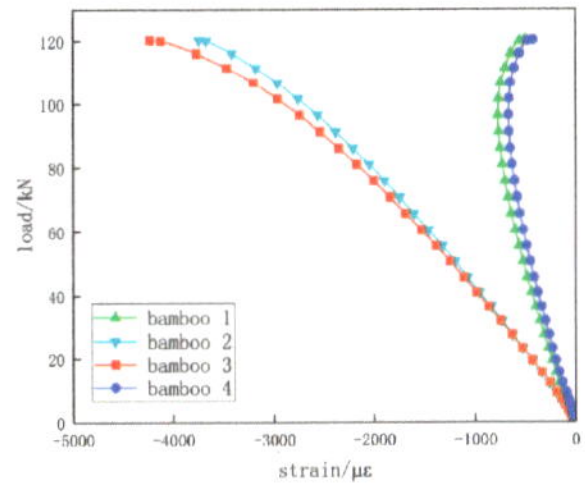

(**b**) S-Z-Z load–strain

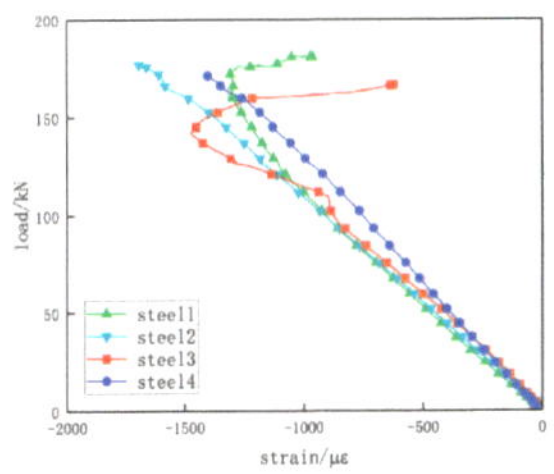

(**c**) S-G-Z-Z steel load–strain

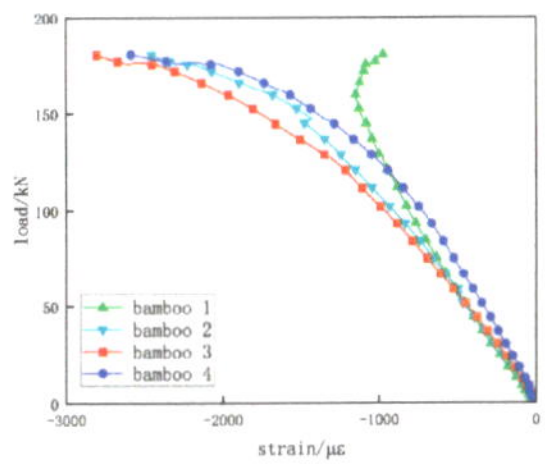

(**d**) S-G-Z-Z bamboo load–strain

Figure 25. Load–strain relationship curve of the cross-shaped composite special-shaped columns.

It can be seen from Figure 25c,d that, at the same stage, the strain of the bamboo scrimber is greater than that of steel. The cross-shaped steel–bamboo composite special-shaped column is in the elastic stage before being loaded to about 50% of the ultimate load, and the strains of all the steels and all the bamboo scrimbers are approximately overlapped, respectively. When the loading is continued, the specimen turns into the elastic-plastic stage, and glue failure constantly occurs in the specimen. During the loading process, the whole specimen is always in the compression state, and all the strain values are negative.

4. Finite Element Analysis

4.1. Establishment of Finite Element Model

The finite element software Abaqus 2021 is used to create finite element models for L-shaped, T-shaped, cross-shaped steel, bamboo, and steel–bamboo special-shaped columns. The components are endowed with material properties according to the specific parameters obtained in the material property test. The material of bamboo scrimber has the natural property of anisotropy [25]. The material of bamboo scrimber has rift grain and cross grain, and the material direction shall be set for it. Set the fiber direction of rift grain as the main direction and that of the cross grain as the secondary direction; the assigned direction of the material is shown in Figure 26. The actual contact surface is a cemented surface, which is set as a surface-to-surface contact type and the slip formula as a small slip; the contact attributes are set as tangential behavior, normal behavior, viscous behavior, and damage. To tightly connect the screw surface with the specimen, set the type as binding.

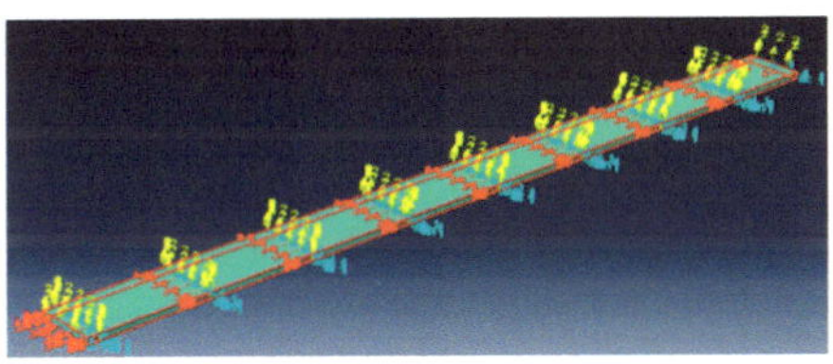

Figure 26. The assignment direction of bamboo scrimber materials.

The first step is to set the elastic buckling analysis and create the analysis step. Select the linear perturbation-buckling analysis as the program type, input 5 for the number of requested characteristic values, set the vector used in each iteration to 10, and the maximum number of iterations at 30. By setting this analysis step, the buckling characteristic value and the corresponding critical load at each stage can be obtained. The second step is to set the non-elastic buckling analysis and create the analysis step. Select the general-static analysis as the program type. In the non-elastic buckling analysis, introduce the initial defect; consider the material and contact of the specimen, and the load value output after the analysis is the load corresponding to the elastic buckling characteristic value.

Set the upper-end constraint of the specimen as translational freedom along the x-axis and y-axis directions and the rotational freedom along the x-axis, y-axis, and z-axis directions. Apply the displacement in the direction z on the reference point of the backing plate and set the lower-end constraint as the translational freedom along the x-axis, y-axis, and z-axis directions and the rotational freedom along the x-axis, y-axis, and z-axis directions. After the setting is completed, conduct the grid division; the model grid division diagram is shown in Figure 27.

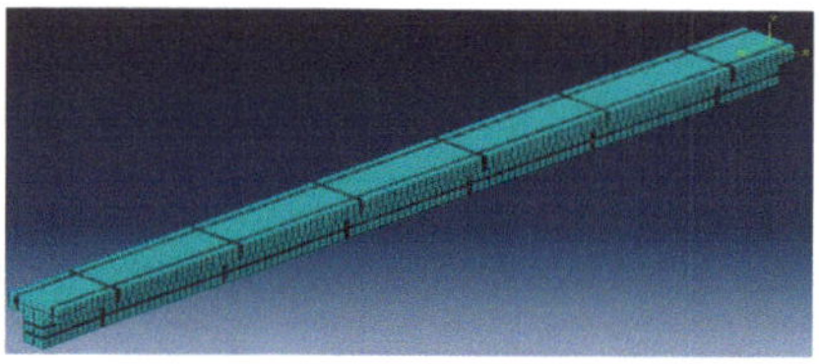

Figure 27. Model grid division diagram.

4.2. Finite Element Results

The stress cloud diagram of the L-shaped column is shown in Figure 28. The middle flange of the L-G-Z specimen is bent, the flange is buckled in a wave shape, and the specimen is bent integrally and has instability failure. The L-Z-Z specimen is bent, the middle part of the long flange is obviously deformed, and the specimen is subject to bending instability failure. The L-G-Z-Z inner steel is buckled in wave shape, and the specimen is obviously bent and has instability failure.

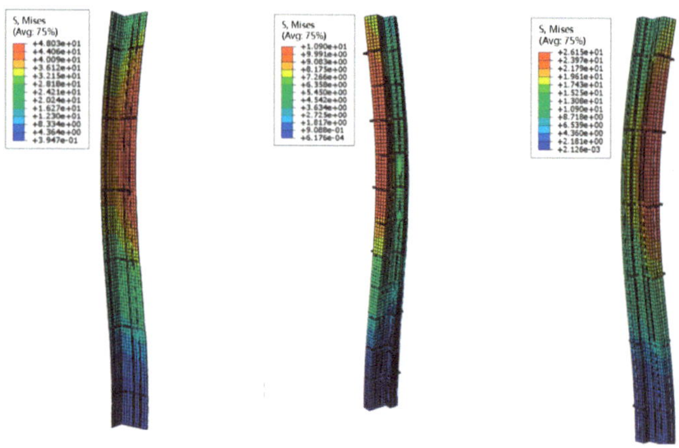

(**a**) L-G-Z cloud diagram (**b**) L-Z-Z cloud diagram (**c**) L-G-Z-Z cloud diagram

Figure 28. Stress cloud diagram of L-shaped column.

Compare the simulated load-axial displacement curve with the test curve, as shown in Figure 29. (1) At the linear stage, the slope of the load-displacement curve in the simulation result is approximately the same as that in the test result, which proves that the rigidity of the finite element model is basically consistent with that of the specimen. (2) For the descending section, the simulation curve and the test curve are relatively flat, which shows that the failure of the specimen is not a brittle failure after reaching the ultimate bearing capacity and has a certain degree of deformation capacity. (3) The simulated ultimate bearing capacity of all the specimens is slightly higher than the ultimate bearing capacity of the test, which indicates that there are some human errors in the components of the test and that the glue failure occurs in the loading process of the test.

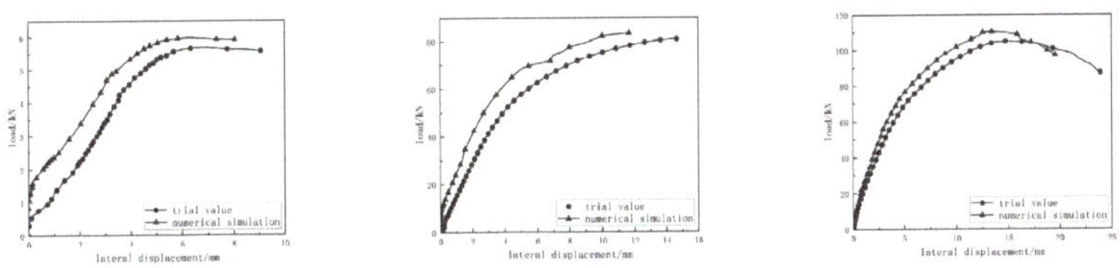

(a) (b) (c)

Figure 29. L-shaped column load-lateral displacement contrast diagram. (**a**) L-G-Z load-lateral displacement; (**b**) L-Z-Z load-lateral displacement; (**c**) L-G-Z-Z load-lateral displacement.

Figure 30 shows the stress cloud diagram of the T-shaped column. The T-G-Z web is bent and twisted towards the flange, and distortional buckling appears in the middle of one flange. The specimen has the failure modes of distortional buckling and flexural-torsional buckling. The T-Z-Z has an obvious bending effect integrally, and the specimen is subject to bending failure integrally. The steel in the middle of T-G-Z-Z has wave-shaped bending, and the specimen is bent integrally; thus, the specimen has instability failure and plate-buckling failure.

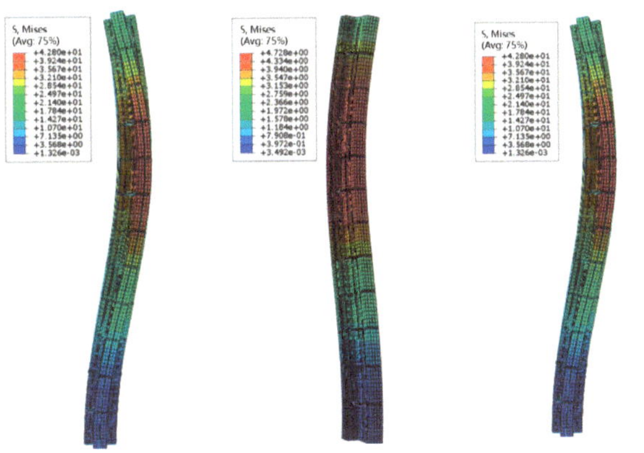

(**a**) T-G-Z cloud diagram(**b**) T-Z-Z cloud diagram(**c**) T-G-Z-Z cloud diagram

Figure 30. T-shaped column stress cloud diagram.

The comparative analysis diagram of the model and the test is shown in Figure 31.

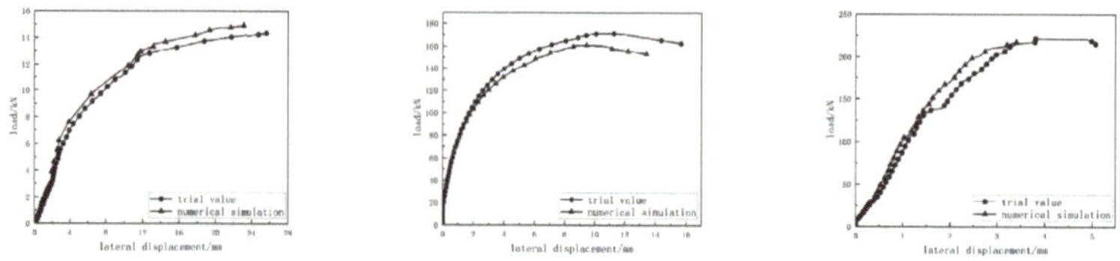

(**a**) (**b**) (**c**)

Figure 31. Load-transverse displacement comparison diagram of T-shaped column. (**a**) T-G-Z load-lateral displacement; (**b**) T-Z-Z load-lateral displacement; (**c**) T-G-Z-Z load-lateral displacement.

(1) The finite element analysis curve and the test curve of all specimens have high similarity, and the general direction is basically the same, which indicates that the finite element model used in this paper can simulate the steel–bamboo composite special-shaped column under the condition of axial compression, verifying that the model has good reliability.

(2) The simulated bearing capacity of all specimens increases faster than that of the test. That is because the elastic modulus and the ultimate bearing capacity of the bamboo scrimber will decrease with the increase of the slenderness ratio in the test process, and the influence of the slenderness ratio is not considered in specific parameters such as the elastic modulus set in the simulation.

Figure 32 shows the stress cloud diagram of the cross-special-shaped column. The front flange of S-G-Z has wave-shaped buckling, it is twisted integrally, and the specimen is subjected to local buckling and flexural-torsional buckling failure. The middle-upper part of S-Z-Z has obvious bending deformation, and finally, the specimen has instability failure. All the internal plates of S-G-Z-Z show wave-shaped buckling; they have obvious bending integrally, and the ultimate failure of the specimen is instability failure and plate buckling.

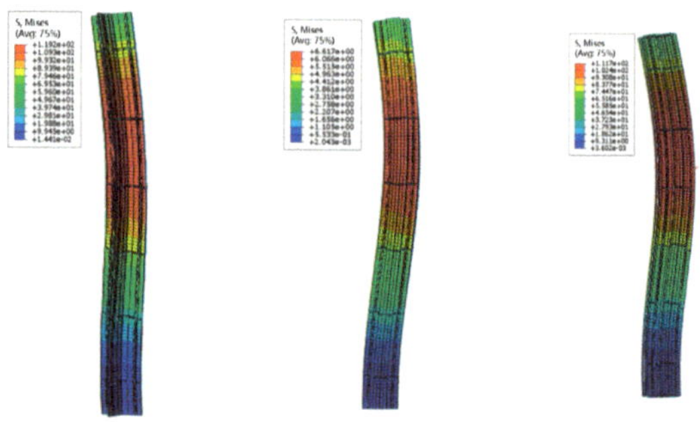

(**a**) S-G-Z cloud diagram(**b**) S-Z-Z cloud diagram(**c**) S-G-Z-Z cloud diagram

Figure 32. Stress cloud diagram of the cross-shaped column.

Compare the simulated load-axial displacement curve with the test curve, as shown in Figure 33. It can be seen that the simulated ultimate bearing capacity of all specimens is slightly higher than the tested ultimate bearing capacity. Due to the problem of the manufacturing process of the specimen, the compressive strength of the specimen cannot be fully developed, but the finite element model can simulate the full compressive strength of the specimen in ideal conditions.

From Table 8, it can be seen that the ultimate bearing capacity of L-G-Z-Z is the sum of L-G-Z and L-Z-Z increased by 23.11%, the ultimate bearing capacity of T-G-Z-Z is the sum of T-G-Z and T-Z-Z increased by 23.43%, and the ultimate bearing capacity of S-G-Z-Z is the sum of S-G-Z and S-Z-Z increased by 14.83%, which indicates that the steel and the bamboo scrimber have a good composition effect, and the bearing capacity of composite specimens can be improved.

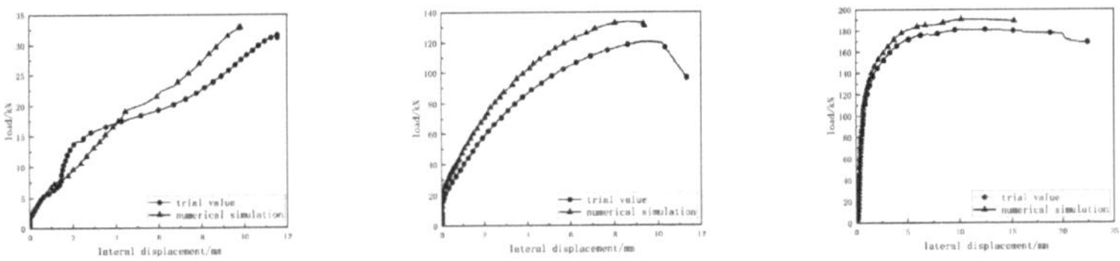

(a) (b) (c)

Figure 33. Comparison of load-transverse displacement of cross-shaped columns. (**a**) S-G-Z load-lateral displacement; (**b**) S-Z-Z load-lateral displacement; (**c**) S-G-Z-Z load-lateral displacement.

Table 8. Comparison of simulation results with experimental results.

Specimen No.	P_A/kN	P_t/kN	P_A/P_t
L-G-Z	6.38 kN	5.68 kN	1.12
T-G-Z	15.34 kN	14.82 kN	1.04
S-G-Z	32.88 kN	31.62 kN	1.04
L-Z-Z	83.73 kN	80.99 kN	1.03
T-Z-Z	160.79 kN	171.51 kN	0.94
S-Z-Z	133.32 kN	120.31 kN	1.11
L-G-Z-Z	110.94 kN	105.18 kN	1.05
T-G-Z-Z	217.39 kN	221.76 kN	0.98
S-G-Z-Z	190.85 kN	181.58 kN	1.05

The maximum value for the ratio of the simulated ultimate bearing capacity to the tested ultimate bearing capacity is 1.12, and the minimum value is 0.94. As there are many factors affecting the actual composite columns, the simulation is in an ideal state, which results in the ultimate bearing capacity of the test being slightly lower than that of the simulation. However, the ratio of the two is very close to 1, which indicates that the simulation results fit well with the test results. The established Abaqus finite element model can simulate well the buckling behaviors of the L-shaped, the T-shaped, and the cross-shaped cold-formed thin-walled steel–bamboo scrimber composite special-shaped columns under axial compression, which has practical significance for engineering applications.

5. Calculations of Bearing Capacity Under Axial Compression

5.1. Basic Assumptions and Calculation Formula

The load–strain is analyzed for three kinds of steel–bamboo composite special-shaped columns as above. From the curve, it can be seen that the strain development trend of cold-formed thin-walled steel and bamboo scrimber is the same during the loading process and is basically maintained in the elastic stage, which indicates that the cold-formed thin-walled steel and the bamboo scrimber work together under the action of epoxy resin adhesive and bolts. When the specimen reaches the ultimate load, the steel reaches the yield state, and the bamboo scrimber material is still in the linear elastic stage without obvious damage. Based on this conclusion, the following three basic assumptions are taken as the basis for deriving the formula:

(1) The cold-formed thin-walled steel–bamboo scrimber composite special-shaped column is suitable for the assumption of a flat section.

(2) When the cold-formed thin-walled steel in the composite special-shaped column reaches the yield state, the specimen reaches the yield state integrally.

(3) Before the specimen reaches the yield state integrally, the cold-formed thin-walled steel and the bamboo scrimber work together in the elastic stage, and they have the same strain change trend.

On the basis of the above-mentioned basic assumptions, the calculation formula for the axial compression capacity of the cold-formed thin-walled steel–bamboo scrimber special-shaped column is derived.

$$N_{cr} = a\varphi(f_y A_s + f_b A_b) = a\varphi(f_y A_s + \frac{E_b}{E_s} f_y A_b) \quad (5)$$

wherein *Ncr* is the bearing capacity of the composite special-shaped column, kN; a is the equation modification coefficient, φ is the overall stability coefficient of the composite special-shaped column, f_y is the yield strength of cold-formed thin-walled steel, f_b is the compressive strength of bamboo scrimber, A_s is the sectional area of cold-formed thin-walled steel, A_b is the sectional area of the bamboo scrimber, E_s is the elastic modulus of the cold-formed thin-walled steel, and E_b is the elastic modulus of the bamboo scrimber.

5.2. Comparison Between Calculation Results and Experimental Results

From Table 9, it can be seen that the error in the ultimate bearing capacity and experimental value of the composite special-shaped column calculated theoretically is within 13.28%. It is considered that the theoretical calculation formulas of the three composite special-shaped columns can be used for reference in practical engineering. The ultimate bearing capacity of the steel–bamboo composite special-shaped column is obviously higher than the sum of the steel composite special-shaped column and the bamboo composite special-shaped column.

Table 9. Comparison of theoretical formula results and experimental results of bearing capacity.

Specimen No.	Theoretical Value for Calculations in Formula/kN	Experimental Value/kN	Error
L-G-Z	6.43 kN	5.68 kN	13.13%
T-G-Z	12.85 kN	14.82 kN	−13.28%
S-G-Z	34.42 kN	31.62 kN	8.84%
L-Z-Z	81.04 kN	80.99 kN	0.06%
T-Z-Z	151.22 kN	171.51 kN	−11.82%
S-Z-Z	135.88 kN	120.31 kN	12.94%
L-G-Z-Z	110.65 kN	105.18 kN	5.20%
T-G-Z-Z	202.95 kN	221.76 kN	−8.48%
S-G-Z-Z	182.55 kN	181.58 kN	0.53%

6. Conclusions

(1) According to the test, the failures of the steel composite special-shaped column include local buckling, flexural-torsional buckling, and distortional buckling; the failures of the bamboo scrimber special-shaped column include instability failure and glue failure; and the failures of the steel–bamboo scrimber include instability failure, glue failure, and steel-plate buckling failure. After the experiment was completed, the bamboo scrimber composite column and the steel–bamboo composite column basically recovered without any external damage, which indicates that the bamboo scrimber material has good elastic recovery capability and toughness.

(2) The bearing capacity of the L-shaped steel–bamboo composite special-shaped column is 21.4% higher than the sum of the L-shaped steel composite special-shaped column and the L-shaped bamboo composite special-shaped column. The bearing capacity of the T-shaped steel–bamboo composite special-shaped column is 18.8% higher than the sum of the T-shaped steel composite special-shaped column and the T-shaped bamboo composite special-shaped column. The bearing capacity of the cross-shaped steel–bamboo composite special-shaped column is 19.5% higher than the sum of the cross-shaped steel composite special-shaped column and the cross-shaped bamboo composite special-shaped column.

(3) The calculation formula for the axial compression bearing capacity of the three kinds of composite special-shaped columns is derived. Compared with the experimental

data, the error in the theoretical value and the experimental value of the ultimate bearing capacity of the composite special-shaped columns is within 13.28%, which proves that the theoretical formula has a certain reliability for calculating the ultimate bearing capacity of the composite special-shaped columns.

(4) In the simulating condition, the composite special-shaped column is in the ideal state, so the simulated ultimate bearing capacity is generally higher than the ultimate bearing capacity in the experiment, but the ratio of both is 0.94–1.12. Meanwhile, the failure process of the specimen is almost the same under the experimental study and the simulation analysis, and the simulation results fit well with the experimental results, which indicate that the finite element model is suitable for simulating the composite special-shaped column.

(5) According to the experimental research, theoretical analysis, and numerical simulation comparison analysis, it can be known that steel and bamboo scrimber work together and have a good composition effect; the steel–bamboo composite special-shaped column has obviously higher ultimate bearing capacity and increased deformation capacity, and the bearing capacity of L-shaped section is improved most obviously.

Author Contributions: Conceptualization, C.L., Y.W. and B.Y.; methodology, J.H. and X.F.; software, Y.W.; validation, C.L. and B.Y.; formal analysis, Y.W. and C.L.; investigation, C.L.; resources, J.H. and B.Y.; data curation, C.L. and Y.W.; writing—original draft preparation, C.L., B.W. and B.Y.; writing—review and editing, Y.W. and C.L.; visualization, C.L. and Y.W.; supervision, J.H., B.W. and X.F.; project administration, J.H.; funding acquisition, J.H. All authors have read and agreed to the published version of the manuscript.

Funding: This research was funded by the National Natural Science Foundation of China (51678237) and (51208171).

Data Availability Statement: The original contributions presented in the study are included in the article, further inquiries can be directed to the corresponding author.

Conflicts of Interest: The authors declare no conflict of interest.

References

1. Yu, R.; Spiesz, P.; Brouwers, H.J.H. Effect of nano-silica on the hydration and microstructure development of Ultra-High Performance Concrete (UHPC) with a low binder amount. *Constr. Build. Mater.* **2014**, *65*, 140–150. [CrossRef]
2. Li, X. Study on Bearing Capacity of Bolted Joints of Bamboo Scrimber. Ph.D. Thesis, China Academy of Forestry Sciences, Beijing, China, 2013.
3. Zhang, Q. *Industrial Utilization of Bamboo in China*; China Forestry Publishing House: Beijing, China, 1995.
4. Song, X.; Liu, X. Industrialized Utilization of Bamboo. *For. Sci. Technol.* **2011**, *36*, 55–57.
5. Huang, Z.; Li, C.; Wu, Y. Application of bamboo in civil engineering. *For. Eng.* **2007**, *22*, 79–80.
6. Yan, S.; Li, Y. Analysis of Application Prospect of Bamboo in Building Structure. *For. Eng.* **2008**, *24*, 62–65.
7. Wu, Y.; Li, Y.; Ge, B. Application and Prospect of Modified Bamboo. *For. Eng.* **2008**, *24*, 68–71.
8. Yall, W.M.; Xie, Z.Q.; Song, L.L.; He, H.-X. Study on the mechallical propeny of self-piercing rivet and its constinltive model in cold-fomed thin-walled steel. *Eng. Mech.* **2017**, *34*, 133–143.
9. Yao, X. Design reliability analysis of cold-formed thin-walled steel members with lipped channel sections considering distortional bucJding. *Open Civ. Eng. J.* **2017**, *11*, 906–918.
10. Wu, M. Study on the Axial Compression Performance of Built-in Steel Reinforced Bamboo Scrimber. Master's Thesis, Northeast Forestry University, Harbin, China, 2022.
11. Ge, Y.; Li, Y.; Tong, K.; Zhang, J. Study on shear performance of thin-walled steel-recombined bamboo composite I-beam. *For. Eng.* **2018**, *34*, 72–79.
12. Zhang, X.; Zeng, Z. Finite element analysis of cold-formed thin-walled steel-recombined bamboo composite columns under eccentric compression. *Shanxi Constr.* **2018**, *44*, 45–46.
13. Mao, M.; Zhang, J.; Tong, K.; Li, Y. Comparative analysis of bending performance of steel-bamboo composite beams based on different kinds of bamboo plates. *Build. Struct.* **2020**, *50*, 107–113.
14. Mahdavi, M.; Cloustion, P.L.; Arw Ade, S.R. Development of laminated bamboo lunber: Review of processing, performance, and economical considerations. *J. Mater. Cival Eng.* **2011**, *23*, 1036–1042. [CrossRef]
15. Hebel, D.E.; Javadian, A.; Helsel, F.; Schlesier, K.; Griebel, D.; Wielopolski, M. Processing-controlled optimization of the tensile srenth of bamboo fiber composites for structural applications. *Compos. Part B Eng.* **2014**, *67*, 125–131. [CrossRef]

16. Zakikhani, P.; Zahari, R.; Sultan, M.T.H.; Majid, D.L. Extraction and preparation of bamboo fiber-reinforced composites. *Materals Des.* **2014**, *63*, 820–828.
17. van der Lugt, P.; van den Dobbelsteen, A.A.J.F.; Janssen, J.J.A. An environmental, economic and practical assessment of bamboo as a building material for supporting structures. *Constr. Build. Mater.* **2006**, *20*, 648–656. [CrossRef]
18. Yu, D.W.; Tan, H.W.; Ruan, Y.G. A future bamboo-structure residential building prototype in China: Life cycle asscssment of energy use and carbon emission. *Energy Build.* **2011**, *43*, 2638–2646. [CrossRef]
19. Liu, S.M.; Liu, J.S. New building material-the development and application of recombinant bamboo. *Adv. Mater. Res.* **2013**, *773*, 441–444. [CrossRef]
20. Hang, W.; Fu, W.; Zhou, J.; Zhang, Z.; Chen, Z. A preliminary study on bamboo original state multi recombination building material. *Wood Process. Mach.* **2014**, *25*, 20+39–41.
21. *GB/T50329-2012*; Standard for Test Methods of Timber Structures. China Construction Industry Press: Beijing, China, 2002.
22. *GB/T40247-2021*; Bamboo Scrimber. China Standards Publishing House: Beijing, China, 2021.
23. *GB/T1938-2009*; Test Method for Tensile Strength Parallel to Grain of Wood. China Standard Publishing House: Beijing, China, 2009.
24. *GB50018-2002*; Technical Code for Cold-Formed Thin-Walled Steel Structures. China Planning Press: Beijing, China, 2002.
25. Zhang, X.; Jing, E.; Li, Y.; Zhang, Y. Experimental study on compressive and flexural mechanical properties of reconstituted bamboo. *Ind. Build.* **2016**, *46*, 7–12.

buildings

MDPI

Article

Predictive Model for Erosion Rate of Concrete Under Wind Gravel Flow Based on K-Fold Cross-Validation Combined with Support Vector Machine

Yanhua Zhao [1,2], Kai Zhang [1,2,*], Aojun Guo [1], Fukang Hao [1] and Jie Ma [1]

1. Civil Engineering Department, Lanzhou Jiaotong University, Lanzhou 730070, China; zhaoyanhua1109@126.com (Y.Z.); guoaojun@yeah.net (A.G.); yangbo4892@yeah.net (F.H.); zhanghl000210@163.com (J.M.)
2. National and Provincial Joint Engineering Laboratory of Road & Bridge Disaster Prevention and Control, Lanzhou Jiaotong University, Lanzhou 730070, China

* Correspondence: zhangkai0212@yeah.net

Abstract: In the Gobi region, concrete structures frequently suffer erosion from wind gravel flow. This erosion notably impairs their longevity. Therefore, creating a predictive model for wind gravel flow-related concrete damage is crucial to proactively address and manage this problem. Traditional theoretical models often fail to predict the erosion rate of concrete (CER) structures accurately. This issue arises from oversimplified assumptions and the failure to account for environmental variations and complex nonlinear relationships between parameters. Consequently, a single traditional model is inadequate for predicting the CER under wind gravel flow conditions in this region. To address this, the study utilized a machine learning (ML) model for a more precise prediction and evaluation of CER. The support vector machine (SVM) model demonstrates superior predictive performance, evidenced by its R^2 value nearing one and a notable reduction in RMSE 1.123 and 1.573 less than the long short-term memory network (LSTM) and BP neural network (BPNN) models, respectively. Ensuring that the training set comprises at least 80% of the total data volume is crucial for the SVM model's prediction accuracy. Moreover, erosion time is identified as the most significant factor affecting the CER. An enhanced theoretical erosion model, derived from the Bitter and Oka framework and integrating concrete strength and erosion parameters, was formulated. It showed average relative errors of 22% and 31.6% for the Bitter and Oka models, respectively. The SVM model, however, recorded a minimal average relative error of just −0.5%, markedly surpassing these improved theoretical models in terms of prediction accuracy. Theoretical models often rely on simplifying assumptions, such as linear relationships and homogeneous material properties. In practice, however, factors like concrete materials, wind gravel flow, and climate change are nonlinear and non-homogeneous. This significantly limits the applicability of these models in real-world environments. Ultimately, the SVM algorithm is highly effective in developing a reliable prediction model for CER. This model is crucial for safeguarding concrete structures in wind gravel flow environments.

Keywords: wind gravel flow; concrete; machine learning; support vector machine; erosion model

1. Introduction

The Lanzhou–Xinjiang high-speed railway crosses five significant wind zones: Anxi, Yandun, Baili, Thirty Mile, and Dabancheng. Together, these zones extend for about 580 km along the railway's route [1]. Notably, they are among the most wind-prone regions in the world [2]. The region is known for intense and long-lasting high winds. Such conditions significantly increase risks, such as train overturning, operational interruptions, and damage to train parts, thereby severely jeopardizing railroad safety [3,4]. During the operation of the Lanzhou–Xinjiang Railway, trains are occasionally blown over, which severely compromises their safe operation, as shown in Figure 1.

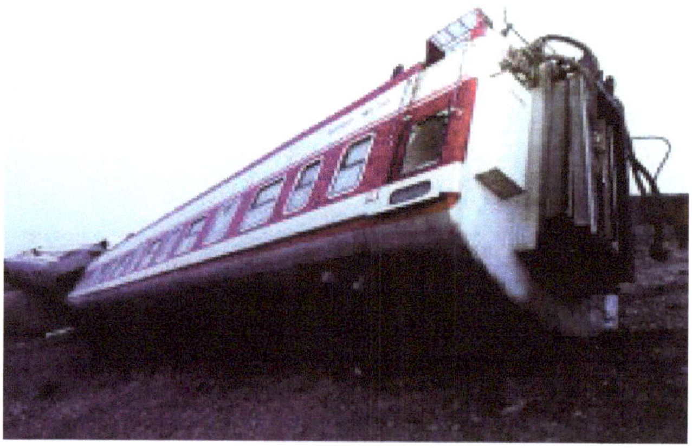

Figure 1. The scene of the Lanzhou–Xinjiang Railway accident in the Gobi windy region.

Additionally, the region, located in the desert, is characterized by Gobi landscapes, predominantly covered with coarse sand and gravel. Such terrain, when coupled with high winds, is conducive to the formation of intense wind gravel flows [5]. Concrete structures are constantly impacted by sand and gravel, leading to an accelerated expansion of microcracks on their surfaces. This progression, in turn, leads to carbonation, freeze–thaw cycles, corrosion, and other concrete material issues, all of which considerably reduce the structure's durability, as indicated in Figure 2 [6].

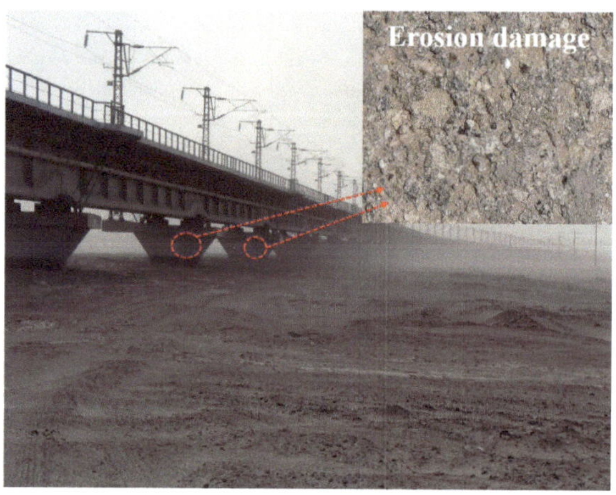

Figure 2. Damage to concrete in Gobi gale zone.

Considering the significant damage to concrete structures in wind–sand environments, a wide range of studies, both nationally and globally, have focused on understanding the erosive wear of concrete caused by gas–solid two-phase flow. It mainly includes indoor experiments and numerical simulation studies. Xue et al. [7] performed orthogonal testing to evaluate the effects of wind–sand erosion wind speed, gravel flow rate, and erosion angle on the erosion rate of aeolian sand concrete. They integrated these data with microscopic three-dimensional depth cloud maps to better understand the erosion mechanisms in concrete. Hao et al. [8] conducted experiments on wind and sand erosion in concrete of various strengths, using similarity theory to link indoor experiments with real-world conditions. Wang et al. [9] merged the wind–sand movement and solid particle erosion models, specific to the Gobi region, to simulate numerically the erosion process on vertical walls. They discovered that both the wind–sand erosion wind speed and gravel coverage critically impact wind–sand jump erosion, noting that erosion volume intensifies with increasing erosion wind speed and gravel coverage. Wang and Yang [10] created a finite element model to analyze erosion and wear in materials, specifically using examples of both brittle and ductile types. This model examined how the erosion angle, wind–sand erosion wind speed, and gravel particle size affect the erosion rate of these materials. A strong correlation was observed between the results of their numerical simulations and the data from existing experiments. Indoor experiments cannot fully replicate the extreme climatic conditions and dynamic wind gravel flow environment of the Gobi region. Furthermore, the accuracy of the finite element model relies on assumptions and simplifications, such as the material's elasticity and the linearity of erosion behavior, which may not hold true in real-world conditions.

Simultaneously, scholars have formulated various theories about material erosion, informed by data from erosion tests. Finnie [11–14] introduced the microcutting theory, which suggests that wear occurs when rigid particles strike plastic materials at certain speeds and angles. This action results in a cutting effect on the material's surface. Levy [15] formulated a theory about extruded flake exfoliation, examining the effects of repeated particle impacts on various materials. He found that erosion particles consistently extrude and forge on the surface, resulting in the formation of highly deformed flakes. Subsequently, these flakes detach from the surface due to ongoing impacts. Oka and Yoshida [16] developed an equation for quantifying erosion damage from solid particle impacts on materials. This equation facilitates the prediction of erosion under different impact conditions, such as wind–sand erosion wind speed, erosion angle, and gravel particle size. Bitter [17,18] formulated a theory of deformation wear in materials, focusing on the erosion process. He determined that erosive wear is due to both particle impact and cutting. Consequently, an erosion equation was developed, considering factors such as particle mass, wind–sand erosion wind speed, EA, and the properties of the impacted material. However, these theoretical models primarily examine relatively uniform environments and may not cover all erosion parameters comprehensively.

Artificial intelligence (AI) is currently opening new avenues for progress in civil engineering. Machine learning (ML), a subset of AI centered on data and algorithms, is gaining significant traction as a research area within this field [19,20]. Notably, ML excels in tasks involving data regression and classification [21,22]. Traditional theoretical models, with their solid theoretical foundation and simplified computational methods, are suitable for situations involving simple parameters and stable environments. However, they have significant limitations when handling complex interactions, nonlinear relationships, and dynamic changes. In contrast, ML models excel due to their flexibility, automated learning ability, and capacity to recognize complex patterns, making them better equipped to manage multifactor interactions, nonlinear relationships, and dynamic changes. These models are especially effective for processing large-scale, complex real-world data. Such capability allows for the development of highly generalizable models [23,24], effectively overcoming the limitations of traditional approaches [25].

A wide range of scholars have employed ML techniques to forecast a variety of concrete properties, covering both mechanical and durability aspects. Mechanical properties often include compressive strength [26–28], flexural strength [29,30], and tensile strength [31,32]. Regarding durability, the emphasis is typically on frost resistance [33,34], resistance to chloride penetration [35,36], and carbonation resistance [37,38].

Support vector machine (SVM) is a classic technique in ML, acclaimed for its strong theoretical foundation. It diverges from traditional methods, which typically move from induction to deduction, by efficiently streamlining the regression process. As a result, a significant number of researchers have employed SVM algorithms for predicting concrete performance. Rong et al. [39] utilized an SVM algorithm to simulate the long-term creep behavior in recycled aggregate concrete. They found that SVM-based predictions were more precise than existing models for this type of concrete. Zhang et al. [40] created a hybrid prediction model that merges the least squares SVM with a meta-vapor-type algorithm to accurately determine the carbonation depth of fly ash concrete. Abd and Abd [41] utilized SVM for predicting the compressive strength of lightweight foam concrete and discovered that the SVM model outperformed traditional regression models in accuracy. Sun et al. [42] applied an evolutionary SVM to estimate both the permeability coefficient and the unconfined compressive strength of pervious concrete, demonstrating its effectiveness in evaluating concrete performance.

However, when it comes to integrating concrete wind damage assessment with ML, current research mainly centers on using ML to analyze images that show areas affected by concrete wind damage. For example, Cui et al. [43,44] created several deep learning-based target detection algorithms to identify concrete wind erosion damage, including MHSA-YOLOv4 and a modified YOLO-v3. Their research showed that these algorithms effectively and accurately pinpointed damage in concrete images affected by wind and sand erosion, validating deep learning's utility in analyzing such damage.

To sum up, there is limited research on the erosion and wear of concrete in the Gobi's wind gravel flow environment. Current theoretical models struggle to predict concrete erosion damage accurately. Meanwhile, ML offers significant potential in this field, although its use has predominantly focused on image analysis. The application of ML in directly modeling concrete erosion damage is notably rare.

Therefore, this study integrates indoor experiments with machine learning (ML) to investigate erosion damage patterns in concrete exposed to wind gravel flow. We developed a specific erosion damage model for the Gobi's wind gravel flow environment. In ML analysis, first, input variables comprise the material composition and erosion parameters of the concrete, and the output variable is defined as the concrete erosion rate (CER). The SVM algorithm has been used to create a predictive model for CER under wind gravel flow conditions. Second, the model's predictions are then compared to those from the BP neural network (BPNN) [45], the long short-term memory network (LSTM) [46], and random forest (RF) [47,48]. Furthermore, the SVM model's effectiveness is assessed by considering the data division ratio and the quantity of input variables. Finally, the accuracy of the SVM model in predicting the CER is further verified by comparing it with the proposed Oka and Bitter theoretical improved erosion model. The model can provide an important basis for the protection of concrete buildings in wind gravel flow environments.

2. Materials and Methods

2.1. Raw Materials

This test examines the raw materials used in constructing bridges and other structures along the Lanzhou–Xinjiang high-speed railway through the Gobi windy region, specifically Gansu Qilian Mountain P.O. 42.5 grade ordinary silicate cement. For the mineral admixture, Class I fly ash and S95-grade mineral powder were utilized (Gansu, China). The coarse aggregate comprised hard gravel, sized 5 to 31.5 mm, while the fine aggregate consisted of well-graded river sand with a fineness modulus of 2.8. To further improve workability, a polycarboxylic acid water-reducing agent was added, achieving a 26.5% reduction in water usage (Sobute New Materials Co., LTD, Nanjing, China). These components were then mixed with tap water to prepare the concrete.

2.2. Concrete Preparation

The laboratory determined the final mix ratios for the concrete by considering the variety and quality of the raw materials. These ratios directly influenced the cubic compressive strength of the concrete specimens, as detailed in Table 1.

Table 1. Concrete mix ratio and compressive strength.

Specimen Number	Water-Binder Ratio	Raw Material Consumption (kg/m^3)						Water-Reducing Agent (%)	Compressive Strength (MPa)
		Water	Cement	Mineral Powder	Fly Ash	Sand	Gravel		
A-1	0.40	138	173	86	86	863	1054	1.5	39.9
A-2	0.39	140	179	90	90	836	1065	1.7	46.0
A-3	0.37	138	187	93	93	831	1058	1.9	50.8
A-4	0.34	140	206	103	103	815	1033	2.1	58.1

2.3. Erosion Test Methods and Equipment

In this study, the wind gravel flow erosion and abrasion test on concrete utilized the airflow sand injection method [8], offering a more realistic simulation of the Gobi wind and sand environment compared to the wind tunnel test. This method boasts several advantages: ease of operation, cost-effectiveness, short testing cycles, and straightforward parameter control. The airflow sand injection method provides enhanced control over test parameters. It uses gravel of varying grain sizes to replicate the gravel surfaces in the Gobi region and allows for precise control of the erosion angle, aligning with the region's wind direction. Additionally, the method can simulate high wind speeds and extended erosion periods, typical of the Gobi's windy conditions, by adjusting wind speeds and erosion time. It also mimics frequent wind, sandy weather, and large-scale sand transport by modulating the gravel flow rate. Moreover, this method can be integrated with numerical simulations and field tests, offering greater flexibility in adjusting test parameters and improving its applicability.

The test device consists of three core components: an air supply system, a sand supply system, and an erosion system. Initially, the air compressor creates high-velocity airflow, which is subsequently blended with sand and gravel in the spray gun. Within the erosion system, a pressure regulator valve finely tunes the erosion wind speed, propelling the mixture through a nozzle to strike the specimen. For precise erosion, the erosion angle is adjusted by altering the nozzle's position in relation to the concrete surface. Post-erosion, the sand and gravel are effectively recaptured and recycled using the specialized recovery system. Figure 3 depicts the detailed operating principle of the airborne sand injection test device.

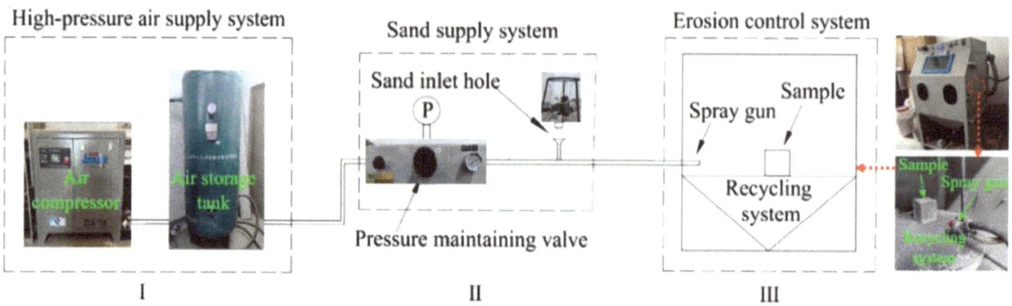

Figure 3. Schematic diagram of airflow sand transport test device.

2.4. Erosion Parameters

In the wind gravel flow environment, erosion and wear of concrete materials are primarily influenced by key erosion parameters. This study identifies five critical parameters: gravel particle size, erosion angle, gravel flow rate, erosion wind speed, and erosion time. Gobi's gale-prone areas are mainly covered with coarse sand and gravel. To replicate these conditions, three gravel particle size ranges of 0.25–0.5 mm, 1–2 mm, and 3–5 mm are selected for the experiment. To investigate the concrete's erosion damage under different angles, six erosion angles of 15°, 30°, 45°, 60°, 75°, and 90° are chosen. Based on the wind conditions in the Baili wind zone, five erosion wind speeds of 20, 25, 30, 35, and 40 m/s are selected, corresponding to wind gusts of 8, 10, 11, 12, and 13, respectively. To simulate the region's frequent sandstorms and substantial sediment transport, four gravel flow rates of 30, 60, 90, and 120 g/min are used. Finally, to assess the impact of erosion duration on concrete, a 10 min period is selected, with concrete quality measured every minute. The specific parameters are listed in Table 2.

Table 2. Erosion test parameters.

Erosion Parameter	Parameter Value
gravel particle size (mm)	0.25–0.5, 1–2, 3–5
erosion angle (°)	15, 30, 45, 60, 75, 90
erosion wind speed (m/s)	20, 25, 30, 35, 40
gravel flow rate (g/min)	30, 60, 90, 120
erosion time (min)	1, 2, 3, 4, 5, 6, 7, 8, 9, 10

2.5. CER

In this paper, the degree of erosive wear on concrete specimens by wind gravel flow is measured by the CER, as shown in Equation (1).

$$\delta = \frac{m_1 - m_2}{A} \tag{1}$$

where δ is the CER; m_1 and m_2 are the mass of the concrete before and after erosion, respectively; A is the lateral area of the concrete.

3. Test Results and Analysis

3.1. Compressive Strength of Concrete

Figure 4 illustrates the variation in CER among materials of different strengths. This variation is observed under specific conditions: a gravel flow rate set to 120 g/min, an erosion angle of 90°, an erosion wind speed of 35 m/s, and an erosion time of 10 min.

The figure uses the symbol 'Δ' to indicate changes in CER, either as an increase or a decrease. Notably, Figure 4 shows that the erosion rate for specimen A-4, when subjected to varying grain sizes of sand and gravel, decreases by 66.1% to 74.1% compared to specimen A-1. As the compressive strength of concrete rises, the CER correspondingly decreases. This phenomenon is due to the increased presence of cementitious material and a lower water-binder ratio in the stronger concrete mix. This composition strengthens the bond between aggregates, which in turn makes the surface cement mortar more resistant to impacts, particularly from gravel. As a result, this stronger bonding significantly improves the concrete's erosion resistance. Compressive strength is strongly linked to the microstructural properties of concrete, especially pore distribution, and plays a crucial role in its erosion resistance. Enhancing compressive strength typically requires optimizing the pore structure, which in turn improves the concrete's ability to withstand erosion caused by wind gravel flow.

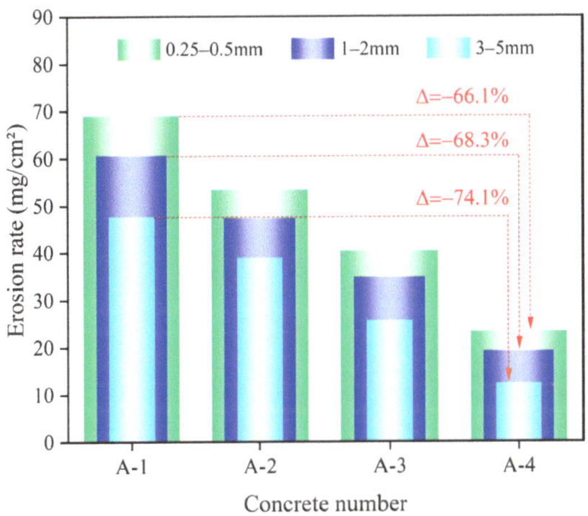

Figure 4. Variation rule of CER with strength.

Similar erosion patterns are observed in specimens A-1, A-2, A-3, and A-4 across different erosion parameters. Therefore, specimen A-3 is chosen for in-depth analysis to better understand the variations in CER due to these parameters.

3.2. Gravel Flow Rate

Figure 5 demonstrates the variation in the erosion rate of specimen A-3 under different gravel flow rate, with the erosion angle fixed at 90°, erosion wind speed of 35 m/s, and an erosion time of 10 min. The data show that at a gravel flow rate of 120 g/min, the erosion rate of A-3 escalates by 134.9% to 335.6% in comparison to a gravel flow rate of 30 g/min, influenced by various gravel grain sizes. This marked increase is attributed to the greater number of gravel particles striking the concrete surface as gravel flow rate rises, thereby significantly enhancing the CER. At high gravel flow rates, collisions between the incident and rebounding gravel reduce the kinetic energy of the incident gravel, slowing the CER increase and resulting in a nonlinear pattern.

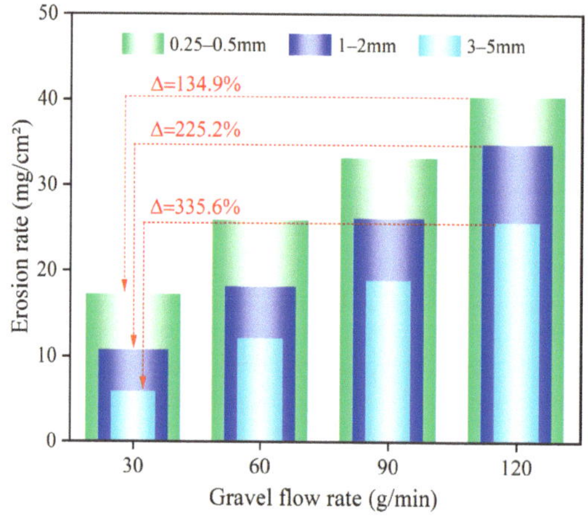

Figure 5. Variation rule of erosion rate with gravel flow rate for specimen A-3.

3.3. Erosion Angle

Figure 6 depicts the variation in erosion rate for specimen A-3 at different erosion angle, maintained under consistent conditions: a gravel flow rate of 120 g/min, an erosion wind speed of 35 m/s, and an erosion time of 10 min. According to the data, the erosion rate of A-3 experiences a substantial increase, ranging from 157.3% to 358.9%, at an erosion angle of 90° compared to 15°. The CER noticeably increases as erosion angle rises, consistent with the erosion behavior observed in brittle materials. In these materials, the normal velocity component of eroded particles significantly contributes to material loss. Consequently, high-angle erosion, characterized by a higher normal velocity component of gravel, results in a substantially higher CER than low-angle erosion due to increased impact energy. At high erosion angles, the CER increases nonlinearly due to stronger stress concentration from particle impacts and faster damage accumulation.

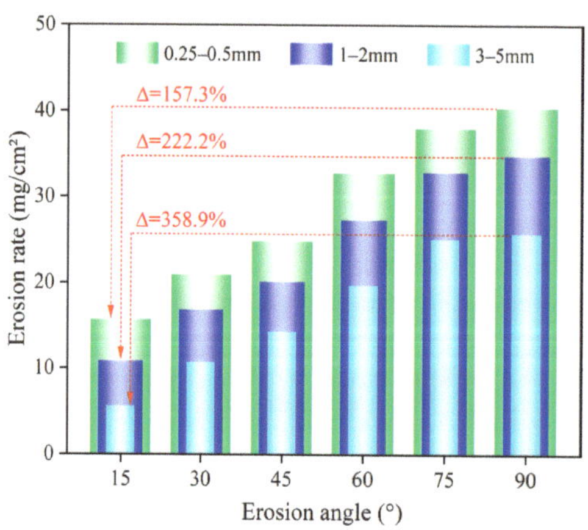

Figure 6. Variation rule of erosion rate with erosion angle for specimen A-3.

3.4. Erosion Wind Speed

Figure 7 illustrates the variation in erosion rate for specimen A-3 across a range of erosion wind speed, with the gravel flow rate fixed at 120 g/min, erosion angle at 90°, and erosion time at 10 min. The figure indicates that at an erosion wind speed of 40 m/s, the erosion rate increases dramatically, from 315.5% to 720.0%, compared to 20 m/s, especially when the specimen is subjected to sand and gravel of different grain sizes. This substantial increase in the CER is due to the enhanced kinetic energy of the gravel particles at higher wind speeds, leading to increased impact energy and consequently a marked rise in CER.

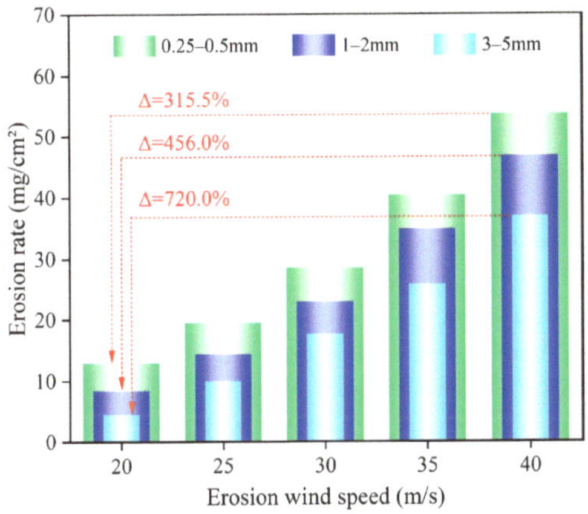

Figure 7. Variation rule of erosion rate with erosion wind speed for specimen A-3.

3.5. Erosion Time

Figure 8 depicts the changes in erosion rate per unit time and the cumulative erosion rate of specimen A-3 over 10 min, subjected to a gravel flow rate of 120 g/min, an erosion angle of 90°, and an erosion wind speed of 35 m/s. The analysis of these data indicates that the erosion process of concrete typically undergoes an initial acceleration phase followed by a phase of stabilization. During the first 1–3 min, the erosion rate per unit time for concrete is elevated, signifying an accelerated phase. This rate then gradually levels off from 3 to 10 min, entering a stabilization phase. A detailed analysis of the cumulative erosion rate demonstrates that for specimen A-3, exposed to sand and gravel of different grain sizes, the rate at an erosion time of 10 min escalates by 634.3% to 692.2% compared to an erosion time of just 1 min. This significant increase indicates that a longer erosion time correlates with a substantial increase in the CER.

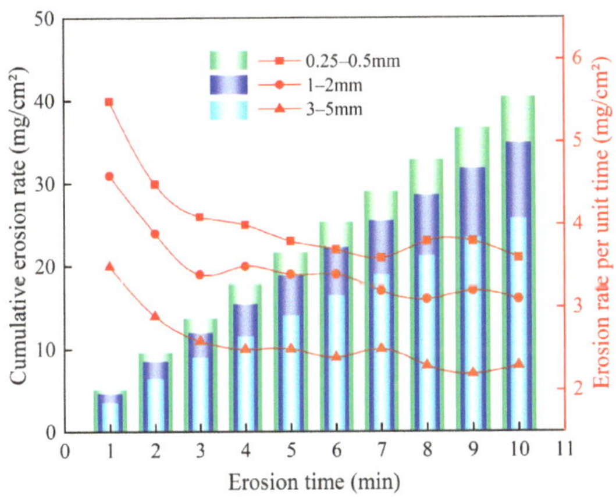

Figure 8. Variation rule of erosion rate with erosion time for specimen A-3.

As erosion wind speed and time increase, concrete damage intensifies, significantly reducing the durability of structures. In areas with high winds, regular inspection and maintenance of concrete facilities are crucial for safety. Additionally, using higher-strength concrete or applying surface coatings should be considered to improve protection.

3.6. Gravel Particle Size

Figures 4–8 indicate that the CER escalates as the gravel particle size decreases. Figure 9 illustrates the micro-erosion morphology and mechanism of concrete eroded by gravel of varying particle sizes, with a gravel flow rate of 120 g/min, an erosion angle of 90°, and an erosion wind speed of 35 m/s. As shown in Figure 9a,b, when the gravel particle size is 0.25–0.5 mm, numerous cracks appear in the mortar on the concrete surface, signaling imminent dislodgement. However, the erosion pits are small. In contrast, with gravel particle sizes of 3–5 mm, the number of erosion pits decreases, and cracks become less frequent. However, the pits that form are larger due to the increased particle size of the gravel. As shown in Figure 9c,d, smaller gravel particles predominantly erode the mortar around the coarse aggregates, thereby significantly exposing them. In contrast, larger gravel particles, due to their size, tend to impact directly onto the coarse aggregates rather than eroding the mortar. This leads to a reduced erosion rate for larger gravel, given that the coarse aggregates are harder than the mortar.

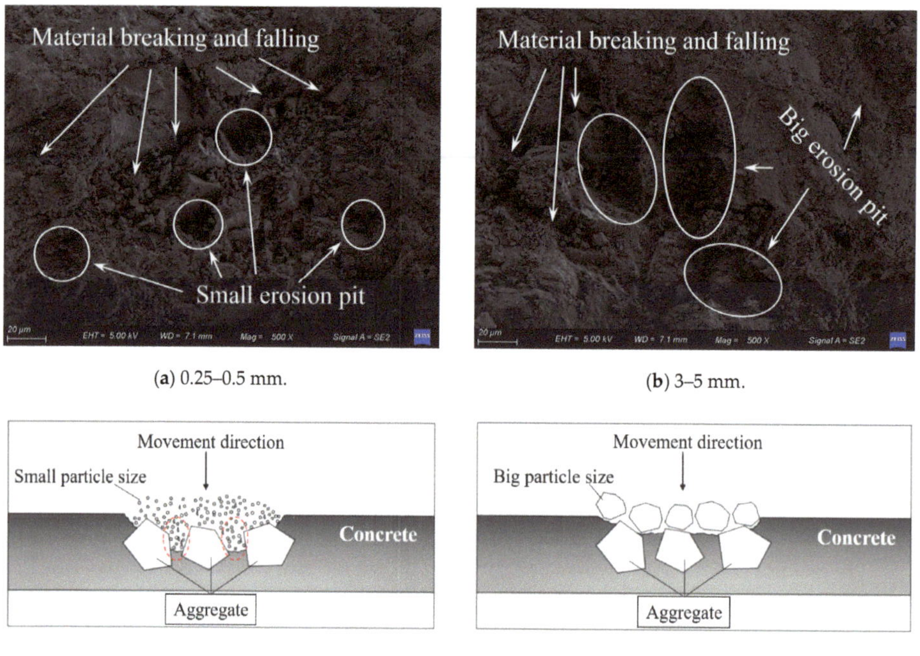

(a) 0.25–0.5 mm. (b) 3–5 mm.

(c) Small particle size erosion. (d) Big particle size erosion.

Figure 9. Damage mechanism of concrete under the erosion of sand and gravel with different particle sizes. Red dashed circles indicate chiseling.

3.7. Macroscopic Morphology Analysis

Figure 10a,b illustrate the macroscopic erosion patterns on concrete surfaces at varying erosion angles under consistent experimental conditions: gravel particle size of 0.25–0.5 mm, gravel flow rate of 90 g/min, erosion wind speed of 35 m/s, and erosion time of 10 min. At an erosion angle of 30°, the damage on the concrete surface is predominantly characterized by cutting scratches, indicating a shear-dominated erosion mechanism. Conversely, at an erosion angle of 90°, the damage is primarily associated with mortar spalling and the development of erosion pits, exposing parts of the internal coarse aggregate. This difference highlights the significant influence of erosion angle on the damage morphology of concrete surfaces.

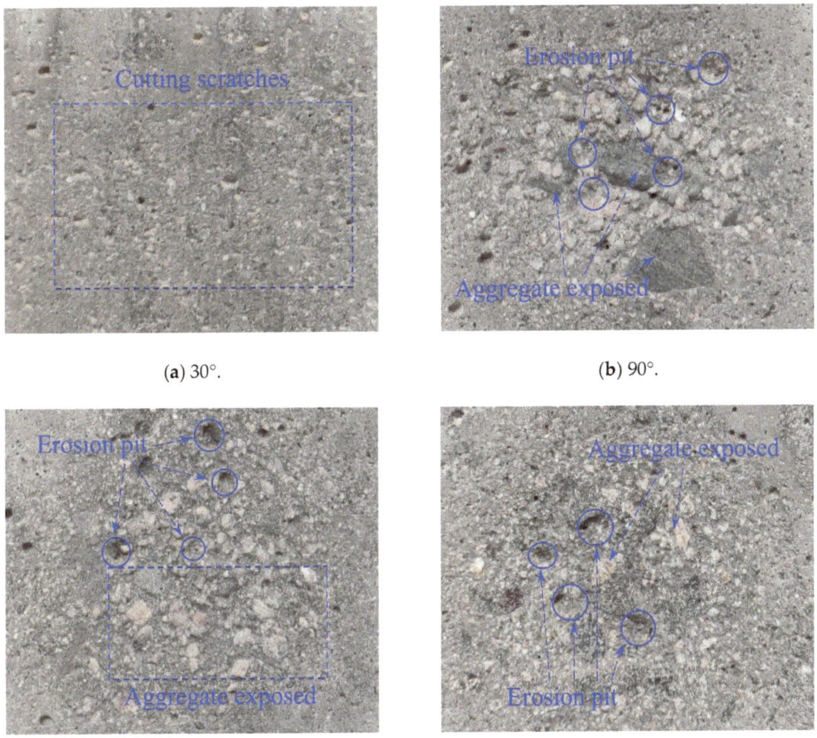

(**a**) 30°. (**b**) 90°.

(**c**) 0.25–0.5 mm. (**d**) 3–5 mm.

Figure 10. Erosion macroscopic morphology of concrete surface under different erosion parameters.

Figure 10c,d depict the macroscopic erosion patterns on concrete surfaces caused by varying gravel particle sizes under the following constant conditions: a gravel flow rate of 90 g/min, an erosion wind speed of 35 m/s, an erosion angle of 90°, and an erosion time of 10 min. When the gravel particle size ranges from 0.25 to 0.5 mm, the surface erosion on the concrete is concentrated, with significant erosion of the cement mortar surrounding the aggregates. This erosion exposes the aggregates clearly. As the gravel particle size increases, the erosion range on the concrete surface gradually widens. However, the degree of aggregate exposure decreases, the erosion depth becomes shallower, and the surface becomes relatively smoother and flatter.

4. SVM Model

4.1. Data Collection and Analysis

This study utilizes a robust dataset of 264 erosion rate measurements from the wind gravel flow erosion test to construct a SVM model. The model analyzes the CER using nine input variables, categorized into two groups. The first group includes variables related to concrete material: water content, cementitious material content, fine aggregate content, and coarse aggregate content. The second group comprises erosion parameters: gravel particle size, erosion angle, erosion wind speed, gravel flow rate, and erosion time. The primary output variable of the SVM model is the CER. Table 3 outlines the range of input and output data in this study, including the minimum, maximum, mean, and standard deviation. The dataset comprises 264 sets, of which 211 (80%) form the training set and the remaining 53 sets (20%) constitute the test set used to assess the model's accuracy. A total of 264 experimental datasets are collected for this study, with the variance of CER measured at 0.671. The dataset comprises two primary categories of input variables: concrete material properties and erosion parameters. These variables are carefully selected to simulate the wind gravel flow environment more accurately, thereby improving the realism and reliability of the simulations.

Table 3. Range of input data and output data.

Input/Output Variables	Unit	Minimum	Maximum	Mean	Standard Deviation	Type
X_1: Water content	kg/m^3	138	140	139	1	Input
X_2: Cementitious material content	kg/m^3	345	412	372.25	24.99	Input
X_3: Fine aggregate content	kg/m^3	815	863	836.25	17.28	Input
X_4: Coarse aggregate content	kg/m^3	1033	1065	1052.5	11.93	Input
X_5: Gravel particle size	mm	0.25–0.5	3–5	1.96	1.51	Input
X_6: Erosion angle	°	15	90	79.77	21.4	Input
X_7: Gravel flow rate	g/min	30	120	111.93	22.45	Input
X_8: Erosion wind speed	m/s	20	40	33.86	3.97	Input
X_9: Erosion time	min	1	10	7.95	2.96	Input
Y: CER	mg/cm^2	2.7	92	23.73	15.93	Output

4.2. Theoretical Methods

The SVM regression algorithm stands out in regression analysis for its unique approach. Unlike traditional methods, SVM adopts a nonlinear model to tackle nonlinear regression issues. It achieves this by nonlinear mapping, which converts data into a high-dimensional space, thereby strengthening the linear regression capabilities of both dependent and independent variables. SVM then effectively addresses nonlinearity by fitting these variable relationships and returning to the original data context. Figure 11 illustrates the nonlinear mapping of sample data from 2D to 3D space. This mapping seeks to maximize the margin between the hyperplane and the training data in three dimensions, ultimately resulting in the creation of the regression model. Assuming a linear functional relationship between input and output factors in the sample, we calculate the regression prediction function *f (x)* as shown in Equation (2) [49].

$$f(x) = \omega^T \varphi(x) + b \tag{2}$$

where ω^T is a vector of weight coefficients for $\varphi(x)$; $\varphi(x)$ is a nonlinear mapping from the sample space to a high-dimensional linear space; b is a scalar parameter.

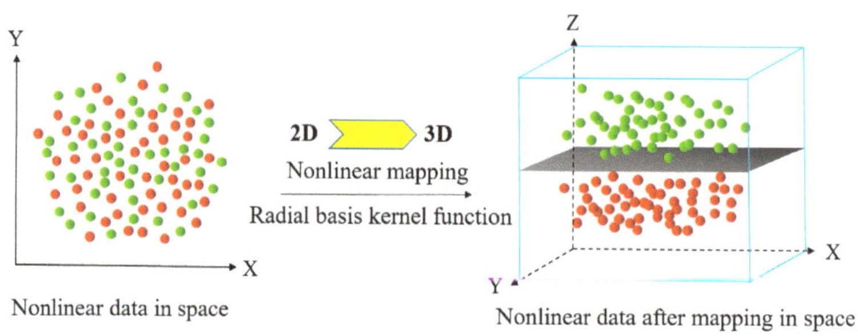

Figure 11. Nonlinear-to-linear mapping of SVM model.

Assuming that the training sample set is $\{(x_i, y_i)|i = 1, 2, \cdots, l\}$, Equation (2) is transformed into a pairwise function by introducing Lagrange multipliers [50]. The pairwise functions and constraints are shown in Equation (3),

$$\min\frac{1}{2}\|\omega\|^2 + c\sum_{i=1}^{l}(\xi_i + \xi_i^*)$$
$$s.t.\begin{cases} y_i - \omega^T\varphi(x_i) - b \le \varepsilon + \xi_i \\ \omega^T\varphi(x_i) + b - y_i \le \varepsilon + \xi_i \\ \xi_i, \xi_i^* \le 0 \end{cases} \tag{3}$$

where l is the number of training samples; ε is the insensitive loss function; c is the penalty parameter, $c > 0$, which is used to balance the function complexity and loss error; ξ_i and ξ_i^* are both slack variables.

Equation (3) is then solved using the Lagrange multiplier method [50] and the result is shown in Equation (4).

$$\min_{\alpha,\alpha*}\frac{1}{2}\sum_{i=1}^{l}\sum_{j=1}^{l}(\alpha_i - \alpha_i^*)(\alpha_j - \alpha_j^*)K(x_i, x_j) + \varepsilon\sum_{i=1}^{l}(\alpha_i - \alpha_i^*) - \sum_{i=1}^{l}y_i(\alpha_i - \alpha_i^*)$$
$$s.t.\begin{cases} \sum_{i=1}^{n}(\alpha_i - \alpha_i^*) = 0 \\ 0 \le \alpha_i, \alpha_i^* \le c, i = 1, 2, \cdots, l \end{cases} \tag{4}$$

where α_i, α_i^* are the Lagrange factors; x_j is the output variable; the kernel function $K(x_i, x_j) = \varphi(x_i)^T\varphi(x_j)$.

The kernel function's role is crucial in mapping data with nonlinear relationships into a high-dimensional feature space, significantly impacting SVM model prediction performance. Presently, the Radial Basis Function (RBF) is the most widely adopted kernel function for SVM models due to its robustness against interference and localization, making it an ideal choice for handling nonlinear problems. Consequently, in this study, RBF is selected as the kernel function for the SVM model, as represented in Equation (5),

$$K(x, x_i) = \exp(-g\|x - x_i\|^2) \tag{5}$$

where g is a parameter.

The functional expression for nonlinear SVM regression is shown in Equation (6).

$$f(x) = \sum_{i=1}^{l}(\alpha_i - \alpha_i^*)K(x, x_i) + b \tag{6}$$

4.3. Data Processing

In certain special cases, irregular interference samples in the data can increase the computational complexity of the model, potentially harming its accuracy and causing convergence problems. Additionally, when building the model, data with a wide range of variation may dominate data with a narrower range. To mitigate this, we normalize the initial data before constructing the model. In this paper, we choose to normalize the data to a range of [0, 1], as determined by Equation (7),

$$\overline{x} = \frac{x_i - x_{\min}}{x_{\max} - x_{\min}}, \tag{7}$$

where $\overline{x}$ is the normalized data; x_i is the input or output data; $x_{\max}$ and $x_{\min}$ represent the maximum and minimum values of the transformed feature data, respectively.

4.4. Determination of Model Parameters

In SVM models, the choice of hyperparameters significantly influences prediction performance. This study focuses on two key hyperparameters: 'c', the penalty parameter, and 'g', the RBF parameter. Setting 'c' and 'g' too high can lead to overfitting, which reduces the model's ability to generalize. Conversely, setting them too low simplifies the model excessively, resulting in underfitting. Therefore, it is vital to find the optimal values for 'c' and 'g'. Currently, there are several methods for optimizing the values of parameters 'c' and 'g', such as the grid search, enumeration, particle swarm, and genetic algorithms. The grid search method is well suited for the smaller hyperparameter space in this study, as it systematically evaluates all possible combinations to identify the optimal solution. Moreover, it is simple to implement, debug, and ideal for preliminary model tuning. The grid search method in particular systematically examines parameter values within predefined ranges by evenly dividing the grid. This approach leads to the identification of the global optimal solution, which presents clear advantages over alternative methods [51].

Cross-validation is a widely used statistical method to assess the performance of SVM models [52]. It involves dividing the initial sample dataset into K subsets, using K-1 subsets for training and reserving one as the test set. This cross-validation process is repeated until each sample subgroup has been tested once. Figure 12 illustrates the K-fold cross-validation process, which effectively prevents both underfitting and overfitting. This is especially beneficial when working with a significant amount of original sample data, leading to more favorable model outcomes. When K is small, it results in a larger training set and a smaller test set, which may lead to unstable evaluations and higher variance. Conversely, a larger K reduces the training set size and increases the test set, raising computational costs and potentially introducing greater bias. A common choice for K is 10, as it effectively balances bias and variance, providing stable and reliable results. Thus, K = 10 is selected for this study.

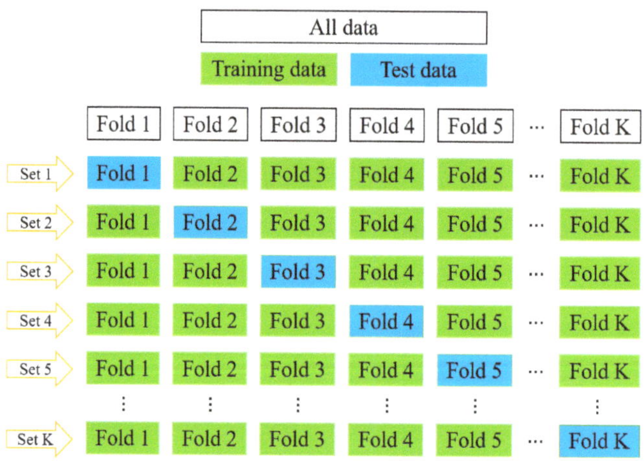

Figure 12. Schematic diagram of K-fold cross-validation procedure.

In this study, we determine the optimal SVM model parameters by employing a combination of the grid search approach and K-fold cross-validation. The outcomes of parameter selection are illustrated in Figure 13, where the RBF parameter (g) and the penalty parameter (c) vary over the range from 2^{-8} to 2^{8}. Through this integration of the grid search approach with K-fold cross-validation, the model achieves optimal values: c = 4 and g = 0.5. Consequently, the model attains a minimum mean square error (MSE) of 0.00079425.

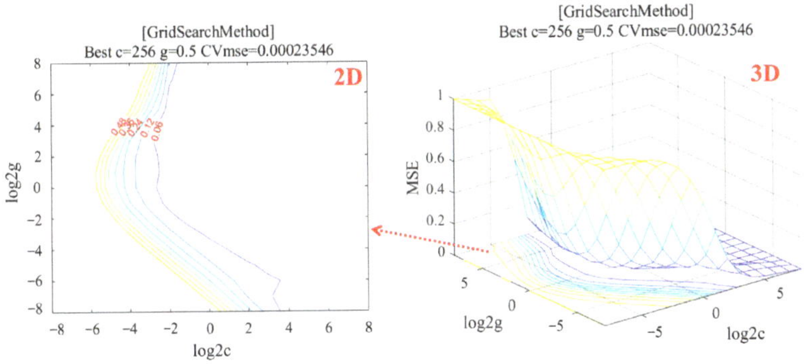

Figure 13. Parameter optimization result.

4.5. SVM Modeling Process

Figure 14 illustrates the SVM model's overall structural flowchart for predicting the CER, encompassing four distinct steps.

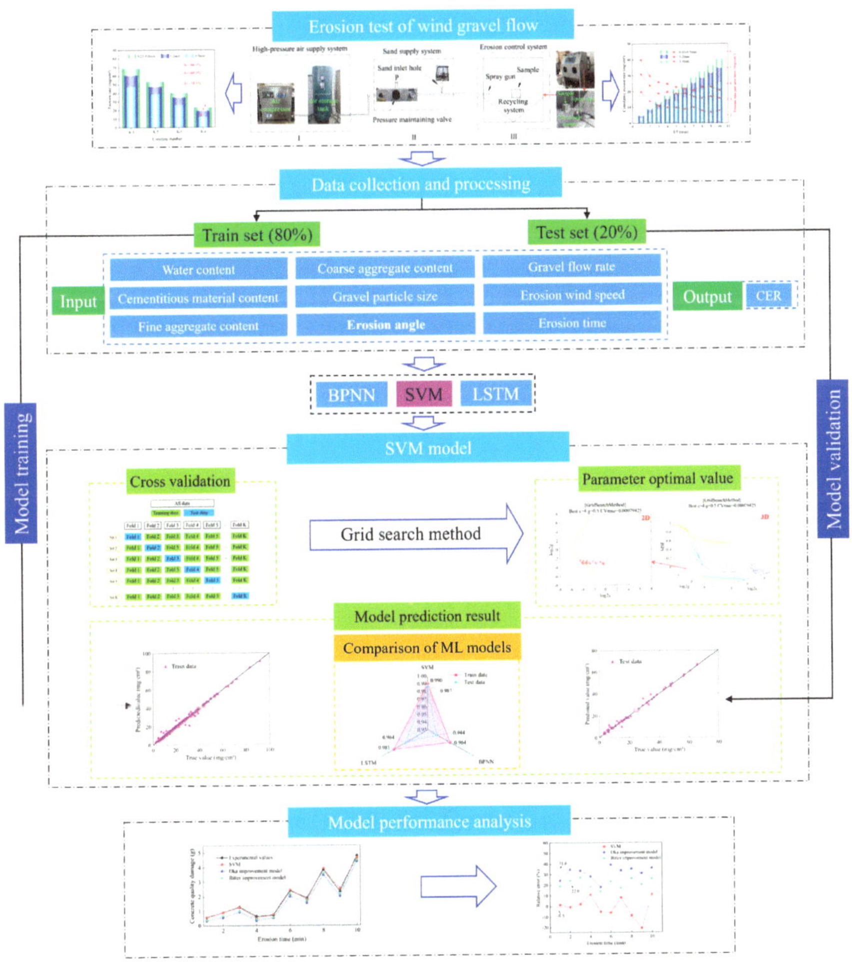

Figure 14. Architecture of the SVM model.

(1) Wind gravel flow erosion test. The test results are used to analyze the correlation between CER changes and erosion parameters. Subsequently, the data are systematically collected and organized.
(2) Data collection and processing. The initial phase consolidates experimental data to pinpoint factors affecting the CER and identifies crucial input and output variables for the ML model. Following this, a sensitivity analysis evaluates the influence of input factors on the CER. The final stage involves training the model using 80% of the dataset and validating it with the remaining 20%.
(3) Model training and validation. First, optimal hyperparameters are identified using a grid search method combined with K-fold cross-validation. The model is then trained on the training set and validated using the test set. Performance is assessed based on four key metrics: R^2, RMSE, MAE, and MBE. Finally, the outcomes are contrasted with predictions from BPNN and LSTM ML models.
(4) Model performance analysis. This analysis evaluates the SVM model's performance, focusing on the data division ratio and input variable count. Additionally, it compares the SVM model's predictions with those from the formula model.

5. Analysis of SVM Model Prediction Results

5.1. Evaluation Index

This paper presents four distinct evaluation indices to precisely assess the SVM model's prediction results. The indices are defined as follows.

The coefficient of determination (R^2) is shown in Equation (8). The approach of R^2 value to one signifies a corresponding increase in the accuracy of model predictions.

$$R^2 = 1 - \frac{\sum_{i=1}^{m} (t_i - p_i)^2}{\sum_{i=1}^{m} (t_i - \bar{t})^2} \tag{8}$$

Root Mean Square Error ($RMSE$) is as shown in Equation (9). It is used to measure the error between the predicted value and the true value.

$$RMSE = \sqrt{\frac{\sum_{i=1}^{m} (t_i - p_i)^2}{m}} \tag{9}$$

Mean absolute error (MAE) is as shown in Equation (10). The average of the sum of the absolute differences between the predicted and true values is determined.

$$MAE = \frac{\sum_{i=1}^{m} |t_i - p_i|}{m} \tag{10}$$

The average bias error (MBE) is as shown in Equation (11). Positive and negative errors can cancel each other out to determine whether there is a positive or negative bias in the model,

$$MBE = \frac{\sum_{i=1}^{m} (t_i - p_i)}{m} \tag{11}$$

where m is the total number of data samples, t is the true value (test value), p is the predicted value (output value), and $\bar{t}$ is the average of all true values.

5.2. SVM Model Prediction Results

The SVM model is trained with optimal hyperparameters on a dataset of 211 entries and subsequently validated using a separate test set comprising 53 datasets. Figure 14 displays a comparative analysis of the SVM model's predictions during both training and testing phases. Notably, Figure 15a highlights the close correlation between the predicted and actual values in the training dataset, as evidenced by the near-overlap of the respective curves. Figure 15b shows that most scatter points align closely with the ideal black line, highlighting the small difference between predicted and actual values. This alignment indicates that the model has successfully learned the decision rule connecting input and output variables, effectively capturing their impact on the CER. The model's generalization ability is assessed by examining its predictive accuracy on test data. Table 4 details the SVM model's prediction accuracy for both training and testing phases. The R^2 value for the test set, as shown in Table 4, is an impressive 0.987, closely approaching 1, and the RMSE stands at a mere 1.868. Such metrics highlight the model's superior predictive and generalization performance in relation to the CER.

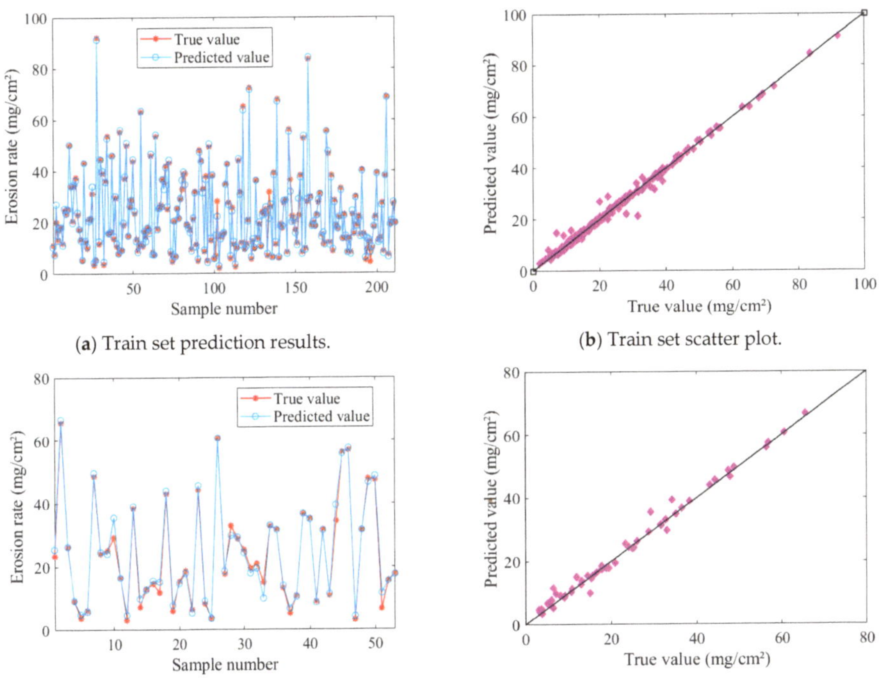

(**a**) Train set prediction results. (**b**) Train set scatter plot.

(**c**) Test set prediction results. (**d**) Test set scatter plot.

Figure 15. Comparison of SVM model prediction results.

Table 4. Comparison of SVM model prediction accuracy.

Date Set	Evaluation Index			
	R^2	RMSE	MAE	MBE
Train set	0.990	1.580	0.944	−0.013
Test set	0.987	1.868	1.232	0.457

5.3. Comparison with Other ML Models

To effectively compare the predictive capabilities of the SVM model, the BPNN and LSTM models are also employed to predict the CER. This approach allows for a direct comparison with the predictions made by the SVM model. All three ML models are developed using the same dataset, providing a uniform foundation for the comparison.

The BPNN, depicted in Figure 16, is a sophisticated multilayer feedforward neural network [45]. In this study, the BPNN is structured into three distinct layers: input, hidden, and output. The input layer, containing nine neurons, mirrors the nine input variables, while the output layer, with a single neuron, corresponds to the output variable. A meticulous process of iterative training leads to the optimization of the hidden layer with 10 neurons. This network adopts the data division ratio used in the SVM model for consistency. To ensure the model's robustness and accuracy, an error threshold of 1×10^{-6} is strategically established, effectively curtailing overfitting risks.

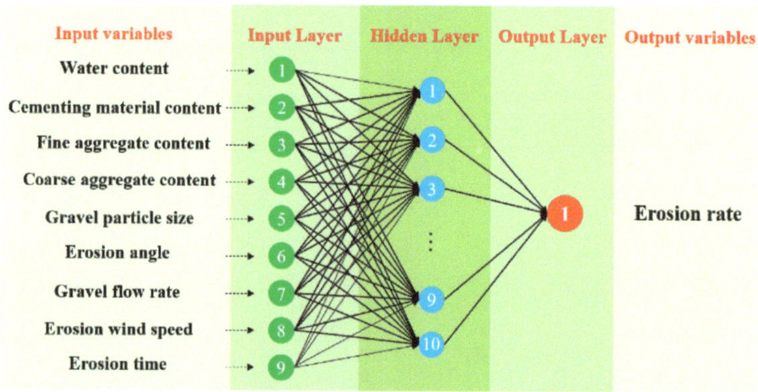

Figure 16. Schematic diagram of BPNN model structure.

LSTM, a distinct variant of recurrent neural networks [46], is notably adept at adapting and scaling during data training, particularly in managing long-term dependencies within sequential data. This model includes three main components: an input gate *i(t)*, a forget gate *f(t)*, and an output gate *o(t)*. Together, these gates determine the processing of input data and how the hidden state from the previous moment is handled. The model utilizes a back-propagation algorithm and a fitting loss function, facilitating the learning of patterns and trends in the sequence for future value predictions. It adheres to the same data division ratio as the SVM model. The model's structure is depicted in Figure 17.

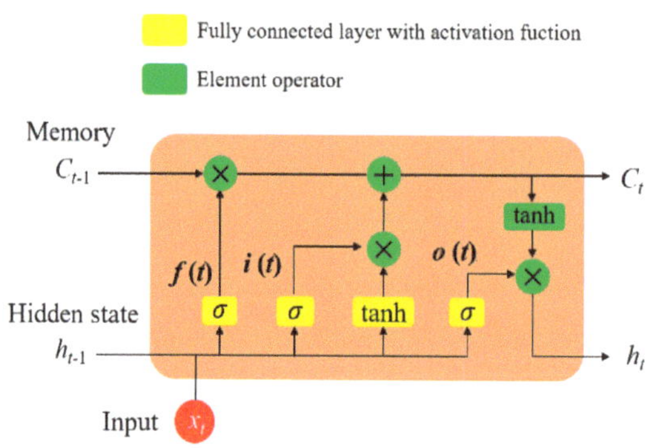

Figure 17. Schematic diagram of LSTM model structure.

RF is an ensemble learning method [47,48] that falls under the bagging category. The RF model's structure is shown in Figure 18. It relies on decision trees and employs two key techniques: bootstrap sampling and random feature selection. To construct a decision tree, the bootstrap method randomly selects M samples from the dataset and n features as sub-nodes. After n iterations, n decision trees are generated, and the final output is the average of their predictions. The number of decision trees and nodes significantly influences the RF model's prediction accuracy. In this study, after several tuning iterations, the number of decision trees is set to 400, with each tree having two nodes.

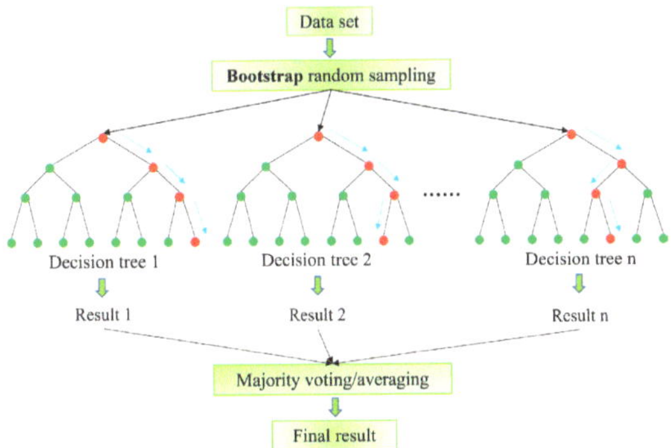

Figure 18. Schematic diagram of RF model structure.

Table 5 shows the main differences among ML models of SVM, BPNN, LSTM and RF.

Table 5. Major differences in ML models.

ML Model	Training Time	Interpretability	Computational Demand
SVM	longer	higher	high
BPNN	longer	lower	high
LSTM	longest	lowest	highest
RF	shorter	higher	intermediate

Figure 19 shows a scatter plot that contrasts the predicted and actual values of four ML models: SVM, BPNN, LSTM, and RF. The 45° line in this figure represents ideal predictive accuracy (100% prediction accuracy). The SVM model's predictions in particular align more linearly with this line, indicating a closer match to the actual values. The LSTM model's training set scatter points are closely grouped, indicating high pre-diction accuracy. Yet, in its test set, these points stray from the ideal black line, denoting limited generalization ability. Conversely, the BPNN model exhibits scatter points in both its training and testing sets that are significantly far from the ideal black line, reflecting struggles in both prediction accuracy and generalization. However, RF has the lowest prediction accuracy in both the training and test sets, with most data points deviating significantly from the ideal black line. This suggests that the RF model is less reliable than other machine learning models for predicting the erosion rate of concrete. Table 6 showcases the prediction accuracy of four ML models: SVM, BPNN, LSTM, and RF. The SVM model consistently surpasses both BPNN, LSTM and RF in all evaluated metrics. In the training set, its R^2 value reaches 0.990, a notable increase from RF's 0.900, and its RMSE lowers by 0.612, 1.518, and 3.215 in comparison to LSTM, BPNN, and RF, respectively. Similarly, in the testing set, the SVM's R^2 value climbs to 0.987 from RF's 0.849, and it achieves RMSE reductions of 1.123, 1.573, and 5.388 when compared to LSTM, BPNN, and RF. The SVM model notably surpasses BPNN, LSTM, and RF models in predictive and generalization capabilities. Its superior performance becomes particularly clear in predicting the CER under wind gravel flow conditions, rendering it a more dependable option compared to other ML models. In this study, the SVM model is constructed with the RBF kernel, which effectively handles nonlinear data, interacting parameters, and outliers in complex environments, such as wind gravel flow erosion in the Gobi region. The SVM's robust nonlinear modeling capabilities, efficient computation, strong generalization, and capacity to process high-dimensional data make it more effective than other ML models for predicting CER.

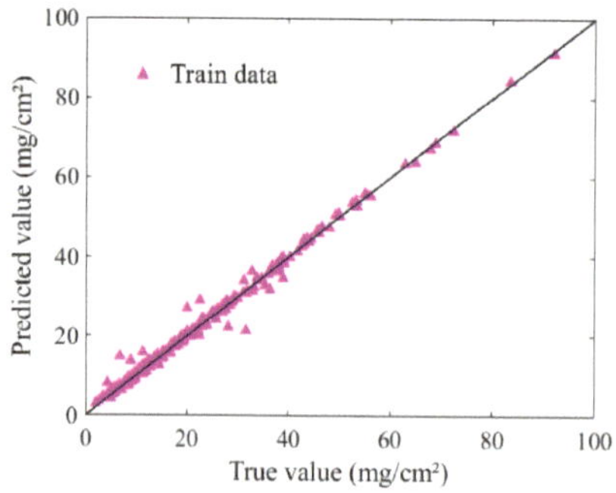

(**a**) SVM model training set.

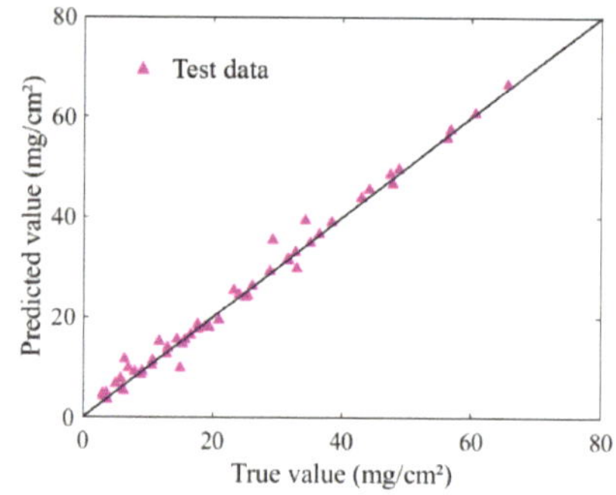

(**b**) SVM model testing set.

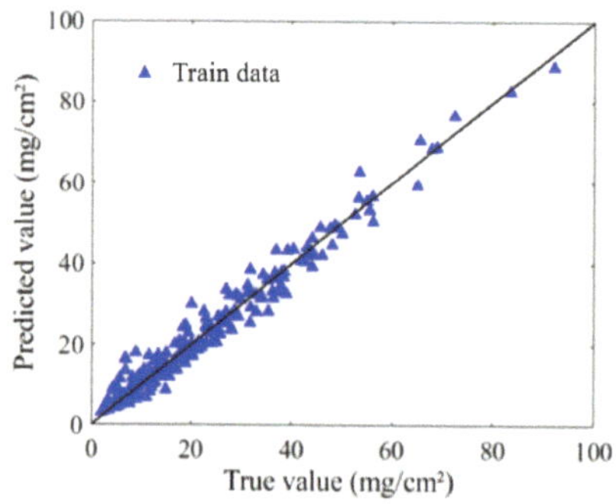

(**c**) BPNN model training.

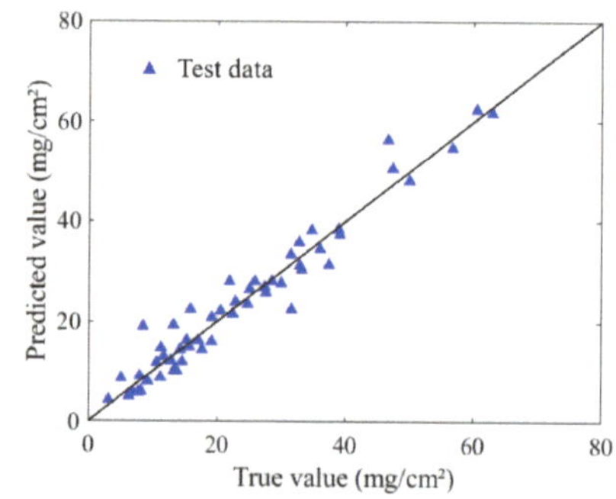

(**d**) BPNN model testing set.

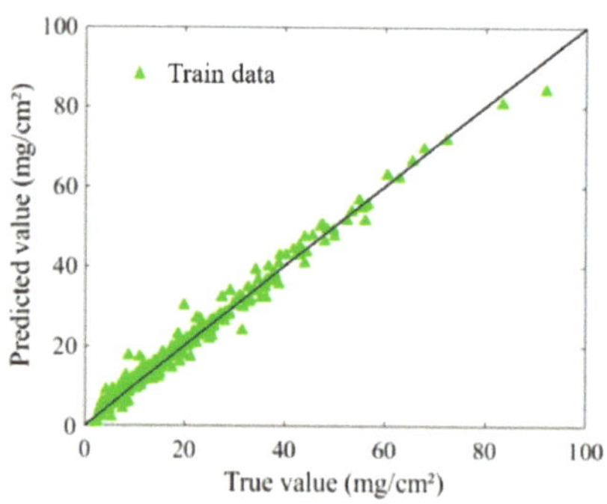

(**e**) LSTM model training set.

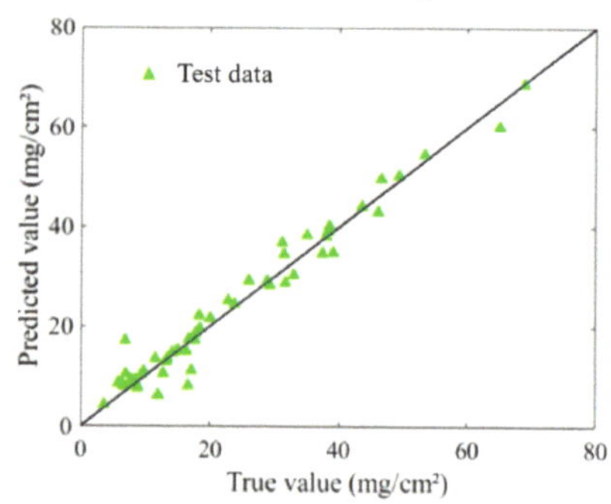

(**f**) LSTM model testing set.

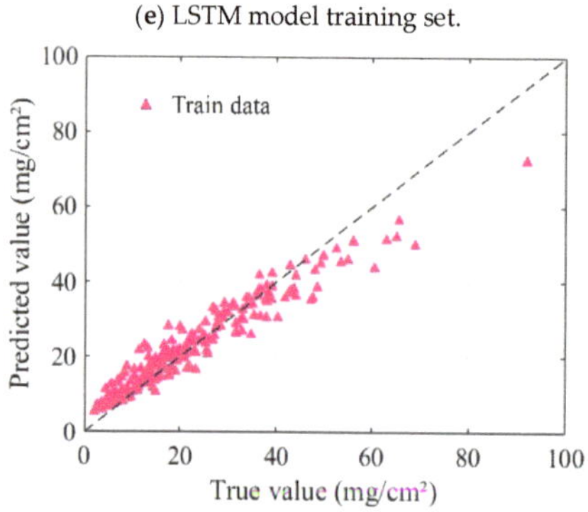

(**g**) RF model training set.

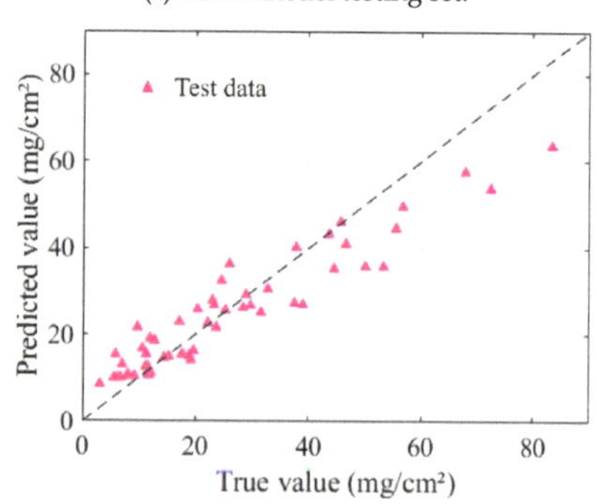

(**h**) RF model testing set.

Figure 19. Comparison of predicted values and true values of different ML models.

Table 6. Comparison of prediction accuracy results of different ML models.

Data Set	ML Models	Evaluation Index			
		R^2	RMSE	MAE	MBE
Train date	SVM	0.990	1.580	0.944	−0.013
	BPNN	0.964	3.098	2.384	0.072
	LSTM	0.981	2.192	1.559	0.166
	RF	0.900	4.795	3.540	0.221
Test date	SVM	0.987	1.868	1.232	0.457
	BPNN	0.944	3.441	2.581	0.150
	LSTM	0.964	2.991	2.136	0.305
	RF	0.849	7.256	5.401	−1.036

Figure 20 features a radar chart that compares the prediction accuracy of four ML models, clearly and intuitively highlighting their respective strengths and weaknesses. Based on the indices R^2, RMSE, and MAE, the models' accuracy ranks as follows: SVM, LSTM, BPNN, and RF, which is consistent with previous analysis. In the context of MBE metrics, the SVM model displays a negative bias in the training set but shifts to a positive bias in the testing set. Conversely, both the LSTM and BPNN models maintain a predominantly positive bias, while the RF model displays significant positive deviation in the training set and significant negative deviation in the test set.

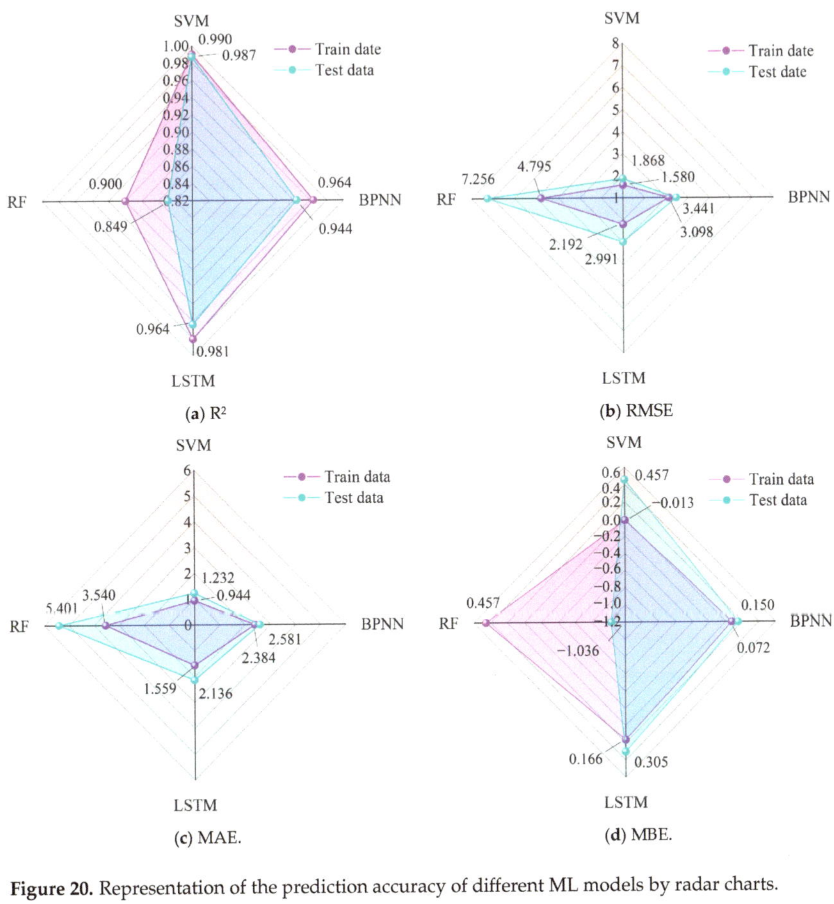

Figure 20. Representation of the prediction accuracy of different ML models by radar charts.

5.4. Interpretive Analysis of SVM Model

This study uses the SHAP method to interpret the SVM model's prediction results. Figure 21 provides the global interpretation based on SHAP analysis. The feature importance, calculated by averaging the SHAP values for each feature across all samples, is shown in Figure 21a. Overall, erosion time has the most significant impact on the CER, with an average SHAP value of 5.84. As erosion time increases, the cumulative impact of each collision gradually causes more severe damage to the concrete. For high-strength concrete, initial impacts may cause minimal damage, but over time, the accumulated energy surpasses the concrete's erosion resistance, leading to significant spalling or surface layer destruction. The amount of cementitious material also significantly affects the CER, with an average SHAP value representing 74.5% of the impact of erosion time. In contrast, the amount of water has the least effect on the CER, with an average SHAP value of only 0.78, or 13.4% of the impact of erosion time. The dataset in this study reveals that the water content values in the input variables are similar, with only minor differences. Consequently, water content has a minimal impact on the CER. Wind speed and gravel particle size interact in influencing concrete erosion. Wind speed directly affects the kinetic energy of gravel particles, which in turn determines their impact on the concrete surface. At higher wind speeds, even small particles can cause significant erosion due to the increased kinetic energy. Additionally, the particle size of gravel influences the strength and effectiveness of its impact on the concrete.

Figure 21b shows a heat map of SHAP value distributions for each characteristic parameter, highlighting their influence. The horizontal axis represents specific SHAP values, which reflect feature influence on the model output, while the vertical axis ranks feature contributions based on the sum of SHAP values across all samples. Each point corresponds to a sample, stacked vertically by sample size, with color indicating the characteristic values (red for high values, blue for low values). As shown in the figure, erosion time is the most influential variable affecting the concrete's erosion rate. As erosion time increases, the SHAP value rises, resulting in a higher erosion rate. The figure also reveals that variables such as erosion time, coarse aggregate content, erosion wind speed, erosion angle, gravel flow rate, and fine aggregate content amount positively impact the CER, while cementitious material, gravel particle size, and water content negatively affect it.

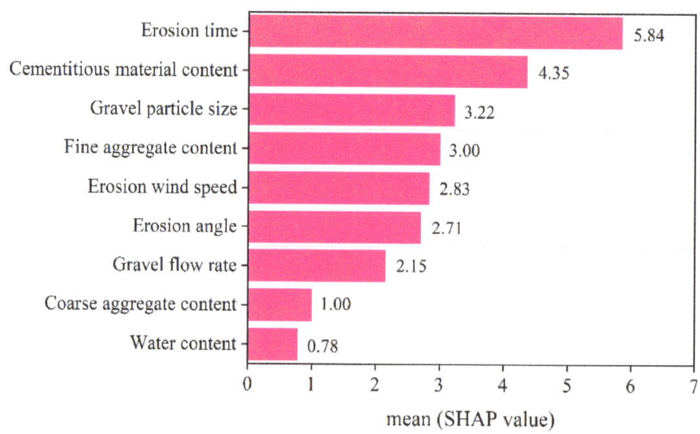

(**a**) Feature importance analysis based on SHAP value.

Figure 21. *Cont.*

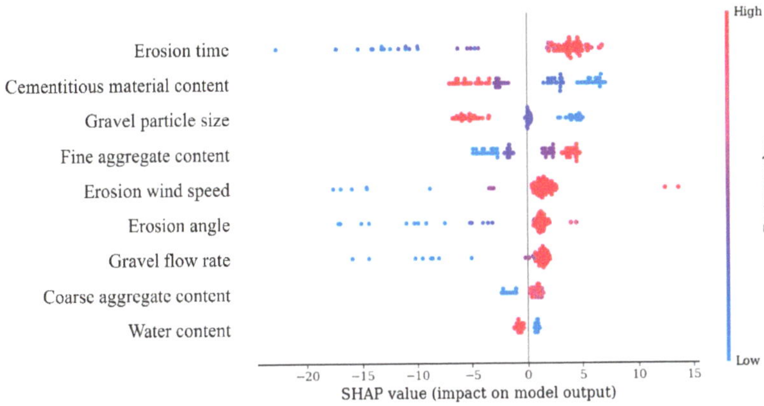

(**b**) SHAP value distribution heat map of 9 characteristic parameters.

Figure 21. SHAP interpretability analysis of SVM model.

6. SVM Model Performance Analysis

6.1. Percentage of Data Division

The performance of a trained model is largely influenced by the proportion of its training set. This research focuses on examining how different training set ratios affect the accuracy of the SVM model. Accordingly, we set varied data ratios for testing and training sets, namely 9:1, 8:2, and 7:3.

Table 7 displays the SVM model predictions across three scales, all of which exhibit high accuracy. Notably, in the training set data, the R^2 values for each scale are near one, signifying that the predictions closely align with the actual values. The SVM model's predictions for the 9:1 and 8:2 scales exhibit comparable R^2 and RMSE values. In contrast, the 7:3 scale sees a rise in RMSE to 1.612, marginally exceeding those of the previous scales. This pattern suggests that decreasing the number of training sets correlates with higher prediction errors. The testing set's prediction results reflect the training set's outcomes. A decrease in the number of training sets leads to diminished performance in the training model's predictions, which in turn impacts the testing set's results. Notably, when the training set constitutes 70% of the total data, the testing set's R^2 value falls to 0.982, significantly lower compared to the other two scales. The RMSE value is 2.053, which is 0.182 and 0.185 higher than that of the 9:1 and 8:2 scaled SVM models, respectively. Therefore, for improved prediction accuracy of the model, it is essential to retain a significant portion of the data in the training set, preferably no less than 80% of the total data.

Table 7. Effect of data division ratio on SVM model prediction results.

Data Set	Percentage of Data Division	Evaluation Index			
		R^2	RMSE	MAE	MBE
Train date	9-1	0.990	1.575	0.936	0.088
	8-2	0.990	1.580	0.944	−0.013
	7-3	0.990	1.612	0.985	0.108
Test date	9-1	0.987	1.871	1.247	0.345
	8-2	0.987	1.868	1.232	0.457
	7-3	0.982	2.053	1.413	0.071

6.2. *Number of Input Variables*

Table 8 details six input combinations for analysis. The first combination uses the original data set. The second and third combinations exclude erosion time and water content, respectively. Significantly, the sixth combination includes only five variables from the erosion parameters. In contrast, the fourth and fifth combinations randomly omit different variables.

Table 8. Prediction accuracy of SVM model under different combinations.

Combination	Evaluation Index			
	R^2	RMSE	MAE	MBE
1: $X_1, X_2, X_3, X_4, X_5, X_6, X_7, X_8, X_9$	0.987	1.868	1.232	0.457
2: $X_1, X_2, X_3, X_4, X_5, X_6, X_7, X_8$	0.644	8.806	5.737	−0.241
3: $X_2, X_3, X_4, X_5, X_6, X_7, X_8, X_9$	0.990	1.798	1.196	−0.484
4: $X_2, X_3, X_4, X_6, X_7, X_8, X_9$	0.837	5.208	4.137	0.173
5: $X_2, X_3, X_4, X_6, X_7, X_8$	0.509	10.468	8.706	−0.656
6: X_5, X_6, X_7, X_8, X_9	0.485	11.038	8.485	3.818

Figure 22 depicts the prediction results of the SVM model for six different input combinations, and Table 8 presents the associated evaluation indices. The model's most accurate predictions are observed with Combination 3, which omits water content, identified as the least significant factor affecting the CER. Omitting water content notably enhances the model's precision, demonstrated by an increase in R^2 from 0.987 to 0.990 and a reduction in RMSE from 1.868 to 1.798. The model's prediction accuracy has seen moderate improvement. However, in Combination 6, the SVM model shows significantly weaker predictive capabilities. This is evident from its low R^2 value of 0.485 and a high RMSE of 11.038. The primary reason for this underperformance is the exclusion of several crucial input variables essential for robust predictions. Interestingly, adding more input variables does not invariably lead to a decrease in the model's accuracy. Combination 2, comprising eight input variables, yields a lower prediction accuracy with an R^2 of 0.644 and an RMSE of 8.806. Conversely, Combination 4, consisting of zeven input variables, displays a notably higher prediction accuracy. This is indicated by its improved R^2 of 0.837 and reduced RMSE of 5.208, surpassing Combination 2's performance. The disparate performances of Combination 2 and Combination 4 primarily stem from their handling of the erosion time variable. Combination 2 omits erosion time, a crucial factor, while Combination 4 includes it, significantly impacting prediction accuracy. This inclusion of erosion time is pivotal, as its absence leads to a substantial drop in prediction accuracy, evidenced by R^2 decreasing from 0.987 to 0.644.

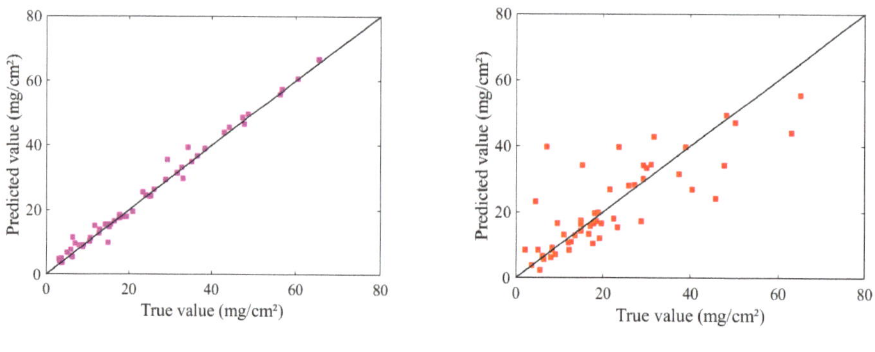

(**a**) Combination 1. (**b**) Combination 2.

Figure 22. *Cont.*

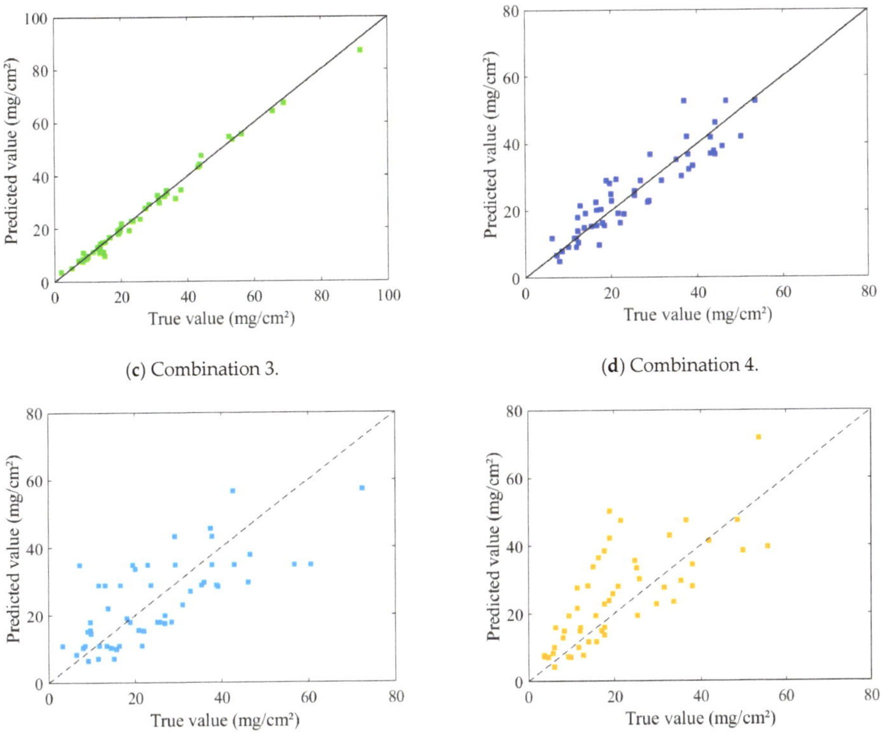

(c) Combination 3.

(d) Combination 4.

(e) Combination 5.

(f) Combination 6.

Figure 22. SVM model prediction results under different combinations.

6.3. Comparison with the Formula Model

In the field of material erosion theory, Oka [16] and Bitter [17,18] proposed erosion theory and deformation wear theory, respectively. These theories provide comprehensive insights into the factors influencing material erosion and have broader applicability. As a result, this paper enhances Oka's erosion theory and Bitter's deformation wear theory, enabling them to describe the erosive wear of concrete influenced by wind gravel flow in the Gobi region [6].

(1) The Oka improvement model:

$$\Delta M = \mathrm{k} \cdot \eta \cdot (F_R \cdot t) D(d) (H_V)^{\mathrm{k}_1} (V)^{\mathrm{k}_2} f(\alpha), \tag{12}$$

$$f(\alpha) = \sin\alpha[1 + H_V(1 - \sin\alpha)], \tag{13}$$

$$D(d) = c \cdot e^{(-d/f)} + g, \tag{14}$$

where ΔM is the material erosion wear; η is the concrete strength factor; F_R is the gravel flow rate; t is the erosion time; $D(d)$ is the particle size function, d is the gravel particle size; H_V is the material hardness; V is the erosion wind speed; k_1, k_2 are exponential factors; $f(\alpha)$ is the erosion angle function; α is the erosion angle; k, c, f, and g are constants.

(2) The Bitter improvement model:

$$\Delta M = W_D + W_C = \frac{F_R \cdot t\eta D(d) \cdot (V \sin\alpha - C)^2}{2\varepsilon} + \frac{F_R \cdot t\eta D(d) \cdot (V \cos\alpha)^2 \sin\alpha}{2\mu}, \quad (15)$$

where W_D and W_C are the deformation and cutting wear, respectively; C is the critical wind speed; ε and μ are the deformation and cutting wear energy consumption coefficients, respectively.

Considering the significant impact of erosion time on CER, we conducted experiments under varying conditions. Specifically, with gravel particle size ranging from 3 to 5 mm, a gravel flow rate of 120 g/min, an erosion angle of 90°, and an erosion wind speed of 35 m/s, we assessed concrete mass loss across different erosion time values. Our calculations utilized both the Oka and Bitter improved models. Figure 23a,b depict the comparison between experimental and computational results, corresponding to the Oka and Bitter improved models, respectively. Both improved models clearly yield more precise predictions of concrete erosion wear. Particularly, the Bitter improved model demonstrates superior prediction capabilities when compared to the Oka improved model. Furthermore, lower concrete strength was associated with reduced prediction errors. These results suggest that both improved models excel in forecasting erosion and wear in low-strength concrete.

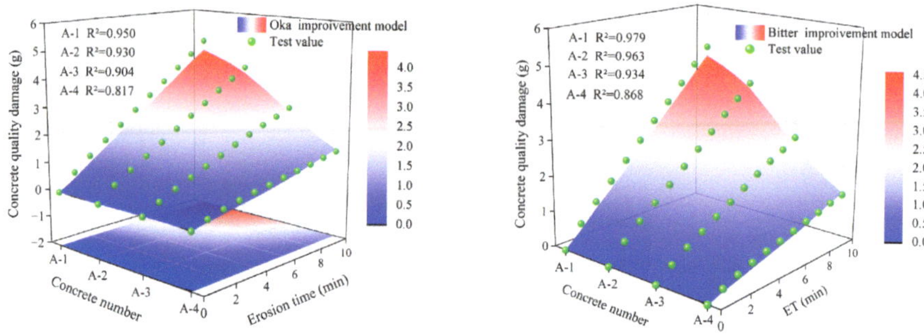

(**a**) Oka improvement model (**b**) Bitter improvement model

Figure 23. Comparison of test results of CER with Oka and Bitter-improved models for different erosion times.

To validate the SVM model's accuracy more effectively, its predictions were compared with those of the two improved models previously discussed. Figure 24a illustrates this comparison, specifically highlighting how each model predicts concrete quality degradation at different erosion time levels. Following this, Figure 24b displays the relative prediction errors of the three models, offering a detailed analysis of their overall performance. The figure analysis indicates that Bitter's improved model and Oka's improved model have average relative errors of 22.0% and 31.6%, respectively. The overall predictions of these two models fall short of the experimental results. In comparison, the SVM model shows significantly higher accuracy, mirroring the test result curves with a minimal average relative error of −0.5%. This underscores the SVM model's exceptional proficiency in accurately predicting concrete quality degradation. The SVM model's prediction performance is significantly better than that of other models. Bitter and Oka's theoretical model for predicting CER struggles in complex natural environments. This is largely due to its simplifying assumptions, neglect of nonlinear and synergistic effects between variables, and lack of flexibility. In wind gravel flow erosion, the relationship between erosion wind speed and gravel particle size is typically nonlinear, particularly in environments with high wind speeds and gravel flow rates. In such cases, the impact and friction effects of the sand grains are highly complex. Oka and Bitter's model oversimplifies these interactions, failing to capture the intricate interplay between erosion wind speed, gravel particle size, and erosion angle. In contrast, the SVM model excels at handling nonlinear relationships, performing automatic feature selection, and offering strong generalization capabilities. These features make it more accurate and effective in predicting wind gravel flow erosion. As a result, SVM modeling is extremely effective for evaluating the erosive wear of concrete in the high-wind regions of the Gobi desert.

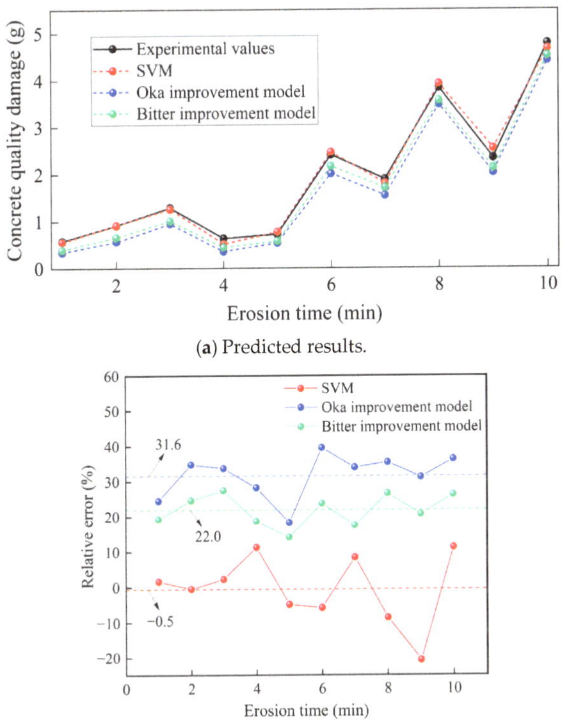

(b) Relative error.

Figure 24. Comparison of SVM model and Oka and Bitter-improved model prediction results.

7. Conclusions

In this study, we conducted a wind gravel flow erosion test to analyze how CER varies with erosion parameters. We collected data to create a comprehensive database and used K-fold cross-validation in combination with the SVM algorithm to build a predictive model for CER in the wind gravel flow environment. The following conclusions were obtained:

(1) Concrete's compressive strength directly correlates with its resistance to erosive wear. The CER rises with higher gravel flow rate, erosion wind speed, erosion angle, and erosion time values. During concrete erosion, distinct accelerating and stabilizing phases are evident. Significantly, concrete incurs more severe erosion damage from small-sized gravel than from large-sized gravel.

(2) Compared to models like LSTM, BPNN, and RF, the SVM model achieves an R^2 close to 1 (0.990 for the training set and 0.987 for the test set) and an RMSE closer to 0 (1.580 for the training set and 1.868 for the test set). These results indicate that the SVM model offers superior prediction accuracy. Consequently, the SVM-based CER prediction model is more reliable than other ML models.

(3) The SHAP method analyzed the SVM model's prediction results, revealing that erosion time is the most significant variable influencing the concrete's erosion rate. In contrast, water content has the least impact. Variables like erosion time, coarse aggregate content, erosion wind speed, erosion angle, gravel flow rate, and fine aggregate content positively affect the erosion rate, while cementation material content, gravel particle size, and water content have a negative effect.

(4) An analysis of the SVM model's performance demonstrates that maintaining a training set with at least 80% of the total data volume ensures the model's prediction accuracy. Furthermore, when erosion time is excluded, the SVM model's R^2 decreases from 0.987 to 0.644. This highlights the significant impact of neglecting erosion time on the SVM model's predictive results, emphasizing the crucial role of erosion time as an input variable. Overall, erosion parameters have a substantially greater influence on CER than the concrete material itself.

(5) CER prediction involves the use of both the theoretically improved erosion model and the SVM model. While the average relative error for the improved Bitter and Oka models stands at 22% and 31.6%, respectively, the SVM model displays an average relative error of just −0.5%. This underscores the SVM model's superior prediction accuracy, whereas the theoretical improved model's generalization ability is restricted due to its more limited considerations.

In the future, laboratory results will be integrated with numerical simulations and field tests to model various climatic conditions, such as seasonal windstorms, and extreme events like sandstorms or sudden changes in wind speed. This approach will enhance the applicability of the research findings. By observing concrete erosion caused by wind gravel flow in the Gobi desert, we can gather the necessary parameters and data. These can be input into the SVM model to quickly predict the erosion rate, assess the concrete's durability, and develop an effective maintenance strategy.

Author Contributions: Y.Z.: Writing—original draft, Methodology, Project administration, Visualization. K.Z.: Writing—review and editing, Writing—original draft, Conceptualization. A.G.: Writing—review and editing. F.H.: Data curation, Validation. J.M.: Investigation. All authors have read and agreed to the published version of the manuscript.

Funding: This study was supported by the National Natural Science Foundation of China (42461011, 52468034, 52405196), and the China Postdoctoral Science Foundation (2021M703466).

Data Availability Statement: The data sets generated or analyzed during this study are available from the corresponding author on reasonable request.

Conflicts of Interest: The authors declare no conflicts of interest.

References

1. Qu, J.; Wang, T.; Niu, Q.; Liu, B.; Tan, L.; Han, Q.; Gao, Y.; Xiao, J. Mechanisms of the formation of wind-blown sand hazards and the sand control measures in Gobi areas under extremely strong winds along the Lanzhou-Xinjiang high-speed railway. *Sci. China Earth Sci.* **2022**, *66*, 292–302. [CrossRef]
2. Cheng, J.; Jiang, F.; Xue, C.; Xin, G.; Li, K.; Yang, Y. Characteristics of the disastrous wind-sand environment along railways in the Gobi area of Xinjiang, China. *Atmos. Environ.* **2015**, *102*, 344–354. [CrossRef]
3. Liu, D.; Liang, X.; Zhou, W.; Zhong, M.; Lu, Z. Fundamental research on the dynamic safety of a high-speed train under strong wind conditions. *Vehicle. Syst. Dyn.* **2023**, *61*, 1602–1620. [CrossRef]
4. Liu, T.; Wang, L.; Gao, H.; Xia, Y.; Guo, Z.; Li, W.; Liu, H. Research progress on train operation safety in Xinjiang railway under wind environment. *Transp. Saf. Environ.* **2022**, *4*, tdac005. [CrossRef]
5. Wang, T.; Qu, J.; Tan, L.; Gao, Y.; Zhang, K.; Shi, B. Aeolian sediment transport over the Gobi with high gravel coverage under extremely strong winds in the Hundred Miles windy area along the Lanzhou-Xinjiang High-Speed Railway. *J. Wind Eng. Ind. Aerod.* **2022**, *220*, 104857. [CrossRef]

6. Zhang, K.; Feng, Z.; Yu, Y.; Yang, B.; Yu, B.; Xie, C. Concrete erosion mechanism and model research under the action of wind gravel flow in Gobi gale area. *Constr. Build. Mater.* **2023**, *409*, 133940. [CrossRef]
7. Xue, H.; Shen, X.; Liu, Q.; Wang, R.; Liu, Z. Analysis of the damage to the aeolian sand concrete surfaces caused by wind-sand erosion. *J. Adv. Concr. Technol.* **2017**, *15*, 724–737. [CrossRef]
8. Hao, Y.; Feng, Y.; Fan, J. Experimental study into erosion damage mechanism of concrete materials in a wind-blown sand environment. *Constr. Build. Mater.* **2016**, *111*, 662–670. [CrossRef]
9. Wang, Y.; Zhang, J.; Dun, H.; Huang, N. Numerical Investigation on Impact Erosion of Aeolian Sand Saltation in Gobi. *Atmosphere* **2023**, *14*, 349. [CrossRef]
10. Wang, Y.; Yang, Z. Finite element model of erosive wear on ductile and brittle materials. *Wear* **2008**, *265*, 871–878. [CrossRef]
11. Finnie, I. Erosion of surfaces by solid particles. *Wear* **1960**, *3*, 87–100. [CrossRef]
12. Finnie, I. Some observations on the erosion of ductile metals. *Wear* **1972**, *19*, 81–90. [CrossRef]
13. Finnie, I.; Mc Fadden, D.H. On the velocity dependence of the erosion of ductile metals by solid particles at low angles of incidence. *Wear* **1978**, *48*, 181–190. [CrossRef]
14. Finnie, I. Some reflection on the past and future of erosion. *Wear* **1995**, *186–187*, 1–10. [CrossRef]
15. Levy, A. *Solid Particle Erosion and Erosion-Corrosion of Materials*; ASM International: Materials Park, OH, USA, 1995.
16. Oka, Y.; Yoshida, T. Practical estimation of erosion damage caused by solid particle impact Part 2: Mechanical properties of materials directly associated with erosion damage. *Wear* **2005**, *259*, 102–109. [CrossRef]
17. Bitter, J. A study of erosion phenomena, part I. *Wear* **1963**, *6*, 5–21. [CrossRef]
18. Bitter, J. A study of erosion phenomena, part II. *Wear* **1963**, *6*, 169–190. [CrossRef]
19. Huang, Y.; Fu, J. Review on application of artificial intelligence in civil engineering. *Comput. Model. Eng. Sci.* **2019**, *121*, 845–875. [CrossRef]
20. Lagaros, N.; Plevris, V. Artificial intelligence (AI) applied in civil engineering. *Appl. Sci.* **2022**, *12*, 7595. [CrossRef]
21. Jordan, M.; Mitchell, T. Machine learning: Trends, perspectives, and prospects. *Science* **2015**, *349*, 255–260. [CrossRef]
22. Janiesch, C.; Zschech, P.; Heinrich, K. Machine learning and deep learning. *Electron. Mark.* **2021**, *31*, 685–695. [CrossRef]
23. Zhou, Z. Open-environment machine learning. *Nati. Sci. Rev.* **2022**, *9*, nwac123. [CrossRef] [PubMed]
24. Hopkins, E. Machine learning tools, algorithms, and techniques. *J. Self-Gov. Manag. Econ.* **2022**, *10*, 43–55.
25. Huang, T.; Liu, T.; Ai, Y.; Ren, Z.; Ou, J.; Li, Y.; Xu, N. Modelling the interface bond strength of corroded reinforced concrete using hybrid machine learning algorithms. *J. Build. Eng.* **2023**, *74*, 06862. [CrossRef]
26. Asteris, P.; Skentou, A.; Bardhan, A.; Samui, P.; Pilakoutas, K. Predicting concrete compressive strength using hybrid ensembling of surrogate machine learning models. *Cem. Concr. Res.* **2021**, *145*, 106449. [CrossRef]
27. Feng, D.; Liu, Z.; Wang, X.; Chen, Y.; Chang, J.; Wei, D.; Jiang, Z. Machine learning-based compressive strength prediction for concrete: An adaptive boosting approach. *Constr. Build. Mater.* **2020**, *230*, 117000. [CrossRef]
28. Shen, Z.; Deifalla, A.; Kamiński, P.; Dyczko, A. Compressive strength evaluation of ultra-high-strength concrete by machine learning. *Materials* **2022**, *15*, 3523. [CrossRef]
29. Qian, Y.; Sufian, M.; Hakamy, A.; Farouk Deifalla, A.; EI-said, A. Application of machine learning algorithms to evaluate the influence of various parameters on the flexural strength of ultra-high-performance concrete. *Front. Mater.* **2023**, *9*, 1114510. [CrossRef]
30. Kang, M.; Yoo, D.; Gupta, R. Machine learning-based prediction for compressive and flexural strengths of steel fiber-reinforced concrete. *Constr. Build. Mater.* **2021**, *266*, 121117. [CrossRef]
31. Wu, Y.; Zhou, Y. Splitting tensile strength prediction of sustainable high-performance concrete using machine learning techniques. *Environ. Sci. Pollut. Res.* **2022**, *29*, 89198–89209. [CrossRef]
32. Albaijan, I.; Mahmoodzadeh, A.; Flaih, L.; Ibrahim, H.; Alashker, Y.; Mohammed, A. Evaluating the Tensile Strength of Reinforced Concrete using Optimized Machine Learning Techniques. *Eng. Fract. Mech.* **2023**, *292*, 109677. [CrossRef]
33. Gao, X.; Yang, J.; Zhu, H.; Xu, J. Estimation of rubberized concrete frost resistance using machine learning techniques. *Constr. Build. Mater.* **2023**, *371*, 130778. [CrossRef]
34. Kahraman, E.; Ozdemir, A. The prediction of durability to freeze–thaw of limestone aggregates using machine-learning techniques. *Constr. Build. Mater.* **2022**, *324*, 126678. [CrossRef]
35. Taffese, W.; Espinosa-Leal, L. Prediction of chloride resistance level of concrete using machine learning for durability and service life assessment of building structures. *J. Build. Eng.* **2022**, *60*, 105146. [CrossRef]
36. Cai, R.; Han, T.; Liao, W.; Huang, J.; Li, D.; Kumar, A.; Ma, H. Prediction of surface chloride concentration of marine concrete using ensemble machine learning. *Cem. Concr. Res.* **2020**, *136*, 106164. [CrossRef]
37. Nunez, I.; Nehdi, M. Machine learning prediction of carbonation depth in recycled aggregate concrete incorporating SCMs. *Constr. Build. Mater.* **2021**, *287*, 123027. [CrossRef]
38. Tran, V.; Mai, H.; To, Q.; Nguyen, M. Machine learning approach in investigating carbonation depth of concrete containing Fly ash. *Struct. Concr.* **2023**, *24*, 2145–2169. [CrossRef]

39. Rong, X.; Liu, Y.; Chen, P.; Lv, X.; Shen, C.; Yao, B. Prediction of creep of recycled aggregate concrete using back-propagation neural network and support vector machine. *Struct. Concr.* **2023**, *24*, 2229–2244. [CrossRef]
40. Zhang, K.; Zhang, K.; Bao, R.; Liu, X. A framework for predicting the carbonation depth of concrete incorporating fly ash based on a least squares support vector machine and metaheuristic algorithms. *J. Build. Eng.* **2023**, *65*, 105772. [CrossRef]
41. Abd, A.; Abd, S. Modelling the strength of lightweight foamed concrete using support vector machine (SVM). *Case Stud. Constr. Mat.* **2017**, *6*, 8–15. [CrossRef]
42. Sun, J.; Zhang, J.; Gu, Y.; Huang, Y.; Sun, Y.; Ma, G. Prediction of permeability and unconfined compressive strength of pervious concrete using evolved support vector regression. *Constr. Build. Mater.* **2019**, *207*, 440–449. [CrossRef]
43. Cui, X.; Wang, Q.; Li, S.; Dai, J.; Xie, C.; Duan, Y.; Wang, J. Deep learning for intelligent identification of concrete wind-erosion damage. *Automat. Constr.* **2022**, *141*, 104427. [CrossRef]
44. Cui, X.; Wang, Q.; Dai, J.; Zhang, R.; Li, S. Intelligent recognition of erosion damage to concrete based on improved YOLO-v3. *Mater. Lett.* **2021**, *302*, 130363. [CrossRef]
45. Chen, M. An improved BP neural network algorithm and its application. *Appl. Mech. Mater.* **2014**, *543*, 2120–2123. [CrossRef]
46. Hochreiter, S.; Schmidhuber, J. Long short-term memory. *Neural. Comput.* **1997**, *9*, 1735–1780. [CrossRef]
47. Gregorutti, B.; Michel, B.; Saint-Pierre, P. Correlation and variable importance in random forests. *Stat. Comput.* **2017**, *27*, 659–678. [CrossRef]
48. Ramosaj, B.; Pauly, M. Consistent estimation of residual variance with random forest Out-Of-Bag errors. *Stat. Probabil. Lett.* **2019**, *151*, 49–57. [CrossRef]
49. Vapnik, V. *The Nature of Statistical Learning Theory*; Springer Science and Business Media: New York, NY, USA, 1999.
50. Jorge, N.; Stephen, J. *Numerical Optimization*; Springer Science and Business Media: New York, NY, USA, 2006.
51. Sun, Y.; Ding, S.; Zhang, Z.; Jia, W. An improved grid search algorithm to optimize SVR for prediction. *Soft. Comput.* **2021**, *25*, 5633–5644. [CrossRef]
52. Berrar, D. Cross-Validation. In *Encyclopedia of Bioinformatics and Computational Biology*, 2nd ed.; Elsevier: Amsterdam, The Netherlands, 2019; Volume 1, pp. 542–545.

MDPI AG
Grosspeteranlage 5
4052 Basel
Switzerland
Tel.: +41 61 683 77 34

Buildings Editorial Office
E-mail: buildings@mdpi.com
www.mdpi.com/journal/buildings

www.ingramcontent.com/pod-product-compliance
Lightning Source LLC
Chambersburg PA
CBHW041358210926
51850CB00013B/3118
* 9 7 8 3 7 2 5 8 4 2 2 1 6 *